Advances and Innovations in Cardiovascular Imaging

Editors

PRASHANT NAGPAL
SANDEEP HEDGIRE

RADIOLOGIC CLINICS OF NORTH AMERICA

www.radiologic.theclinics.com

Consulting Editor
FRANK H. MILLER

May 2024 • Volume 62 • Number 3

ELSEVIER

1600 John F. Kennedy Boulevard • Suite 1800 • Philadelphia, Pennsylvania, 19103-2899

http://www.theclinics.com

RADIOLOGIC CLINICS OF NORTH AMERICA Volume 62, Number 3
May 2024 ISSN 0033-8389, ISBN 13: 978-0-443-13019-9

Editor: John Vassallo (j.vassallo@elsevier.com)
Developmental Editor: Malvika Shah

Radiologic Clinics of North America (ISSN 0033-8389) is published bimonthly by Elsevier Inc., 360 Park Avenue South, New York, NY 10010-1710. Months of issue are January, March, May, July, September, and November. Periodicals postage paid at New York, NY and additional mailing offices. Subscription prices are USD 561 per year for US individuals, USD 100 per year for US students and residents, USD 643 per year for Canadian individuals, USD 754 per year for international individuals, USD 100 per year for Canadian students/residents, and USD 315 per year for international students/residents. For institutional access pricing please contact Customer Service via the contact information below. To receive student and resident rate, orders must be accompanied by name of affiliated institution, date of term and the signature of program/residency coordinatior on institution letterhead. Orders will be billed at individual rate until proof of status is received. Foreign air speed delivery is included in all *Clinics* subscription prices. All prices are subject to change without notice. **POSTMASTER:** Send address changes to *Radiologic Clinics of North America*, Elsevier Health Sciences Division, Subscription Customer Service, 3251 Riverport Lane, Maryland Heights, MO63043. **Customer Service: Telephone: 1-800-654-2452** (U.S. and Canada); **1-314-447-8871** (outside U.S. and Canada). **Fax: 1-314-447-8029. E-mail: journalscustomerservice-usa@ elsevier.com (for print support); journalsonlinesupport-usa@elsevier.com (for online support)**.

Reprints. For copies of 100 or more of articles in this publication, please contact the Commercial Reprints Department, Elsevier Inc., 360 Park Avenue South, New York, New York 10010-1710. Tel.: +1-212-633-3874; Fax: +1-212-633-3820; E-mail: reprints@elsevier.com.

Radiologic Clinics of North America also published in Greek Paschalidis Medical Publications, Athens, Greece.

Radiologic Clinics of North America is covered in *MEDLINE/PubMed (Index Medicus), EMBASE/Excerpta Medica, Current Contents/Life Sciences, Current Contents/Clinical Medicine, RSNA Index to Imaging Literature, BIOSIS, Science Citation Index,* and *ISI/BIOMED.*

Contributors

CONSULTING EDITOR

FRANK H. MILLER, MD, FACR, FSAR, FSABI
Lee F. Rogers, MD Professor of Medical
Education, Chief, Body Imaging Section,
Medical Director, MRI, Professor, Department
of Radiology, Northwestern Memorial Hospital,
Northwestern University Feinberg School of
Medicine, Chicago, Illinois, USA

EDITORS

PRASHANT NAGPAL, MD, FSCCT
Section Chief, Cardiovascular Imaging,
Associate Professor of Radiology, University of
Wisconsin–Madison, Madison, Wisconsin,
USA

SANDEEP HEDGIRE, MD, FSCCT
Section Chief, Cardiovascular Imaging,
Assistant Professor of Radiology,
Massachusetts General Hospital, Harvard
Medical School, Boston, Massachusetts, USA

AUTHORS

PRACHI P. AGARWAL, MBBS
Clinical Professor, Department of Radiology,
Division of Cardiothoracic Radiology, Michigan
Medicine, Ann Arbor, Michigan, USA

AYAZ AGHAYEV, MD
Assistant Professor, Department of Radiology,
Cardiovascular Imaging Program, Brigham and
Women's Hospital, Harvard Medical School,
Boston, Massachusetts, USA

CHIEMEZIE AMADI, MD
Clinical Associate Professor, Department of
Radiology, Michigan Medicine, Ann Arbor,
Michigan, USA

VITALIY ANDROSHCHUK, MBChB
Cardiovascular Directorate, Department of
Cardiology, Guy's and St Thomas' Hospital,
London, United Kingdom

VINIT BALIYAN, MBBS, MD
Radiologist, Division of Cardiovascular
Imaging, Instructor, Department of
Radiology, Massachusetts General Hospital,
Harvard Medical School, Boston,
Massachusetts, USA

JORDI BRONCANO, MD
Head of Cardiothoracic Imaging Unit, Radiology
Department, Hospital San Juan de Dios,
Hospital Cruz Roja, HT Medica, Córdoba, Spain

JINJIN CAO, MD
Fellow, Division of Abdominal Imaging,
Department of Radiology, Massachusetts
General Hospital, Boston, Massachusetts, USA

THOMAS CLIFFORD, MBChB
Medical Doctor, Department of Radiology,
Royal Papworth Hospital, Cambridge, United
Kingdom

CARLO N. DE CECCO, MD, PhD
Professor of Radiology and Biomedical
Informatics, Director, Cardiothoracic Imaging
Division, Department of Radiology and Imaging
Sciences, Emory University, Atlanta, Georgia,
USA

ISHAN GARG, MD
Resident Physician, Department of Internal
Medicine, University of New Mexico Health
Sciences Center, Albuquerque, New Mexico,
USA

GABRIELLE GERSHON, BSc
Medical Student, Translational Laboratory for Cardiothoracic Imaging and Artificial Intelligence, Department of Radiology and Imaging Sciences, Emory University, Atlanta, Georgia, USA

BRIAN GHOSHHAJRA, MD, MBA
Associate Professor, Department of Radiology, Cardiovascular Imaging, Department of Radiology, Massachusetts General Hospital, Harvard Medical School, Boston, Massachusetts, USA

SUMIT GUPTA, MD, PhD
Instructor, Department of Radiology, Cardiovascular Imaging Program, Brigham and Women's Hospital, Harvard Medical School, Boston, Massachusetts, USA

KATE HANNEMAN, MD, MPH, FRCPC
Associate Professor, Department of Medical Imaging, Toronto General Hospital, Peter Munk Cardiac Center, University Health Network (UHN), University of Toronto, Toronto, Ontario, Canada

SANDEEP HEDGIRE, MD
Chief, Division of Cardiovascular Imaging, Division Chief and Assistant Professor, Department of Radiology, Massachusetts General Hospital, Boston, Massachusetts, USA

ELIZABETH LEE, MD
Clinical Associate Professor, Department of Radiology, Michigan Medicine, Ann Arbor, Michigan, USA

CIAN P. McCARTHY, MB, BCh, BAO, SM
Cardiologist, Division of Cardiology, Department of Medicine, Massachusetts General Hospital, Boston, Massachusetts, USA

ERIBERTO MICHEL, MD
Cardiac Surgeon, Division of Cardiac Surgery, Department of Surgery, Massachusetts General Hospital, Boston, Massachusetts, USA

EMANUELE MUSCOGIURI, MD
Fellow, Translational Laboratory for Cardiothoracic Imaging and Artificial Intelligence, Department of Radiology and Imaging Sciences, Emory University, Atlanta, Georgia, USA; Radiologist, Division of Thoracic Imaging, Department of Radiology, University Hospitals Leuven, Leuven, Belgium

GIUSEPPE MUSCOGIURI, MD, PhD
Radiologist, Department of Diagnostic and Interventional Radiology, Papa Giovanni XXIII Hospital, Bergamo, Italy

PRASHANT NAGPAL, MD
Section Chief, Division of Cardiovascular Imaging, Associate Professor, Department of Radiology, University of Wisconsin-Madison, Madison, Madison, USA

CARLOTTA ONNIS, MD
Fellow, Translational Laboratory for Cardiothoracic Imaging and Artificial Intelligence, Department of Radiology and Imaging Sciences, Emory University, Atlanta, Georgia, USA; Resident, Department of Radiology, Azienda Ospedaliero Universitaria (A.O.U.), Cagliari, Italy

ANUSHRI PARAKH, MBBS, MD
Radiologist, Division of Cardiovascular Imaging, Department of Radiology, Massachusetts General Hospital, Boston, Massachusetts, USA

THEODORE T. PIERCE, MD, MPH
Division of Abdominal Imaging, Assistant Professor, Department of Radiology, Massachusetts General Hospital, Harvard Medical School, Boston, Massachusetts, USA

VINAY PRABHU, MD, MS
Clinical Assistant Professor, Department of Radiology, NYU Langone Health, New York, New York, USA

SARV PRIYA, MD
Clinical Assistant Professor, Director of Cardiac Imaging, Medical Director of 3D Lab, Department of Radiology, University of Iowa Carver College of Medicine, Iowa City, Iowa, USA

RONAK RAJANI, DM, MD, FRCP, FESC, FACC, FSCCT, FRCR
Professor, School of Biomedical Engineering and Imaging Sciences, King's College London, London, United Kingdom

PRABHAKAR SHANTA RAJIAH, MD
Professor, Department of Radiology,
Mayo Clinic, Rochester, Minnesota,
USA

MANGUN K. RANDHAWA, MD
Postdoctoral Research Fellow, Division of
Cardiovascular Imaging, Department of
Radiology, Massachusetts General Hospital,
Boston, Massachusetts, USA

LUCA SABA, MD
Dean of the School of Medicine, Professor and
Chairman, Department of Radiology, Azienda
Ospedaliero Universitaria (A.O.U.), Cagliari,
Italy

JAKUB M. SIEMBIDA, MD
Assistant Professor, Department of Radiology,
University of Wisconsin-Madison, Madison,
Wisconsin, USA

MICHAEL STEIGNER, MD
Associate Professor, Department of Radiology,
Cardiovascular Imaging Program, Brigham and
Women's Hospital, Harvard Medical School,
Boston, Massachusetts, USA

MATTHEW T. STIB, MD
Cardiothoracic Radiologist, Division of
Cardiothoracic Imaging, Department of
Radiology, Mayo Clinic Hospital, Phoenix,
Arizona, USA

SADIA SULTANA, MD
Radiologist, Division of Cardiovascular
Imaging, Department of Radiology,

Massachusetts General Hospital, Boston,
Massachusetts, USA

TIMOTHY P. SZCZYKUTOWICZ, PhD
Associate Professor of Radiology, Medical
Physics, and Biomedical Engineering,
University of Wisconsin Madison, Madison,
Wisconsin, USA

MARLY VAN ASSEN, PhD
Assistant Professor, Translational Laboratory
for Cardiothoracic Imaging and Artificial
Intelligence, Department of Radiology and
Imaging Sciences, Emory University, Atlanta,
Georgia, USA

JONATHAN R. WEIR-McCALL, MBChB, PhD
Assistant Professor, Department of Radiology,
School of Clinical Medicine, University of
Cambridge, Cambridge, United Kingdom

**MICHELLE C. WILLIAMS, MBChB, BSc Med
Sci, PhD, BA, MRCP, FRCR, FSCCT**
Senior Clinical Research Fellow, Centre for
Cardiovascular Science, University of
Edinburgh, Edinburgh, The Queen's Medical
Research Institute, Edinburg BioQuarter,
Edinburgh, United Kingdom

EVAN J. ZUCKER, MD
Department of Radiology, Divisions of Pediatric
and Cardiovascular Imaging, Massachusetts
General Hospital, Harvard Medical School,
Boston, Massachusetts, USA

Contents

This review describes current state-of-the-art computed tomography technology required to address human-physiology–based challenges unique to angiographic imaging. Challenges are based on the need to image a bolus of contrast agent traversing inside rapidly moving structures. This article reviews the latest methods to optimize contrast timing and minimize motion.

In this review, the authors summarize the role of coronary computed tomography angiography and coronary artery calcium scoring in different clinical presentations of chest pain and preventative care and discuss future directions and new technologies such as pericoronary fat inflammation and the growing footprint of artificial intelligence in cardiovascular medicine.

 Video content accompanies this article at http://www.radiologic.theclinics.com.

Valvular heart disease (VHD) is a significant clinical problem associated with high morbidity and mortality. Although not being the primary imaging modality in VHD, cardiac computed tomography (CCT) provides relevant information about its morphology, function, severity grading, and adverse cardiac remodeling assessment. Aortic valve calcification quantification is necessary for grading severity in cases of low-flow/low-gradient aortic stenosis. Moreover, CCT details significant information necessary for adequate percutaneous treatment planning. CCT may help to detail the etiology of VHD as well as to depict other less frequent causes of valvular disease, such as infective endocarditis, valvular neoplasms, or other cardiac pseudomasses.

The range of potential transcatheter solutions to valve disease is increasing, bringing treatment options to those in whom surgery confers prohibitively high risk. As the range of devices and their indications grow, so too will the demand for procedural planning. Computed tomography will continue to enable this growth through the provision of accurate device sizing and procedural risk assessment.

Computed tomography (CT) has emerged as a leading imaging modality in the evaluation of congenital heart disease (CHD). With ever-faster acquisition speed, decreasing radiation exposure, impeccable anatomic detail, optional functional data, and numerous post-processing tools, CT offers broad utility in CHD diagnosis, preoperative planning, and postoperative assessment. In this article, the far-reaching role of CT in CHD is reviewed, focusing on technical imaging considerations and key clinical applications.

Heart transplantation is a pivotal treatment of end-stage heart failure, and recent advancements have extended median posttransplant life expectancy. However, despite the progress in surgical techniques and medical treatment, heart transplant patients still face complications such as rejection, infections, and drug toxicity. CT is a reliable tool for detecting most of these complications, whereas MR imaging is particularly adept at identifying pericardial pathologies and signs of rejection. Awareness of these nuances by radiologists, cardiologists, and surgeons is desired to optimize care, reduce morbidities, and enhance survival.

Artificial intelligence (AI) is having a significant impact in medical imaging, advancing almost every aspect of the field, from image acquisition and postprocessing to automated image analysis with outreach toward supporting decision making. Noninvasive cardiac imaging is one of the main and most exciting fields for AI development. The aim of this review is to describe the main applications of AI in cardiac imaging, including CT and MR imaging, and provide an overview of recent advancements and available clinical applications that can improve clinical workflow, disease detection, and prognostication in cardiac disease.

With the increasing prevalence of arrhythmias, the use of electrophysiology (EP) procedures has increased. Recent advancements in computed tomography (CT) technology have expanded its use in pre-assessments and post-assessments of EP procedures. CT provides high-resolution images, is noninvasive, and is widely available. This article highlights the strengths and weaknesses of cardiac CT in EP.

Aortic pathologies encompass a heterogeneous group of disorders, including acute aortic syndrome, traumatic aortic injury , aneurysm, aortitis, and atherosclerosis. The clinical manifestations of these disorders can be varied and non-specific, ranging from acute presentations in the emergency department to chronic incidental findings in an outpatient setting. Given the non-specific nature of their clinical presentations, the reliance on non-invasive imaging for screening, definitive diagnosis, therapeutic strategy planning, and post-intervention surveillance has become paramount. Commonly used imaging modalities include ultrasound, computed tomography (CT), and MR imaging. Among these modalities, computed tomography angiography (CTA) has emerged as a first-line imaging modality owing to its excellent anatomic detail, widespread availability, established imaging protocols, evidence-proven indications, and rapid acquisition time.

This comprehensive article reviews the complex realm of aortic surgical and endovascular interventions, focusing on the aortic root, ascending aorta, aortic arch, descending aorta, and abdominal aorta. It outlines the nuances of various procedures, emphasizing the importance of computed tomography angiography acquisition for an accurate assessment. Detailed discussions encompass expected postsurgical/endovascular findings and complications, covering various scenarios, from hematoma and infection to pseudoaneurysms and graft-related issues. This article serves as a crucial resource for radiologists, offering invaluable insights into the complexities of aortic interventions and their subsequent imaging, fostering a comprehensive understanding of diagnostic and management strategies.

The visceral vasculature is inextricably intertwined with abdominopelvic disease staging, spread, and management in routine and emergent cases. Comprehensive evaluation requires specialized imaging techniques for abnormality detection and characterization. Vascular pathology is often encountered on nondedicated routine imaging examinations, which may obscure, mimic, or confound many vascular diagnoses. This review highlights normal arterial, portal venous, and systemic venous anatomy and clinically relevant variants; diagnostic pitfalls related to image-acquisition technique and disease mimics; and characteristics of common and rare vascular diseases to empower radiologists to confidently interpret the vascular findings and avoid misdiagnosis.

RADIOLOGIC CLINICS OF NORTH AMERICA

SERIES OF RELATED INTEREST

Advances in Clinical Radiology
Available at: https://www.advancesinclinicalradiology.com/
Magnetic Resonance Imaging Clinics
Available at: https://www.mri.theclinics.com/
Neuroimaging Clinics
Available at: www.neuroimaging.theclinics.com
PET Clinics
Available at: www.pet.theclinics.com

THE CLINICS ARE AVAILABLE ONLINE!
Access your subscription at:
www.theclinics.com

PROGRAM OBJECTIVE

The objective of the *Radiologic Clinics of North America* is to keep practicing radiologists and radiology residents up to date with current clinical practice in radiology by providing timely articles reviewing the state of the art in patient care.

TARGET AUDIENCE

Practicing radiologists, radiology residents, and other healthcare professionals who provide patient care utilizing radiologic findings.

LEARNING OBJECTIVES

Upon completion of this activity, participants will be able to:

1. Describe the significance of the Radiologist's knowledge surrounding imaging patterns of aortic diseases and post-treatment complications.
2. Discuss how computed tomography (CT) has emerged as a leading imaging modality in the evaluation of congenital heart disease (CHD).
3. Recognize cardiac computed tomography (CCT) provides both relevant and detailed significant information necessary for adequate treatment planning.

ACCREDITATION

The Elsevier Office of Continuing Medical Education (EOCME) is accredited by the Accreditation Council for Continuing Medical Education (ACCME) to provide continuing medical education for physicians.

The EOCME designates this journal-based CME activity for a maximum of 11 *AMA PRA Category 1 Credit*(s)™. Physicians should claim only the credit commensurate with the extent of their participation in the activity.

All other healthcare professionals requesting continuing education credit for this enduring material will be issued a certificate of participation.

DISCLOSURE OF CONFLICTS OF INTEREST

The EOCME assesses conflict of interest with its instructors, faculty, planners, and other individuals who are in a position to control the content of CME activities. All relevant conflicts of interest that are identified are thoroughly vetted by EOCME for fair balance, scientific objectivity, and patient care recommendations. EOCME is committed to providing its learners with CME activities that promote improvements or quality in healthcare and not a specific proprietary business or a commercial interest.

The planning committee, staff, authors, and editors listed below have identified no financial relationships or relationships to products or devices they or their spouse/life partner have with commercial interest related to the content of this CME activity:

Prachi P. Agarwal, MBBS; Ayaz Aghayev, MD; Chiemezie Amadi, MD; Vitaliy Androshchuk, MBChB; Vinit Baliyan, MBBS, MD; Jordi Broncano, MD; Jinjin Cao, MD; Thomas Clifford, MBChB; Ishan Garg, MD; Gabrielle Gershon, BSc; Brian Ghoshhajra, MD, MBA; Sumit Gupta, MD, PhD; Kate Hanneman, MD, MPH, FRCPC; Sandeep Hedgire, MD; Kothainayaki Kulanthaivelu, BCA, MBA; Elizabeth Lee, MD; Michelle C. Littlejohn; Eriberto Michel, MD; Emanuele Muscogiuri, MD; Giuseppe Muscogiuri, MD, PhD; Prashant Nagpal, MD; Carlotta Onnis, MD; Anushri Parakh, MBBS, MD; Vinay Prabhu, MD, MS; Sarv Priya, MD; Ronak Rajani, DM, MD, FRCP, FESC, FACC, FSCCT, FRCR; Prabhakar Rajiah, MD; Mangun K. Randhawa, MD; Luca Saba, MD; Jakub M. Siembida, MD; Michael Steigner, MD; Matthew T. Stib, MD; Sadia Sultana, MD; Sadia Sultana, MD; Jonathan R. Weir-McCall, MBChB, PhD; Evan J. Zucker, MD

The planning committee, staff, authors, and editors listed below have identified financial relationships or relationships to products or devices they or their spouse/life partner have with commercial interest related to the content of this CME activity:

Carlo N. De Cecco, MD, PhD: Research Support: Siemens Healthineers; Consultant: Bayer, Xeos

Cian P. McCarthy, MB, BCh, BAO, SM: Consultant: Abbott Laboratories, Roche Diagnostics

Theodore T. Pierce, MD, MPH: Consultant & Equity: AutonomUS Healthcare; Research Support: General Electric

Timothy P. Szczykutowicz, PhD: Research Support: Canon Medical Systems, GE HealthCare; Consultant: Alara Imaging, Imalogix, Aidoc, Asto CT/Leo Cancer Care; Royalties related to intellectual property: Qaelum; Founder: RadUnity

Marly van Assen, MSc, PhD: Research Support: Siemens Healthineers

Michelle C. Williams, MBChB, BSc Med Sci, PhD, BA, MRCP, FRCR, FSCCT: Speaker: Canon Medical Systems, Siemens Healthineers, Novartis

UNAPPROVED/OFF-LABEL USE DISCLOSURE

The EOCME requires CME faculty to disclose to the participants:

1. When products or procedures being discussed are off-label, unlabelled, experimental, and/or investigational (not US Food and Drug Administration [FDA] approved); and

2. Any limitations on the information presented, such as data that are preliminary or that represent ongoing research, interim analyses, and/or unsupported opinions. Faculty may discuss information about pharmaceutical agents that is outside of FDA-approved labelling. This information is intended solely for CME and is not intended to promote off-label use of these medications. If you have any questions, contact the medical affairs department of the manufacturer for the most recent pre-scribing information.

TO ENROLL

To enroll in the *Radiologic Clinics of North America* Continuing Medical Education program, call customer service at 1-800-654-2452 or sign up online at http://www.theclinics.com/home/cme. The CME program is available to subscribers for an additional annual fee of USD 340.00.

METHOD OF PARTICIPATION

In order to claim credit, participants must complete the following:
1. Complete enrolment as indicated above.
2. Read the activity.
3. Complete the CME Test and Evaluation. Participants must achieve a score of 70% on the test. All CME Tests and Evaluations must be completed online.

CME INQUIRIES/SPECIAL NEEDS

For all CME inquiries or special needs, please contact elsevierCME@elsevier.com.

Preface
Advances in Cardiovascular Imaging

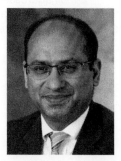
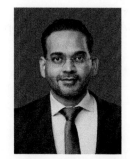

Prashant Nagpal, MD, FSCCT   Sandeep Hedgire, MD, FSCCT

Editors

Cardiovascular diseases are the leading cause of death worldwide. Imaging has become a cornerstone for various cardiovascular diseases and is needed for diagnosis, treatment planning, follow-up, and prognostication of patients. Cardiovascular system imaging can be challenging due to physiologic factors, like differences in cardiac output, breathing, and cardiac motion. Technical advances in computed tomographic (CT) hardware and software have now allowed rapid imaging with minimal need for case supervision. This has led to a steady increase in the use of imaging for cardiovascular diseases. Furthermore, research on imaging biomarkers has established tools like CT-based fractional flow reserve that now enable robust anatomic and physiologic imaging of coronary vessels.

In this special issue of the *Radiologic Clinics of North America*, international experts in the field of cardiovascular imaging have summarized various topics focusing on the ever-expanding role of CT imaging in cardiovascular diseases. This issue highlights the "latest" technical advances in CT hardware and protocols as well as the "greatest" innovations on the horizon for imaging, like artificial intelligence.

Readers will discover an in-depth review of CT technology and physics by Dr Szczykutowicz, followed by a detailed examination of coronary imaging by Drs Lee, Agarwal, and their team. Dr Broncano and colleagues offer an insightful review

of cardiac CT in assessing native heart valves. CT has emerged as the test of choice for planning and monitoring advanced cardiovascular interventions and surgeries. Drs Clifford, Weir-McCall, and their team discuss the growing importance of cardiovascular CT in the planning and follow-up of percutaneous cardiac valve interventions. This is complemented by Dr Zucker's thorough review of cardiac CT in congenital heart disease. Dr Randhawa and colleagues, including the co-editors, explore the role of cardiovascular CT in heart transplant patients. Drs Onnis, De Cecco, and their team provide an excellent analysis of the emerging role of artificial intelligence in cardiovascular imaging. Dr Sultana and colleagues focus on the role of CT in cardiac electrophysiology procedures.

Among the vascular system–specific reviews, you will find a comprehensive review on aortic imaging by the co-editors and their team. Continuing with the theme of the role of CT for postprocedure follow-up, Dr Aghayev and colleagues have done a very image-rich review on the role of CTA after transcatheter and surgical aortic interventions, followed by imaging of visceral vessels by Dr Pierce and colleagues. The diversity of these topics and discussions highlights how CT angiography is playing a central role in improving the anatomic evaluation of multiorgan vascular systems.

From the breadth of these reviews, we aim to enrich readers from all realms: clinical, educational, and research perspectives. It has been a pleasure

Radiol Clin N Am 62 (2024) xiii–xiv
https://doi.org/10.1016/j.rcl.2024.02.001
0033-8389/24/© 2024 Published by Elsevier Inc.

and honor to serve as Guest Editors for this issue. We hope you enjoy reading this issue as much as we enjoyed working on it.

Prashant Nagpal, MD, FSCCT
Cardiovascular Imaging
University of Wisconsin–Madison
Madison, WI, USA

Sandeep Hedgire, MD, FSCCT
Cardiovascular Imaging
Massachusetts General Hospital
Harvard Medical School
Boston, MA, USA

E-mail addresses:
pnagpal@wisc.edu (P. Nagpal)
hedgire.sandeep@mgh.harvard.edu (S. Hedgire)

Computed Tomography Angiography
Principles and Advances

Timothy P. Szczykutowicz, PhD

KEYWORDS

- CT technology • Computed tomography • CCTA acquisition • CT protocol • Cardiac gating
- Prospective gating • Retrospective gating • Heart rate adaptation

KEY POINTS

- The newest computed tomography (CT) acquisition modes for cardiovascular imaging adapt to a patient's size, heart rate, heart rate variability, and likelihood of irregular beats.
- Modern CT systems can automatically facilitate robust coronary computed tomography angiography (CCTA) protocols accounting for heart rate variability/irregularity via adjusting the amount and phase of data acquisition during the cardiac cycle.
- Because of differences in scanner geometry (wide axial vs dual source) and gating options (automatic irregularity adaptation), harmonizing the technical acquisition of CCTA protocols between different scanner makes and models can be a challenge, albeit the end result may be similar: low-motion high-contrast coronaries.

INTRODUCTION

Historically, cardiac imaging has been the most challenging task for computed tomography (CT).[1] Several factors make imaging of the heart difficult. In later discussion, the challenges and technological solutions are itemized. In many cases, differences exist in technology, as different solutions are better suited for different clinical situations (eg, prospective gating using axial/sequential scanning vs slow helical/spiral pitch retrospective gating). Furthermore, different CT vendors have developed diverging technologies in some cases (eg, dual source vs wide axial).

Superior-Inferior Coverage Needs

The heart is a relatively large organ, often spanning more than 14 cm in size in the superior-inferior direction. One can understand the historical development of coverage needs for cardiac imaging by focusing on collimation and pitch requirements to cover this roughly 14-cm range. Modern scanners use either wide-beam collimations or higher- (ie, 3.2:1) pitch values combined with prospective electrocardiographic (ECG) gating. These techniques can acquire the heart within a single cardiac cycle. Before the community had wide collimations or dual-source CT scanners, data from multiple cardiac cycles were stitched together across the superior-inferior range of the heart acquired using retrospective or prospective scanning modes. When CT was introduced in the 1970s,[2] it only had a few millimeters of coverage. Not until the 2000s were 16-cm coverage detectors commercially available. To image the entire heart in a single gantry rotation in an axial (ie, sequential) mode, a large collimation detector is required, and multiple CT vendors have commercialized 16-cm detectors for this purpose.[3,4] Coronary computed tomography angiography (CCTA), however, was being performed before the advent of large-area CT detectors through the use of multiple CT couch bed positions and helical (ie, spiral) gated acquisitions in which CT projection data from multiple beats were stitched

University of Wisconsin Madison, 1005 WIMR, 1111 Highland Avenue, Madison, WI 53705, USA
E-mail address: tszczykutowicz@uwhealth.org
Twitter: @Prof_TimStick (T.P.S.)

Radiol Clin N Am 62 (2024) 371–383
https://doi.org/10.1016/j.rcl.2024.01.005
0033-8389/24/© 2024 Elsevier Inc. All rights reserved.

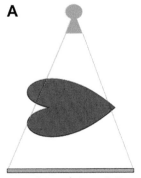
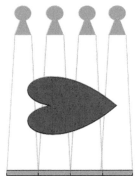
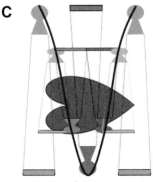

A

"wide axial mode"
Single rotation, 1 couch
position

B

"step and shoot mode"
1 rotation per couch
position, time spent moving
between positions

C

"helical/spiral mode"
Continuous data collection

Superior-Inferior direction
←——————————→

Fig. 1. The 3 main ways cardiac CT data are acquired. (*A*) A wide axial collimation scanner (ie, a collimation of ~16 cm in the superior-inferior patient direction) capable of acquiring heart coverage in a single rotation using an axial/sequential scan mode (ie, the patient couch does not translate during data acquisition). (*B*) A scanner with a beam collimation not large enough to cover the entire heart in a single rotation; hence, entire heart coverage is obtained using multiple couch positions. In other words, in panel B, the patient is scanned using an axial/sequential mode at multiple couch positions where the scanner couch remains still during data acquisition and quickly moves between scanning locations. (*C*) A helical/spiral acquisition. The helical pitch values used in cardiac CT vary greatly from low pitches around 0.1:1 (ie, the scanner moves very slowly and acquired many rotations of data over each part of the heart) commonly used for retrospective gating to very high pitches (eg, 3.2:1) used for prospective gating (eg, Siemens Healthineers Turbo Flash mode).

together to create a single composite image.[5] Dual-source scanners enable smaller than 16 cm detectors to be used in conjunction with high-pitch values to image the entire heart within a single beat.[6] A dual-source scanner operating at 3.2:1 pitch corresponds to a table speed of 737 mm/s, which covers 16 cm in 0.217 seconds. **Fig. 1** reviews the various methods used to acquire the superior-inferior range required to image the heart.

Contrast Dynamics

Blood flow through the human body varies, but in the large elastic arteries of the heart, blood flow will exceed tens of centimeters per second.[7] This means a bolus of contrast agent will reach a peak in the coronary vessels for a limited amount of time.[8] Timing a scan to overlap with peak coronary enhancement is therefore important to maximize image quality. This timing is prone to error given the peak enhancement persists for a matter of seconds. Today, 2 methods are used to achieve patient-specific cardiac contrast timing[9]: (1) bolus tracking uses a real-time intermittent CT scan mode, which measures contrast agent enhancement and triggers the scan when the contrast

reaches a threshold; and (2) a timing bolus method in which a small bolus of contrast agent is delivered and a time-enhancement curve is measured using an intermittent CT scan mode from which the peak is determined and used to time a subsequent CT scan where a full bolus of contrast agent is delivered. Each of these methods have pros and cons, which are described in **Table 1**. For an excellent review of the factors effecting contrast administration in CCTA, see Cademartiri and colleagues.[11]

Motion

When CT was introduced to medicine in the 1970s, scan times were on the order of tens of minutes.[2] The head was an ideal body region for these early scans because motion in the head can be easily controlled and is largely voluntary. Imaging the vessels and chambers of the heart was one of the last organs to be well visualized by CT because it exhibits fast involuntary motion. The right coronary artery, for example, can move at a velocity of 69.5 mm/s.[12] Consider how much motion this is in terms of the resolution of a CT scanner. For a typical cardiac reconstruction field of view of

Table 1
Comparison of bolus tracking and timing bolus contrast timing methods for coronary computed tomography angiography

	Bolus Tracking	Timing Bolus
Typical protocol	A small slice of the patient is scanned (usually extending <10 mm in length). The CT scanner will scan intermittently after a preprogrammed delay (ie, "monitoring delay") at a user-adjustable interval (usually 1–2 s) and plot in real time the ROI value of enhancement. When the ROI reaches a predetermined threshold, the scan is triggered.	A small bolus of contrast agent (eg, 20 mL) is administered to the patient. An ROI is defined, and after a short delay to wait for contrast arrival, the scanner acquires intermittent CT images and produces a plot of CT enhancement over time. The ideal bolus tracking run will include a peak of contrast enhancement.
ROI placement	Typical placement is in the ascending aorta or left ventricle. Enhancement in the left side of the heart (ie, left ventricle or ascending aorta) corresponds to contrast, making it from the venous injection location through the right side of the heart and lungs where it is pumping or about to be pumped into the aorta and coronaries. Choosing the coronaries themselves would be less than ideal given their tiny size and likelihood of motion.	
Typical duration of bolus tracking	The scan is triggered once a threshold is reached. Typical durations can last for 1–3 images corresponding to a scan time of 2–6 s for an interscan delay 2 s. This duration increases as the monitoring delay decreases.	~20 s
Scan delay math	The scan will start after: (1) the bolus tracking monitoring delay (ie, a fixed time patient to patient), (2) the time to reach contrast enhancement (ie, the patient-specific time, which depends on the patient's heart function and contrast administration flow rate), and (3) the time delay between triggering and actual scanning (ie, no scanner can immediately start scanning once the threshold is reached; usually a finite amount of time is needed on the order of a few seconds to increase the beam collimation and move the patient for the subsequent volumetric acquisition).	(Time delay before bolus tracking monitoring) + time to peak from initiation of bolus tracking monitoring to peak enhancement) + (fixed time of usually 4–6 s to account for the smaller volume of contrast agent used in the bolus tracking injection compared with a full diagnostic injection). It is important to understand the peak enhancement from a small volume of contrast will always occur sooner in time than the larger diagnostic dose. For this reason, protocols add time to the peak obtained from a bolus tracking scan.[10] Typically, sites account for this by adding 4–6 extra seconds to the time to peak from the bolus tracking run.
Radiation dose	For both methods, radiation dose is much lower than the subsequent CCTA scan. Dose will usually be higher for a bolus tracking method because the scan duration is longer. Note, the scanner reported CTDIvol may appear quite high (eg, in the tens or hundreds of mGy), but the absorbed dose to the patient is quite small given the beam collimation used for these types of scans is very narrow. Typically, bolus tracking accounts for a few percent of a patient's total effective dose.	

(continued on next page)

Table 1
(continued)

	Bolus Tracking	Timing Bolus
Cons	If the patient has extraordinarily slow or fast cardiac function, it is possible their enhancement may occur outside the window the scanner is programmed to monitor the contrast on, causing a missed bolus. If the patient moves during the scan, the ROI location can move off the prescribed location, which could result in erroneous or useless timing information.	A separate injection is needed, making examination times longer. The patient's cardiac output may change between the bolus tracking run and the diagnostic phase of the examination. The peak of injection from a small volume of contrast agent will always be sooner in time than a larger bolus of contrast agent, so extra time must be added to the peak to predict the peak enhancement in the subsequent full contrast scan.

Abbreviations: ROI, region of interest.

25 cm, with 512 pixels, there is a pixel size of 0.48 mm. If a scan has a duration of 1 second (eg, 1 s*69.5 mm/s = 69.5 mm), the amount of motion blur would be many times the voxel size! For this reason, CT scanners performing cardiac scanning use faster rotation times and special gated acquisitions to avoid imaging at peak vessel motion. **Table 2** discusses technology used to address coronary motion. **Figs. 2–4** depict minimum data acquisition needs for single- and dual-source cardiac and describe the interplay between tube location and vessel motion direction's effect on artifact magnitude.

Spatial Resolution

Visualization and assessment of the coronary vessels is usually the goal for imaging of the heart. These vessels (the left main coronary artery, the left anterior descending coronary artery, the left circumflex coronary artery, and the right coronary artery) vary in size at their proximal end from 3 to 5 mm.[25,26] Although objects of this size are easily visualized on CT, quantification of obstruction within a vessel requires separation of coronary artery plaque from blood within a vessel and is the primary task required from a CT data set by a radiologist.[27] Characterization of plaque within a vessel is therefore a relatively high-resolution task for CT. Readers new to cardiac CT should be aware of "calcium blooming." Calcium blooming refers to the apparent enlargement of coronary calcium on CT. There is nothing unique about cardiac CT imaging nor calcium that enlarges calcium containing plaques. All objects reconstructed in CT are blurred; blurring is inherent to CT data acquisition and reconstruction. Objects with a high CT number, like calcium, also get blurred, and because they started with a high CT number, the size of the calcium appears larger than it really is.[28] Lower-resolution kernels are used in cardiac CT, so this issue could be mitigated by using higher-resolution kernels, but then the noise would prohibitively increase, making assessment of the coronaries difficult.

RADIATION DOSE IN CORONARY COMPUTED TOMOGRAPHY ANGIOGRAPHY

Radiation dose in gated coronary acquisitions is just as complicated as one would suspect, based on **Fig. 5**. Because vendors have implemented so many different methods for controlling the tube current, and this control is often related to a patient's heart rate, predicting radiation dose in CCT is difficult. For example, **Fig. 6** shows how a scanner can literally double the dose when it detects an irregular beat. Furthermore, tube current

(ie, milliampere [mA]) and beam energy (ie, kilovolt [kV]) on most modern CT scanners can also be set to automatically adjust to patient size. The result is that the radiation dose in CCTA can be a function of the CT scanner gating mode, patient heart rate, patient heart rate variability, and patient body size.

There is a difference between the amount of radiation dose contributing to a specific cardiac phase image and the total radiation dose delivered to the patient. Because CCTA uses a short scan reconstruction, which uses a subset of view angles from a tube rotation to minimize motion artifacts (see **Fig. 2**) and is commonly acquired using data acquisition wider in time than a short scan, some radiation dose is acquired but not used for image reconstruction. **Fig. 7** explains the relationship between image dose and patient examination dose. This extra radiation dose may be used to create nonoptimal cardiac phase images, or to feed a motion compensation algorithm extra data to estimate motion fields, or to provide a physician with a range of cardiac phase images to interpret. This can be frustrating to a physician who may have a CCTA examination with a high dose (eg, the patient had a variable heart rate causing the scanner to acquire extra beats worth of data, which could double or triple the radiation dose) but with image noise qualities as if the dose were lower.

Typically, dose values in cardiac CT are reported using CTDIvol (CT dose volume index) in milligray (mGy), dose length product (DLP) in mGy*cm, and effective dose in millisievert (mSv). CTDIvol represents the CT scanner's output of dose delivered to a 32-cm phantom. DLP represents the CTDIvol times the scan range (ie, one can divide the DLP by the scan range and approximate the CTDIvol used for an acquisition), and effective dose represents the risk of developing cancer and genetic effects. Only effective dose can be compared across imaging modalities; CTDIvol and DLP are "CT-only" dose metrics. It is hoped that it is apparent after reading the rest of this article that gated cardiac dose is not easily determined on a modern CT scanner that adjusts to so many patient-specific variables. However, at a high level, the potential dose savings of prospective gating versus retrospective gating can be understood. Because, in prospective gating, the author tries to only irradiate the patient when their heart cycle is in a specific phase, prospective gating inherently delivers a smaller dose than retrospective gating in most cases (ie, exception would be if the scanner detects an irregular beat and rescans the patient). An analysis of 30 publications, including 3330 patients by Menke and

Table 2
Technology developments aimed at reducing the effect of coronary motion artifacts in coronary computed tomography angiography

Technology	Description	Comments
Rotation time decreases	Rotation time in CT is analogous to a photograph's shutter speed. The longer the shutter is open, the more motion blur one sees in a photograph for any objects that are moving during the acquisition of the photograph. In CT, the rotation time defines the time for data collection. The longer the rotation time, the more motion blur present in the projection data. Technically, a CT projection data set is composed of hundreds to thousands of individual projections; each projection measurement would have a very small amount of motion blur because a typical CT projection is acquired in ~1 ms. The movement of an object over the time span of hundreds to thousands of projection measurements is what causes motion artifact in CT.	As rotation time decreases, the amount of photon fluence used to generate an image decrease. Therefore, for large patients imaged with very small rotation times in cardiac imaging, noise can be an issue. For example, a bariatric patient receiving a thoracic spine examination where motion is not a concern may be scanned using 0.5:1 pitch, and 1-s rotation. If that same patient is scanned in a cardiac mode in an axial scan mode at 0.25-s rotation time, their photon fluence would be 8 times smaller for the cardiac scan relative to the spine scan! Current state-of-the-art CT scanners enjoy rotations times around 0.23–0.28 s. Vendors may claim temporal resolutions less than the rotation time because <360° of data are usually used for cardiac CT image reconstruction via partial angle reconstruction and/or the use of dual-source scanning geometry (see Fig. 3).
Partial angle reconstruction	All modern CT scanners use a fan beam geometry. In a fan beam geometry, the x-ray tube needs to circle about the patient for at least 180° plus the fan angle to reconstruct an image[13] (see Fig. 1). Usually, outside of cardiac CT (eg, a diagnostic helical abdomen examination), at least 360° of data are used. A short scan view angular range corresponds to <360°, which means the time for minimum data collection is always less than the rotation time. Because the data near the center of a short scan range are more unique than data at the edges, the effective temporal resolution of a short scan reconstruction is less than the time required for the tube to rotate through 180 plus the fan angle degrees. A rule of thumb (ie, you will see this in a vendor's marketing literature and specification sheets) is to benchmark a scanner's temporal resolution at one-half the rotation time, even though a common short scan angular range would correspond to two-thirds the rotation time (eg, a typical fan angle is ~60° and (180 + 60)/360 = 2/3).	All routine axial scanning in nongated modes will almost always use 360° of scanning. Most helical scanning for pitches below 1:1 will use data acquired from more than 360° of rotation.[14] Only in gated cardiac modes and in some vendor's implementations of CT fluoroscopy images are seen that are made using short scan reconstruction techniques to minimize the effects of motion.

| Dual-source acquisition | Currently, only a single vendor has commercialized CT scanners offering dual-source data acquisition. In a dual-source data acquisition, the angular range needed for a short scan reconstruction is nearly half that of a single x-ray tube system (see Fig. 3). Dual-source cardiac CT represents the best temporal resolution using hardware alone and should theoretically provide the best temporal resolution in ideal heart rate and heart irregularity conditions. | The use of both x-ray tubes on a dual-source system is the default for cardiac-gated scanning but also common for nongated scanning when scan times need to be made shorter via faster CT couch feed speeds, or higher tube outputs are required for bariatric patients. Dual-energy CT cannot be combined with dual-source high-pitch imaging, as the "second" tube must be either used to enable pitches > ~1.5:1 or for DECT. Failure to control a patient's heart rate can make the use of prospectively triggered high-pitch cardiac scanning difficult, because high-pitch prospective cardiac gating is an "all-or-nothing" type of acquisition that is not robust to irregular heart rates like a wide axial scanner. A wide axial scanner can dwell over the same anatomy for a longer period, padding data collection to be robust to irregular beats. Each of these designs has their pros and cons, with dual source offering the best temporal resolution, via giving up some robustness in spanning all patient heart rate presentations. Dual-source scanners will usually default to a retrospectively low-pitch scan mode for patients with high and/or irregular heart rates. |
| Motion mitigation via reconstruction | Most vendors will use algorithms that detect and correct for coronary motion. At a high level, all these methods use some means for estimating coronary vessel motion and then adjust the reconstruction such that the motion can be removed from the projection data. One method is illustrated for obtaining an estimate of vessel motion. If one reconstructs 3 images, each with a different and monotonically increasing ECG phase, the position of a vessel in each image can be determined and the displacement between these positions provides an estimate for the speed and direction of the vessel movement. This information can then be applied during the backprojection step to modify where the vessel signal is placed. Many methods for motion correction exist in the literature,[15–17] and one should expect a modern state-of-the-art CT scanner to come with a commercial motion mitigation solution (eg, GE Healthcare has snapshot freeze; Canon Medical has Adaptive Motion Correction; Philips has Precise Cardiac).[18–21] | Benchmarking 2 scanners against each other in terms of cardiac temporal resolution is a challenge. To the author's knowledge, there is no consensus on performing a head-to-head temporal resolution evaluation between 2 scanners. The ability of an algorithm to mitigate motion is highly nonlinear and will be a function of the relative position of the x-ray tube to the direction of vessel motion during the scan, and the contrast level of the vessel. This can be frustrating in the clinic when patient-to-patient motion levels may appear drastically different even for similar heart rates (see Fig. 4). |

(continued on next page)

Table 2
(continued)

Technology	Description	Comments
ECG-gated acquisition	All regions of the heart are in almost constant motion throughout a single cardiac cycle, with the velocity of motion changing by orders of magnitude for most structures in the heart.[22] Cardiac-gated CT takes advantage of the reproducibility from patient to patient in relatively small movement of the heart during specific cardiac phases.[23] Details on specific structure movement with phases can be found in the literature based on MR imaging[22] and electron beam CT.[12] Cardiac-gated acquisitions record a patient's ECG signal during data acquisition. This allows for 2 things: (1) if desired, data acquisition can be triggered to begin at a specific cardiac phase (ie, prospective cardiac gating); and (2) each projection view angle can be assigned to a specific cardiac phase allowing for phase-specific reconstructions (ie, one may acquire data for a few heart beats and then use a subset of the data acquired near a specific phase to create a phase-specific reconstruction; see **Fig. 5** for a more detailed description of how cardiac-gated CTA acquisition and reconstruction works).	Understanding how a CT scanner may automatically adapt, or how one should manually adapt a CT protocol to account for a patient's heart rate and possible heart variability is described in **Fig. 5**. Many different vendor solutions exist in this space, making a vendor-specific review difficult. This is a changing space as hardware and software advancements constantly change the solutions for cardiac-gated image acquisition. **Fig. 5** reviews the major concepts allowing the reader to understand a vendor's specific solutions.
Beam collimation	Historically, cardiac CT became a reality when CT technology developed large enough beam collimations (ie, collimation great than or equal to roughly 2 cm[24]) to make scan times possible within a few heart beats or within a single contrast bolus and or breath hold. Typical cardiac beam collimations today offer 0.5–0.625-mm slice thicknesses across a superior-inferior range of 6–16 cm.	Today, it appears beam collimations have hit a maximum of 16 cm, with several vendors offering 16-cm scanners. Dual-source CT does not currently offer a 16-cm detector, albeit on a dual-source scanner the optimal cardiac acquisition mode uses a high-pitch imaging mode where a 16-cm detector is not required for single-beat cardiac imaging.

Abbreviations: DECT, dual energy computed tomography.

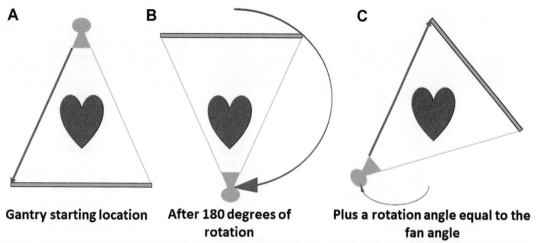

Gantry starting location

After 180 degrees of rotation

Plus a rotation angle equal to the fan angle

Fig. 2. Central to cardiac image reconstruction is the concept of a short scan. In a short scan, only the data within an angular range of 180 plus the fan angle of the beam are required for image formation. Because this is less than 360°, when a short scan reconstruction is used, the temporal window of data acquisition is smaller than if 360° were used. This is critical in cardiac CT to reduce the effect of heart motion. To understand why 180 + the fan angle are needed, consider the blue ray shown at the edge of the fan beam in panel A. The tube must rotate through 180 + the fan angle until it is at the location shown in panel C where the edge of the fan angle is again lined up with the original blue ray. In other words, once the tube rotates from (A), to (B), to (C), it has collected all the nonredundant projections of the patient.

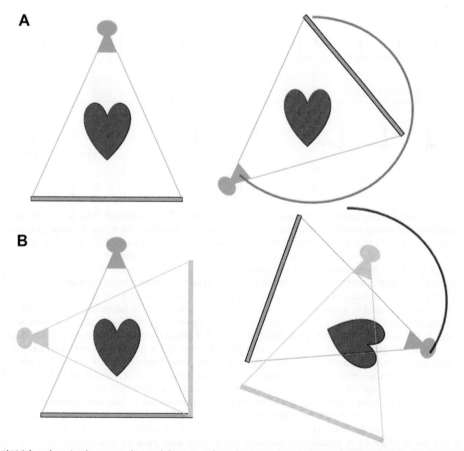

Fig. 3. (A) With only a single x-ray tube and detector, the tube must rotate through 180° + the fan angle, as discussed in **Fig. 2.** However, for scanners using a dual-source geometry, a second tube and detector are presently offset by roughly 90° from the first. (B) This effectively cuts the arc of tube travel needed in half. This corresponds to an increase in the temporal resolution (ie, the time for data acquisition is roughly halved) by roughly a factor of 2.

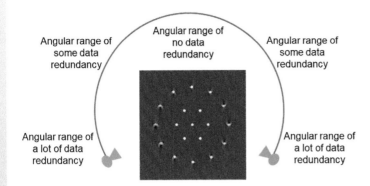

Angular range of some data redundancy

Angular range of no data redundancy

Angular range of some data redundancy

Angular range of a lot of data redundancy

Angular range of a lot of data redundancy

Fig. 4. Motion artifacts in cardiac scans are largely a function of the direction and speed of the vessel motion relative to the location of the x-ray tube and detector during data acquisition. All the circles in the outer ring of circles were simulated to move with the same velocity in an outward tangential direction. Clearly, the degree of artifact observed for each of the circles is quite variable. These results demonstrate that it may be "luck" that produces a good-looking cardiac coronary in a vendor's advertising materials or in a colleague's slide set. In other words, if your vessel is at the 3 o'clock position as shown, it may turn out looking relatively artifact-free compared with whether the tube happened to be shifted 90° during the examination (eg, the 9 o'clock position). (Figure reprinted from Szczykutowicz, T. (2020). The CT handbook: optimizing protocols for today's feature-rich scanners. Medical Physics Publishing.[28])

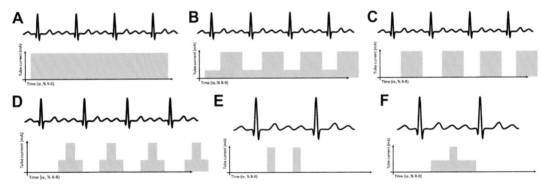

Fig. 5. (*A–F*) Different cardiac gating strategies in the clinic today. These methods can be combined with the various acquisition geometry methods depicted in **Figs. 1** and **3B**, resulting in many different possible gating modes. Usually, a specific CT scanner in one's fleet will only be capable of a subset of the combinations of scanner geometries in **Figs. 1** and **3B** and tube current control shown here. (*A*) A retrospective gating acquisition where the tube current is only for many heart beats. In a usual retrospective gated acquisition, a helical/spiral acquisition is used, and the pitch value is set to a very low value (ie, ~0.1:1) so many rotations of data are obtained over each position within the heart at many different cardiac phases. (*B*) An example of a retrospective acquisition where the tube current is modulated in a prospective manner (this is counterintuitive based on the name, as one would assume a retrospectively gated acquisition would not make prospective guesses as to the timeliness of the heart cycle). In panel B, the user would usually prescribe the target R-R phase for the higher tube current data and the amount to decrease the tube current over the nontargeted phases. (*C*) A prospective multiple beat acquisition where the tube current is modulated on and off, on over a user-prescribed target R-R phase and off otherwise. (*D*) Similar to panel C, a prospective acquisition but here the tube current profile is widened and reduced to allow some robustness to heart rate variability albeit at a lower level of image quality if the optimal reconstruction is off the anticipated higher tube current temporal location. (*E*) A prospective acquisition in which more than one R-R window was prescribed. One should be aware that when 2 windows are prescribed as shown here, eventually these regions will "touch" as the heart rate increases or the windows are increased in size. (*F*) Essentially the same as panel D but for a single-beat acquisition, perhaps for a wide axial type of acquisition where whole heart coverage is obtained in a single heartbeat. The widths of the higher tube current regions observed in panels D, E, and F correspond to a short scan angular range. In panels D, E, and F, a single phase is desired, but a finite amount of the patient's R-R interval must be collected to allow the x-ray tube to collect a short scan's worth of projection data.

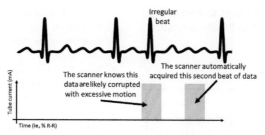

Fig. 6. Advanced cardiac gating modes will be robust to issues at scan time with a patient's heart rate "throwing" an irregular beat. Depicted here is an example of a scanner that sensed an irregular beat during the acquisition and immediately acquired a second window of data. Some scanners will have prebuilt profiles allowing this behavior and may allow the user to control if this feature is active or not. Some scanners may automatically prescribe an additional 2 beats, for a total of 3 beats in certain situations of highly irregular heart patterns. These adaptation to a specific patient's heart patterns can make predicting cardiac radiation dose difficult. One should be aware radiation dose is a function of heart rate and variability when reviewing dosimetry data for gated examinations.

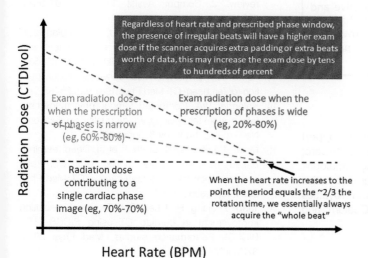

Fig. 7. he radiation dose used to image a single cardiac phase will not vary with a patient's heart rate or heart rate variability. This is because when a short scan reconstruction is used, the same amount of view angle projections always goes into producing the image. Mathematically, in the $Image\ Dose \propto \frac{240}{360} * Tube\ Current * Rotation\ Time$, the factor of 240/360 corresponds to the angular range needed for a short scan cardiac reconstruction. This will not be the scanner reported dose, however, because the scanner reported dose will include any extra padding of data acquisition required to make the examination robust to heart rate irregularities. As the amount of cardiac phase requested for acquisition increases, the radiation dose will increase in a linear manner. As the heart rate increases, the radiation dose will decrease for a given prescription of cardiac window R-R cycle until the heart period equals roughly two-thirds of the rotation time (ie, the condition of a short scan). As the heart rate decreases, the same R-R prescription will take a longer time to elapse, which means examination dose will increase as heart rate creases should be increases. One should be careful when extrapolating the concepts in this plot and caption to a commercial scanner. A vendor may add extra padding and impose limitations to their cardiac gating, which do not behave as described here.

colleagues,[29] found that the effective radiation doses with prospective triggering was lower than retrospectively triggered studies (3.5 mSv in prospective group vs 12.3 mSv in the retrospective group). In terms of CT dose metrics, Menke and colleagues reported a CTDIvol difference of 15.4 to 46.4 mGy between studies reporting prospective and retrospective doses, respectively, and for DLP 205 to 673 mGy*cm, respectively. These values can be used as a reference point to understand radiation dose on your particular cardiac technology, with the caveat of your vendor's implementation of patient-specific dose, and cardiac gating modulation may result in observed doses lower or higher than these reported values.

SUMMARY

In summary, the methods for acquiring cardiac-gated imaging are varied. Because so many variations exist in patient presentation of heart rate and heart irregularity, no single approach for cardiac imaging will be optimal. Modern CT scanners will come with automatic adjustment features allowing the technology they possess to be best used to mitigate cardiac motion. State-of-the-art today comes in many different configurations, which also means 2 scanners sitting next to each other may image the same patient in 2 different ways, producing similar results.

CLINICS CARE POINTS

- Radiation exposure will change from patient to patient on advanced scanners for coronary computed tomography angiography because the scanner adapts for patient size and heart rate/variability.
- Image noise may not decrease with irradiation dose increases because a constant amount of data goes into a cardiac reconstruction, regardless of how much of a patient's cardiac cycle was sampled.
- The difference between a retrospective and prospective cardiac acquisition is hard to define on state-of-the-art systems owing to the high degree of automated patient-specific adaptation.

DISCLOSURE

T.P. Szczykutowicz receives research support from Canon Medical Systems and GE HealthCare; consulting fees from Alara Imaging, Imalogix, Aidoc, and Asto CT/Leo Cancer Care; royalties from Medical Physics Publishing and royalties related to intellectual property from Qaelum; and is founder of RadUnity.

REFERENCES

1. Toia P, La Grutta L, Sollami Giulia, et al. Technical development in cardiac CT: current standards and future improvements—a narrative review. Cardiovascular diagnosis and therapy 2020;10(6):2018.
2. Hounsfield GN. Computerized transverse axial scanning (tomography): Part 1. Description of system. Br J Radiol 1973;46(552):1016–22.
3. Rybicki FJ, Hansel J, Otero ML, et al. Initial evaluation of coronary images from 320-detector row computed tomography. Int J Cardiovasc Imag 2008;24:535–46.
4. So A, Imai Y, Nett B, et al. Evaluation of a 160-mm/256-row CT scanner for whole-heart quantitative myocardial perfusion imaging. Med Phys 2016;43(8):4821–32.
5. Woodhouse CE, Janowitz WR, Viamonte M Jr. Coronary arteries: retrospective cardiac gating technique to reduce cardiac motion artifact at spiral CT. Radiology 1997;204(2):566–9.
6. Morsbach F, Gordic S, Desbiolles L, et al. Performance of turbo high-pitch dual-source CT for coronary CT angiography: first ex vivo and patient experience. Eur Radiol 2014;24:1889–95.
7. Rice University. Anatomy and physiology. OpenStax CNX; 2016.
8. Bae KT. Intravenous contrast medium administration and scan timing at CT: considerations and approaches. Radiology 2010;256(1):32–61.
9. Cademartiri F, Nieman K, van der Lugt A, et al. Intravenous contrast material administration at 16–detector row helical CT coronary angiography: test bolus versus bolus-tracking technique. Radiology 2004;233(3):817–23.
10. Bae KT. Test-bolus versus bolus-tracking techniques for CT angiographic timing. Radiology 2005;236(1):369–70.
11. Cademartiri F, van der Lugt A, Luccichenti Giacomo, et al. Parameters affecting bolus geometry in CTA: a review. J Comput Assist Tomogr 2002;26(4):598–607.
12. Achenbach S, Ropers D, Holle J, et al. In-plane coronary arterial motion velocity: measurement with electron-beam CT. Radiology 2000;216(2):457–63.
13. Parker DL. Optimal short scan convolution reconstruction for fan beam CT. Med Phys 1982;9(2):254–7.
14. Kalender WA. Computed tomography: fundamentals, system technology, image quality, applications. New York: John Wiley & Sons; 2011.
15. Maier J, Lebedev S, Erath J, et al. Deep learning-based coronary artery motion estimation and compensation for short-scan cardiac CT. Med Phys 2021;48(7):3559–71.
16. Tang J, Jiang H, Chen GH. Temporal resolution improvement in cardiac CT using PICCS (TRI-PICCS): Performance studies. Med Phys 2010;37(8):4377–88.
17. Jandt U, Schäfer D, Grass Michael, et al. Automatic generation of time resolved motion vector fields of coronary arteries and 4D surface extraction using rotational x-ray angiography. Phys Med Biol 2008;54(1):45.
18. Liang J, Wang H, Xu L, et al. Impact of SSF on diagnostic performance of coronary computed tomography angiography within 1 heart beat in patients with high heart rate using a 256-row detector computed tomography. J Comput Assist Tomogr 2018;42(1):54–61.
19. Matsumoto Y, Fujioka C, Yokomachi K, et al. Evaluation of the second-generation whole-heart motion correction algorithm (SSF2) used to demonstrate the aortic annulus on cardiac CT. Sci Rep 2023;13(1):3636.
20. Precise Cardiac. Available at: https://www.philips.com/c-dam/b2bhc/master/resource-catalog/landing/precise-suite/incisive_cardiac.pdf. [Accessed 31 August 2023].
21. Canon AMC. Available at: https://us.medical.canon/products/computed-tomography/cardiac-excellence/. [Accessed 31 August 2023].

22. Hofman MBM, Wickline SA, Lorenz CH. Quantification of in-plane motion of the coronary arteries during the cardiac cycle: implications for acquisition window duration for MR flow quantification. J Magn Reson Imag 1998;8(3):568–76.

23. Husmann L, Leschka S, Desbiolles L, et al. Coronary artery motion and cardiac phases: dependency on heart rate—implications for CT image reconstruction. Radiology 2007;245(2):567–76.

24. Flohr TG, Joseph Schoepf U, Kuettner A, et al. Advances in cardiac imaging with 16-section CT systems. Acad Radiol 2003;10(4):386–401.

25. Dewey M, Hoffmann H, Hamm B. Multislice CT coronary angiography: effect of sublingual nitroglycerine on the diameter of coronary arteries. In: RöFo-Fortschritte auf dem Gebiet der Röntgenstrahlen und der bildgebenden Verfahren. New York: © Georg Thieme Verlag KG Stuttgart·; 2006. p. 600–4.

26. Chernoff DM, Ritchie CJ, Higgins CB. Evaluation of electron beam CT coronary angiography in healthy subjects. AJR. American journal of roentgenology 1997;169(1):93–9.

27. Shaw LJ, Blankstein JJ, Ferencik BM, et al. Society of Cardiovascular Computed Tomography/North American Society of Cardiovascular Imaging–expert consensus document on coronary CT imaging of atherosclerotic plaque. Journal of Cardiovascular Computed Tomography 2021;15(2):93–109.

28. Szczykutowicz T. The CT handbook: optimizing protocols for today's feature-rich scanners. Madison, WI: Medical Physics Publishing; 2020.

29. Menke J, Unterberg-Buchwald C, Staab W, et al. Head-to-head comparison of prospectively triggered vs retrospectively gated coronary computed tomography angiography: Meta-analysis of diagnostic accuracy, image quality, and radiation dose. Am Heart J 2013;165(154–163):e3. https://doi.org/10.1016/j.ahj.2012.10.026.

Coronary Artery Disease
Role of Computed Tomography and Recent Advances

Elizabeth Lee, MD[a],*, Chiemezie Amadi, MD[b],
Michelle C. Williams, MBChB, BSc Med Sci, PhD, BA, MRCP, FRCR, FSCCT[c],
Prachi P. Agarwal, MBBS[d]

KEYWORDS

- Coronary CT angiography • Coronary calcium scoring • Coronary artery disease
- Computed tomography

KEY POINTS

- Coronary computed tomography angiography (CCTA) has emerged as a first-line examination for the assessment of patients with both acute and stable chest pain.
- Theadvantages of CCTA over functional ischemia testing include its ability to assess the presence and severity of atherosclerotic plaque, identify high-risk plaque features, and reliably rule out left main stem disease, which all provide prognostic information. In addition, CCTA can identify alternative causes of chest pain that have similar presentations.
- Coronary calcium scoring in asymptomatic patients has incremental value over classic cardiovascular risk factors and enables better prognostication and reclassification in intermediate-risk patients.
- Emerging CT techniques include functional assessment of coronary stenoses by CT perfusion and CT fractional flow reserve, new applications with the potential to improve precision medicine by targeting detection of pericoronary adipose tissue inflammation and complementing the growing role of artificial intelligence in coronary artery disease imaging.

INTRODUCTION

Coronary artery disease (CAD) remains the leading cause of death despite advances in diagnostic and therapeutic options. Based on the National Health and Nutrition Examination Survey data for the period 2015 to 2018, it is estimated that more than 20 million adults (>20 years of age) in the United States have CAD and 3% have suffered from a myocardial infarction.[1] The 2021 American College of Cardiology (ACC)/American Heart Association (AHA) chest pain guidelines highlight the role of coronary computed tomography angiogram (CCTA) as a test with several class 1 (level of evidence A) indications, favoring CCTA in patients less than the age of 65 years or with low probability of obstructive CAD as well as in those with prior inconclusive or mildly abnormal functional testing.[2] Of note, CCTA is the only noninvasive testing modality with a "Class I" endorsement by the ACC/AHA for patients with acute or stable chest pain, supported by "Level A" quality of evidence. Other modalities also received

[a] Department of Radiology, Michigan Medicine, 1500 East Medical Center Drive, TC B1-148, Ann Arbor, MI 48109-5030, USA; [b] Department of Radiology, Michigan Medicine, 1500 Medical Center Drive, Room 5481, Ann Arbor, MI 48109-5868, USA; [c] Centre for Cardiovascular Science, University of Edinburgh, Edinburgh, The Queen's Medical Research Institute, Edinburg BioQuarter, 47 Little France Crescent, Edinburgh EH16 4TJ, UK; [d] Department of Radiology, Division of Cardiothoracic Radiology, Michigan Medicine, 1500 East Medical Center Drive SPC 5868, Ann Arbor, MI 48109, USA
* Corresponding author.
E-mail address: echaripa@med.umich.edu

Radiol Clin N Am 62 (2024) 385–398
https://doi.org/10.1016/j.rcl.2023.12.017
0033-8389/24/© 2023 Elsevier Inc. All rights reserved.

radiologic.theclinics.com

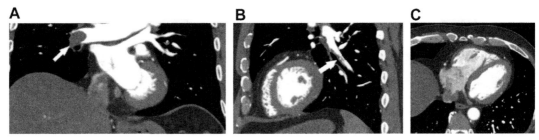

Fig. 1. CCTA in a 58-year-old man with stable chest pain and dyspnea on exertion who underwent assessment for coronary artery disease (CAD) evaluation. Coronary calcium score was 0 and CCTA ruled out CAD. However, CCTA revealed acute on chronic pulmonary embolism explaining the patient's symptoms. Note the centrally located filling defect with acute angles consistent with acute embolism (*A*, coronal *arrow*) superimposed on chronic (*B*, sagittal *arrow*) pulmonary emboli seen as eccentric linear defects with calcification. Pulmonary hypertension is noted with right ventricular hypertrophy and dilatation (*C*).

a Class I endorsement but "Level B" quality of evidence. CCTA may also provide additional benefits compared with functional imaging including the ability to assess other anatomic structures enabling the diagnosis of alternative causes of symptoms (**Fig. 1**), reliably exclude left main disease, and provide prognostically useful information from plaque extent and high-risk plaque (HRP) features. This is in the context of overall low radiation dose that is now easily achievable with contemporary technological advancements. These advancements in detector rows, gantry rotation speed, dual-source scanners, and photon-counting CTs have also dramatically improved spatial and temporal resolution as well as image quality of CCTA. The protocols vary depending on the institutional workflow, scanner type, and baseline patient heart rate and regularity of the rhythm.

The warranty period for CCTA is longer (2 years) than functional imaging (1 year) due to the low number of events in patients with no plaque or stenosis on CT in contrast to functional imaging which cannot evaluate nonobstructive CAD burden.[3] In addition to the role of CT in symptomatic CAD, decades of evidence support the use of coronary artery calcium (CAC) scoring in select asymptomatic patient populations. Multiple treatment guidelines including the ACC/AHA and the European Atherosclerosis Society/European Society of Cardiology guidelines for the management of atherosclerotic disease endorse the use of CAC scoring in intermediate- and borderline-risk patients, thereby providing a more personalized risk assessment for preventative measures.

Recent advancements in CT imaging technology including perfusion imaging and fractional flow reserve derived from CCTA (FFR-CT) allow not only assessment of luminal stenosis severity and overall plaque burden but also assessment of lesion-specific ischemia which can improve the diagnosis and management of patients with

CAD. In this review, the authors summarize the role of CCTA and CAC scoring in different clinical presentations of chest pain and for preventative care. Following this, the authors discuss future directions and new technologies such as pericoronary fat inflammation and the growing footprint of artificial intelligence (AI) in cardiovascular medicine.

ACUTE CHEST PAIN

Evidence from randomized controlled trials (RCTs) has shown that CCTA can be used in patients with acute chest pain presenting to the emergency department for the detection of clinically significant CAD (**Fig. 2**). Most of the studies have focused on patients with low to intermediate risk and have demonstrated that those undergoing

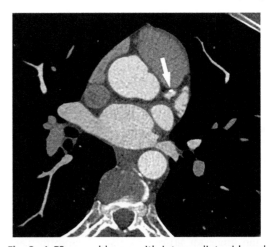

Fig. 2. A 53-year-old man with intermediate risk and no previous history of CAD presented to the emergency room with acute chest pain. CCTA showed a calcified plaque in the proximal left anterior descending artery with minimal (<25%) stenosis (*arrow*). There was no obstructive CAD allowing for rapid discharge from the emergency room.

CCTA versus usual care do not have differences in adverse events.[4,5] This included the 2012 multi-center Rule Out Myocardial Infarction using Computer-Assisted Tomography (ROMICAT) II trial which randomly assigned acute chest pain patients presenting to the emergency room with normal troponins and a nonischemic electrocardiography (EKG) to either CCTA or standard of care.[6] There was no difference between groups in adverse cardiac events, although CCTA arm showed a reduction in length of stay. The efficiency of CCTA, without a compromise in patient outcomes, for patients with acute chest pain has also been confirmed in several meta-analyses.[7,8]

The multicenter Coronary Computed Tomographic Angiography for Systematic Triage of Acute Chest Pain Patients to Treatment trial specifically compared nuclear myocardial perfusion imaging with CCTA. Low-risk acute chest pain patients were randomly assigned to CCTA or perfusion imaging[9] with a similar occurrence of adverse cardiac events in both groups, although CCTA provided advantages like quicker time to diagnosis and lower cost. Additional RCTs that have compared CCTA with perfusion imaging have reinforced and supported the safe use of CCTA in patients with acute chest pain.[10]

CCTA has also been compared with other types of functional tests for the assessment of patients with acute chest pain. For instance, CT coronary angiography compared to exercise ECG (electrocardiogram) (CT-COMPARE) looked at CCTA versus stress EKG in low-to-intermediate risk patients with acute chest pain.[11] They found a higher rate of additional testing in the CCTA group but a lower cost (20% reduction) and 35% relative reduction in length of stay. Another single-center study compared CCTA with stress echocardiography in low-to-intermediation risk acute chest pain patients and found no differences in adverse outcomes, although length of stay was longer for the CCTA group.[12] Of note, the long-term value was assessed in the "Cardiac CT in the treatment of acute Chest pain" study. This study of 600 acute chest pain patients with normal EKG and troponins randomized patients to CCTA or functional testing and found that the composite endpoint for MACE (including cardiac death, myocardial infarction, hospitalization for unstable angina, and late symptom-driven revascularization) to be less frequent in CCTA arm compared with functional testing (5 vs 14 events, $P = .04$) when followed for a median duration of 18.7 months.[5]

These studies establish the value of CCTA for the rapid triage of low- to intermediate-risk acute chest pain patients presenting to the emergency department. However, with the advent of high-sensitivity troponin (hs-cTn) testing, which is now commonly used and preferred over conventional troponin assays due to its efficiency and accuracy for the detection of myocardial injury, it becomes important to reassess the role of CCTA in this context. The BEACON (Better Evaluation of Acute Chest Pain with Computed Tomography Angiography) trial randomized 500 patients to early CCTA versus standard care following hs-cTn testing and found no differences in obstructive CAD requiring revascularization in both study arms.[13] However, CCTA was associated with less outpatient testing (4% vs 10%, $P < .01$) and lower direct medical costs. The PROTECT (Prospective RandOmised Trial of Emergency Cardiac Computerized Tomography) trial looked at patients with indeterminate troponins and nonischemic EKG and randomized them to CCTA versus standard of care.[14] At 1-year adverse cardiac events were the same in each group. Unlike prior studies, there was no reduction in length of stay or costs in the CCTA group, although there was a significant reduction in subsequent outpatient investigations and cardiology referrals with the CCTA strategy. The Rapid Assessment of Potential Ischaemic Heart Disease with CTCA randomized 1748 patients with suspected acute coronary syndrome (ACS) (with at least one of the following: previous coronary heart disease, raised cardiac troponin, or an abnormal EKG) to either CCTA or standard of care.[15] They found that in this intermediate-risk group of patients, early CCTA did not alter outcomes and increased length of stay but reduced the rates of invasive angiography. Some studies have also assessed CCTA in high-risk patients with acute chest pain. As an observational part of the VERDICT (Very Early vs Deferred Invasive Evaluation Using Computerized Tomography in Patients with Acute Coronary Syndromes) trial, CCTA was performed in patients with non-ST segment elevation myocardial infarction randomized to very early (within 12 hours) or standard (48–72 hours) invasive coronary angiography.[16] CCTA had a high diagnostic accuracy and was able to exclude significant stenosis, comparable to that of invasive cardiac catheterization. Such studies provide evidence that CCTA may be of potential benefit in select high-risk patients when an invasive strategy may not be preferred for clinical reasons. Together these studies show the evolving role of CCTA in patients with acute chest pain as treatment pathways develop.

Adding functional assessment to anatomic assessment by using FFR-CT or CT myocardial perfusion imaging (CTP) in the emergency department has also been assessed. A post hoc analysis of ROMICAT II showed that the relative risk of ACS and revascularization in patients with positive FFR-CT ≤0.80 was 4.03 (95% CI 1.56–10.36) and 3.50 (95% CI 1.12–10.96) respectively, and FFR-CT ≤0.80 was associated with the presence of HRP after adjustment for stenosis severity.[17] Similarly, a single-center study reaffirmed that no deaths or myocardial infarctions occurred in acute chest pain patients with a negative FFR-CT when revascularization was deferred.[18]

The potential role of CAC scoring has been evaluated in acute chest pain patients. In a prospective observation cohort study, patients with acute chest pain in the emergency setting underwent stress testing and CAC scoring.[19] Two patients with CAC score of 0 suffered an ACS which was identified by an elevation in troponins during their admission, although they did not experience additional cardiac events during 6 months of follow-up. A meta-analysis in acute chest pain patients without history of CAD and negative troponins and EKG showed that most patients had a CAC score of 0 (60%) and the event rate in patients with a CAC score of 0 is significantly lower compared with those with coronary calcification.[20] However, a CAC score of 0 cannot exclude CAD in low- to intermediate-risk patients with acute chest pain. One study found that 0.7% of patients with acute chest pain and a CAC score of 0 had obstructive CAD on CCTA.[21] For these reasons, CAC is not clinically used or endorsed by societal guidelines in the acute chest pain setting.

The ACC/AHA chest pain guidelines recognize the role of CCTA, which has been given a class 1 recommendation in patients with acute chest pain and intermediate risk.[3] No testing is recommended in patients with acute chest pain and low risk.

STABLE CHEST PAIN

Multiple RCTs have conclusively shown the value of CCTA in stable chest pain patients. The PROMISE RCT randomized 10,003 patients with symptoms suggesting CAD to CCTA or functional testing[22] and found no difference in death or myocardial infarction between the two groups. After 2 years of follow-up, rates of invasive catheterization were higher in the CCTA group; however, the rate of nonobstructive CAD on invasive catheterization was lower in the CCTA group, suggesting the role of CCTA as an effective gatekeeper to invasive testing. Similarly, the RESCUE trial found comparable rates of adverse cardiac events in patients with stable angina randomized to either CCTA or perfusion single photon emission computed tomography (SPECT).[23] CCTA findings of a stenosis≥50%

were found to be a better predictor for subsequent myocardial events than the percent reversible defect size on SPECT. Meta-analyses including various trials have confirmed similar mortality rates for CCTA versus functional testing, although have shown increased additional downstream diagnostic testing in those undergoing CCTA.[24,25] In contrast, the SCOT-HEART trial randomized patients with stable chest pain referred to outpatient cardiology clinics to either standard of care or CCTA.[26] Death from CAD and nonfatal myocardial infarction were halved in the CCTA arm, along with reduced use of invasive catheterization and increased use of preventative therapies in the CCTA group. Unlike other studies, over a 5 year follow-up, the rates of invasive catheterization and revascularization were similar, showing that CCTA does not necessarily lead to increased investigations. Recently, the Diagnostic Imaging Strategies for Patients with Stable Chest Pain and Intermediate Risk of Coronary Artery Disease (DISCHARGE) RCT showed that in 3561 patients with stable chest pain referred for invasive coronary angiography, a CCTA first strategy was associated with similar rates of cardiovascular events and a reduction in major procedure-related complications.[27] These studies establish the role of CCTA to guide the management of patients with suspected CAD.

Additional analysis from both the SCOT-HEART and PROMISE trial as well as other studies have highlighted the incremental prognostic information that CCTA can provide compared with other forms of CAD imaging. Importantly, CCTA can provide an assessment of the plaque burden in the coronary tree and the subtypes of atherosclerotic plaque. In the SCOT-HEART trial, patients experiencing fatal or nonfatal myocardial infarction had a higher burden of quantitatively assessed plaque and all subtypes of plaque. In particular, the presence of a high burden of low-attenuation noncalcified plaque, the imaging characteristics of a thin cap fibroatheroma with a large lipid core, was associated with an increased risk of cardiac events, independent of cardiovascular risk score, stenosis severity, or calcium score.[28] Studies of other patient cohorts have found similar findings, with total plaque and noncalcified plaque associated with adverse cardiac events.[29,30] Based on the growing evidence of the prognostic information which can be provided from plaque assessment with CCTA, CAD-RADS 2.0, the standardized reporting system for CCTA, now incorporates plaque burden severity into its assessment with the new P modifier[31](**Fig. 3**). It provides flexibility to easily incorporate an overall assessment of plaque burden based on methods that are already being used

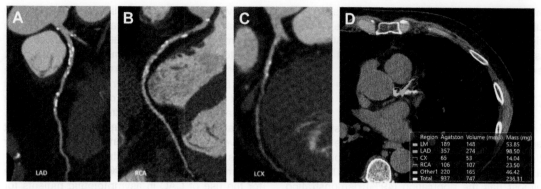

Fig. 3. CAD RADS 4 B/P4. Three-vessel severe coronary artery disease with extensive plaque burden (P4). Plaque burden can be categorized into mild, moderate, severe, or extensive based on various methods including visual assessment and segment-involved score (SIS) on CCTA (A–C) or calcium scoring, if performed (D).

within departments for CT reporting. Plaque is graded as P1 (mild), P2 (moderate), P3 (severe), or P4 (extensive) based on simple visual estimation or quantification with segment involved score from CCTA or CAC scoring, if performed. However, if CAC scoring is used it must be remembered that this does not take noncalcified plaque into account.

Studies in stable chest pain patients have also highlighted the association of HRP features detectable on CCTA with poor clinical outcomes. These include visually assessed spotty calcification, positive remodeling, low-attenuation plaque (<30 HU), and the napkin ring sign (Fig. 4). In CADRADS 2.0 reporting, the modifier HRP is used when two or more high-risk features are present on CCTA. In secondary analysis from the PROMISE trial, adverse events (defined as death, myocardial infarction, or unstable angina) were higher in those with HRP (hazard ratio, 2.73; 95% CI, 1.89–3.93) even after adjusting for cardiovascular risk and severity of stenosis (adjusted hazard ratio 1.72; 95% CI, 1.13–2.62).[32] Similarly, in a nested case control study of 25,251 patients undergoing CCTA, HRP increased the hazard ratio for ACS with most events occurring in those with nonobstructive CAD.[33] Additional studies have

also confirmed these findings that when HRPs are present, there is an increased risk for ischemia or ischemia-related events.[28,34–39] Potentially, the specific type of HRP may be of prognostic significance. In a study of 1430 low- to intermediate-risk patients undergoing CCTA with an almost 11 years of follow-up, low-attenuation plaque and the napkin ring sign predicted major cardiac events but not all cause mortality, whereas spotty calcifications and positive remodeling did not predict future cardiac events.[40]

The prognostic role of CAC scoring in patients with stable chest pain has also been assessed. In one study, a group of stable chest pain patients with low pretest probability of CAD underwent no testing, CAC scoring or CCTA (which included a CAC score as well).[41] The rate of a CAC score of 0 was high at 56.8%. Of those with a CAC 0 who also underwent CCTA most had no atherosclerosis, however, 1.9% had obstructive disease. In the SCOT-HEART trial, among patients with a calcium score of zero, 14% had nonobstructive CAD, 2% had obstructive CAD, and 2% had visually assessed HRP.[42]

Based on the above studies, societal strong class 1 recommendations include the use of CCTA as a first-line testing in intermediate and high-risk patients with stable chest pain along

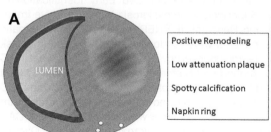
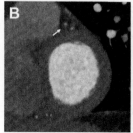
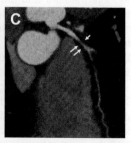

Positive Remodeling

Low attenuation plaque

Spotty calcification

Napkin ring

Fig. 4. High-risk plaque (HRP) features on CCTA are shown in the schematic diagram (A). CT images in cross-sectional view of the LAD (B) and curved planar reformat (C) demonstrate a noncalcified plaque (arrows) with positive remodeling and low attenuation. Because the plaque fulfills two features, this is designated a modifier of HRP in CAD RADS 2.0. LAD, left anterior desecending.

with other modalities including stress testing (with ultrasound [US], MR, or nuclear medicine).[3] In low-risk patients without history of CAD, CAC scoring is reasonable with moderate strength of evidence supporting its use.

ASYMPTOMATIC PATIENTS

Many patients with CAD do not exhibit symptoms and this has been highlighted by multiple observation studies. In the MiHeart study, a cohort of 2359 asymptomatic patients underwent CCTA[43] with almost half the population (49%) demonstrating CAD including 16% of patients with a CAC of 0. A similarly high rate of CAD was found in an intermediate Framingham risk group of 185 asymptomatic patients where 60.5% individuals had CAD.[44]

Although CCTA could be used for the identification of CAD in asymptomatic individuals, registry studies have to date failed to demonstrate the additive value of CCTA to clinical risk factor and CAC scoring stratification. In the multicenter observational Coronary CT Angiography Evaluation for Clinical Outcomes: An International Multicenter Registry (CONFIRM), 7590 asymptomatic individuals underwent CCTA and CAC scoring.[45] The C statistical for the risk factor model for composite outcomes of all-cause mortality and nonfatal myocardial infarction was 0.71 and was raised to 0.75 when CAC score was included. However, the addition of CCTA information to the risk factor plus CAC scoring model only increased the C statistical by 0.02 when using the Framingham risk model and by less than 0.01 when using individual risk factors. Even at 6 year follow-up, there was no incremental value of adding CCTA to a model including CAC scoring and clinical factors in this cohort.[46] However, there may be subsets of asymptomatic patients who may benefit from CCTA. In the CONFIRM registry, the 2018 ACA/AHA cholesterol guidelines were used to place individuals into low, borderline, statin recommended/intermediate and statin recommended/high-risk groups.[47] Those at low or high risk had no improvement in risk classification from CCTA, whereas there was a net reclassification index of 0.27 for borderline and intermediate-risk individuals by using CCTA.

To date, there are no large RCTs on the impact of CCTA on management and outcomes in asymptomatic patients with intermediate or low risk of CAD. In high-risk patients with diabetes, the FACTOR-64 RCT showed that there was no difference in patients undergoing CCTA or standard of care in terms of all-cause mortality, nonfatal myocardial infarction (MI), or unstable angina requiring hospitalization.[48]

However, many of the patients included in this study were already taking preventative therapies before enrollment. The ongoing SCOT-HEART 2 RCT aims to assess whether asymptomatic patients at risk for CAD may benefit from CCTA. In this trial, patients 6000 middle-aged asymptomatic individuals at risk of CAD will be randomized to CCTA versus the standard of care with clinical risk calculation, and patients will be followed up to assess the impact on investigations, medication use, cardiovascular events, and all-cause mortality.[49]

Compared with CCTA, there is strong evidence for the use of CAC in asymptomatic patients for the detection of subclinical CAD. Following the publication of smaller cohort studies, the Multi-Ethnic Study of Atherosclerosis (MESA) and Heinz Nixdorf Recall studies provide strong evidence of the prognostic value of CAC scoring. The MESA study performed CAC scoring in more than 6500 individuals who had no clinical evidence of CAD.[50] They found an increased risk of cardiac events with increasing severity of CAC at 4 years, with those having a score of 101 to 300 having an over 7-fold risk while those with a CAC score of above 300 at almost 10-fold risk. The Heinz Nixdorf study included more than 4000 individuals and looked at the reclassification of risk of cardiac events based on CAC score compared with clinical risk calculators including the Framingham Risk Score and National Cholesterol Education Panel Adult Treatment Panel III guidelines.[51] CAC scoring allowed for the reclassification of a significant proportion of intermediate risk patients at 5 years, with nearly 22% of patients reclassified compared with the National Cholesterol Education Panel Adult Treatment Panel III guidelines and slightly more than 30% when using the Framingham Risk Score. Additional registry studies have verified these findings as well as the increased ability to improve risk stratification specifically in intermediate-risk groups if CAC scoring is applied to clinical risk factors.[52–55]

CAC scoring may also impact patient management. In the randomized Early Identification of Subclinical Atherosclerosis by Noninvasive Imaging Research (EISNER) trial, 2137 asymptomatic patients were randomized to CAC scoring or risk factor counseling.[56] Those who underwent CAC scoring had better management of systolic blood pressure and cholesterol. In addition, the CAC score group had no change in their Framingham risk score over time, whereas those without CAC scoring had a mean increase in the score. Overall, there is a wealth of studies showing a low risk of future cardiac events in asymptomatic individuals with CAC scores of 0, which may obviate the need for preventative medications in select individuals. The results of the Risk Or Benefit IN Screening for CArdiovascular disease RCT are eagerly awaited. They randomized more than 25,000 asymptomatic patients at risk for CAD to CAC scoring versus a clinical risk calculator.[57] CAC scoring identified more patients at low risk and in whom medical therapy was not indicated, and the impact of this on cardiovascular events is awaited.

Multiple society guidelines support the use of CAC scoring in asymptomatic patients who based on clinical risk assessment are borderline to intermediate risk. CAC scoring in these patients allows for better risk stratification and preventative medications. Apart from dedicated ECG-gated coronary calcium examinations, there is an opportunity to use other thoracic scans regardless of original indication as a means to improve cardiovascular preventative care. This can provide a unique opportunity for risk stratification given the high correlation between CAC scoring from gated and non-gated examinations.[58]

PREOPERATIVE RISK ASSESSMENT

Preoperative coronary evaluation may be needed before noncardiac surgery or before noncoronary cardiac surgery.

Evaluation Before Noncardiac Surgery

The 2014 AHA guidelines for preoperative risk assessment for non-emergent, noncardiac surgery recommend pharmacologic stress testing for those undergoing intermediate to high-risk surgeries and in whom there is an unknown or poor functional capacity.[59] The 2014 European Societies of Cardiology and Anesthesiology (ESC/ESA) cite insufficient evidence for the use of CCTA in the perioperative period.[60] Although current guidelines do not recommend CT, its role has been assessed in this scenario. A meta-analysis of 11 studies found a negative predictive value of 96% for cardiac events in the perioperative period in those without multivessel disease on CTA.[61]

Evaluation Before Noncoronary Cardiac Surgery

In most patients greater than 40 years of age undergoing noncoronary cardiac surgery, invasive angiography is recommended by current guidelines.[62] CCTA has been shown to be non-inferior to invasive coronary angiography and results in lower costs.[63] CT is also advantageous when invasive angiography can be risky as in patients with vegetations or with acute dissection. Patients undergoing structural heart evaluation such as before transcatheter

aortic valve implantation routinely get a cardiac CT. Although these patients with aortic stenosis are generally older and have concomitant atherosclerotic disease, CT can rule out CAD in a proportion of these preprocedural scans.[62]

ADVANCES IN COMPUTED TOMOGRAPHY IMAGING FOR CORONARY ARTERY DISEASE
Functional Significance of Anatomic Stenosis

Fractional flow reserve derived from coronary computed tomography angiogram

Using the anatomic data acquired from CCTA, FFR-CT can be calculated as a simulated metric using computational fluid dynamic or machine learning techniques. This allows for the assessment of the physiologic impact of a stenosis without the need for additional investigations. Images from CCTA can be post-processed with computational fluid dynamic techniques which create a patient-specific model of the coronary arteries reflecting alterations of vessel pressure similar to those which can be obtained during invasive coronary catheterization. Compared with CCTA alone, the addition of FFR-CT can provide better identification of hemodynamically significant stenosis and risk of future cardiac events.[64–67] Patients with FFR-CT less than 0.80 have higher rates of adverse cardiac events and need for revascularization.[68,69] Results of FFR-CT can decrease the number of patients undergoing invasive cardiac catheterization resulting in lower overall radiation exposure and costs. In the Prospective Longitudinal Trial of FFR-CT Outcome and Resource Impacts trial, invasive coronary angiography (ICA) was canceled in 77% of patients who underwent CCTA plus FFR-CT compared with usual care.[70] Similar reductions in the number of patients undergoing ICA were documented in the IMPACT FFR study where the rate of ICA in the CCTA group was just more than 50% while in the FFR-CT group was near 20%.[71] Randomized studies looking at patients with stable chest pain using CCTA plus selective FFR-CT versus standard of care have found similar costs in the United States and in the UK National Health System when either strategy is used.[72,73] However, a real-world audit of clinical data with cost analysis comparing FFR-CT to other stress imaging in the United Kingdom showed higher costs for FFR-CT due to higher rates of ICA and revascularization and low FFR-CT positive predictive value (35% to 50% over a range of stenoses).[74] In addition, FFR-CT may not provide additive information compared with a comprehensive description and quantification of plaque severity, HRP, and overall plaque burden

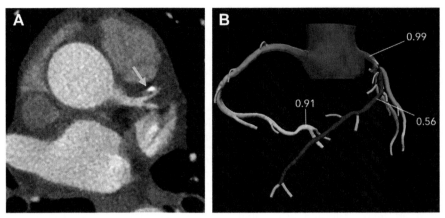

Fig. 5. CCTA and FFR-CT images from a 68-year-old man with chronic exertional chest pain. CCTA showed a moderate stenosis in the proximal LAD (*A, arrow*). FFR-CT (*B*) was positive for lesion-specific ischemia. The CAD-RADS 2.0 classification for this patient was CAD-RADS 3/P2/I+. LAD, left anterior desecending.

based on CCTA alone.[75,76] Overall, further studies are needed to determine the cost-effectiveness as well as best use for FFR-CT.

FFR-CT has been incorporated into CAD-RADS 2.0. The "I" modifier can be added when ischemic imaging has been performed either by FFR-CT or other methods including CT perfusion. When using FFR-CT, lesion-specific ischemia is assessed by looking at FFR-CT at 1 to 2 cm beyond the distal aspect of the stenosis of concern.[77] When FFR-CT is below 0.75, this is considered positive for ischemia and given the designation I+, whereas values of 0.76 to 0.80 are indeterminant (I−/+) and above 0.80 are considered negative for lesion-specific ischemia (I−) (Fig 5).

Computed tomography myocardial perfusion imaging

The myocardium can also be assessed using CT, and protocols have been developed for both single shot "static" and multi-phase "dynamic" CT myocardial perfusion imaging. Similar to myocardial perfusion imaging performed using other imaging modalities, both rest and pharmacologic stress imaging are performed to identify normal, ischemic, and infarcted myocardium. Abnormalities can be identified due to their reduced contrast enhancement, either visually or with quantitative analysis (Fig. 6). The Combined Non-invasive Coronary Angiography and Myocardial Perfusion Imaging Using 320 Detector Computed Tomography (CORE360) study showed that the identification of flow-limiting disease was improved with combined CCTA and CT perfusion, compared with CCTA alone. CT myocardial perfusion imaging has good diagnostic accuracy compared with gold standard assessments including invasive coronary angiography and fractional flow reserve, single-photon emission computed tomography or absolute myocardial blood flow from oxygen-15 after PET.[78,79] Dynamic CT myocardial perfusion imaging can enable the quantification of myocardial blood flow from CT images, which further improves the diagnostic

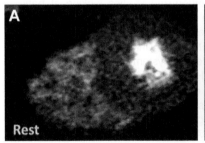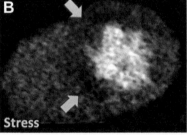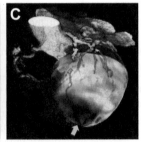

Fig. 6. CT myocardial perfusion imaging from a male patient with suspected angina due to coronary artery disease showing (*A*) rest and (*B*) stress imaging of the apical left ventricle myocardium, and (*C*) a 3D reconstruction of CCTA and quantitative stress perfusion assessment. A reversible perfusion defect indicating ischemia is identified as subendocardial hypoattenuation on the stress imaging (*B, yellow arrows*) and blue/purple color on the 3D image.

accuracy.[79] New methods for assessing CT myocardial perfusion include radiomic analysis and fractal analysis of the myocardium.[80,81]

CT myocardial perfusion imaging could be used to guide management in cases where stenosis severity on CT is uncertain, particularly in those with moderate to severe disease, heavy coronary artery calcification, or intracoronary stents. Small, randomized studies have shown that management based on combined dynamic CT perfusion and CCTA is superior to CCTA alone in terms of reducing the rates of invasive coronary angiography and invasive coronary angiography without revascularization, without affecting outcomes in short-term follow-up.[82] The Comprehensive Cardiac CT versus Exercise Testing in Suspected Coronary Artery study assessed a tiered cardiac CT protocol incorporating calcium score, CCTA if calcium was present, and CT myocardial perfusion imaging if a stenosis of 50% or greater was present. They found that compared with functional testing (95% exercise electrocardiogram), the tiered CT approach led to a reduction in invasive coronary angiograms without revascularization, a similar adverse event rate but a slightly higher radiation dose.[83] Ongoing larger randomized studies seek to assess in a prospective manner the impact of CT myocardial perfusion in terms of subsequent management and outcomes.

ARTIFICIAL INTELLIGENCE COMPUTED TOMOGRAPHY FOR CORONARY ARTERY DISEASE

The applications of AI for imaging of CAD using CT span multiple arenas including plaque detection, plaque characterization, improving risk stratification, and clinical decision-making. AI has been applied to both CAC scoring and CCTA. Studies have shown the ability of AI to detect hemodynamically significant stenosis across a broad range of imaging parameters and its potential ability to decrease the time needed for analysis of images for stenosis.[84,85] AI can significantly reduce the time to perform quantitative plaque analysis, an important barrier to its application in clinical practice.[86] One trial of AI-based CCTA interpretation in patients with stable chest pain referred for ICA found a lower cost compared with conventional interpretation due to lower rates of referral for ICA, without impacting the occurrence of cardiac events.[87] A comprehensive review of all potential applications for AI in CT imaging of CAD is beyond the scope of this review; however, AI is certain to

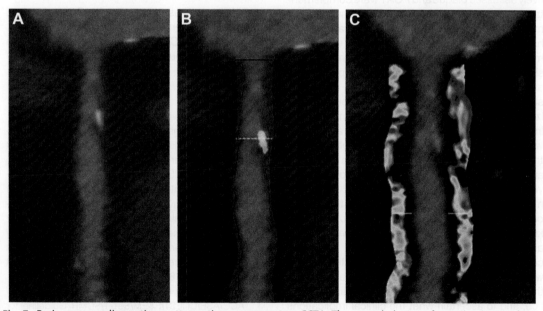

Fig. 7. Pericoronary adipose tissue attenuation assessment on CCTA. The curved planar reformation image shows the presence of a minimal stenosis (>25%) in the proximal right coronary artery (*A*). Quantitative plaque analysis (*B*) shows the presence of noncalcified plaque (*red*) and calcified plaque (*yellow*). Pericoronary adipose tissue (PCAT) attenuation assessment (*C*) in the proximal right coronary artery assesses all adipose tissue-containing voxels within an outer radial distance from the vessel wall of 3 mm which have with an attenuation between −190 Hounsfield units (HU) and −30 HU. More abnormal PCAT attenuation (less negative) is shown in red, compared with the more normal PCAT attenuation in yellow (Analysis performed with Autoplaque 2.5, Cedars Sinai Medical Center, Los Angeles).

change how imaging is ordered, performed, and interpreted in the near future.

PERICORONARY ADIPOSE TISSUE

The fat immediately surrounding the coronary arteries is called the pericoronary adipose tissue (PCAT), and recently, clinical and preclinical research has suggested that it may play an important role in cardiovascular disease. The PCAT is a metabolically active, structure which interacts with the coronary arteries and is involved in inflammation and atherosclerosis in particular, as shown in histologic studies. On CCTA, the attenuation (in Hounsfield units) of the PCAT can be measured with dedicated software (Fig. 7), and this can be indexed for technical factors such as tube voltage and clinical factors such as body mass index and cardiovascular risk factors.

Antonopoulos and colleagues showed that abnormal PCAT could be used as a noninvasive method to assess coronary inflammation and atherosclerosis.[88] The Cardiovascular RISk Prediction using Computed Tomography study demonstrated that PCAT metrics could be used to identify patients at risk of all-cause and cardiac mortality, over and above standard metrics.[89,90] In the SCOT-HEART trial, both low attenuation quantitatively assessed plaque and PCAT were complementary markers of patients at risk of subsequent myocardial infarction.[91] Abnormal PCAT attenuation has been identified in culprit lesions with acute myocardial infarction compared with non-culprit lesions and controls with stable CAD, supporting its association with active inflammation. However, studies assessing associations with general or localized inflammation have been inconsistent. Interestingly, these findings are predominantly associated with right coronary artery PCAT, possibly because this is easier to measure than the more limited fat around the other coronary arteries, or for other, as yet unknown, reasons. Assessment of PCAT radiomic characteristics may further improve the identification of high-risk lesions.[92] We do not currently know what changes in PCAT attenuation represent and possibilities include inflammation, microvascular disease, or focal ulceration/dissection. Future work in this area seeks to automate analysis so that it can be incorporated into routine clinical practice, and to ascertain what the clinical implications and response to treatment is in larger cohorts.

SUMMARY

The use of CT in symptomatic and asymptomatic patients allows for identification of CAD and can guide management and improve prognosis. Beyond CCTA and CAC scoring, emerging CT imaging techniques including quantitative plaque analysis, FFR-CT, and perfusion imaging may allow for better identification of patients who would benefit from more aggressive management.

CLINICS CARE POINTS

- Coronary computed tomography angiography (CCTA) has the highest level of evidence supporting its use in patients with acute and stable chest pain.
- CCTA can identify high-risk plaque features and quantify overall plaque burden, providing important prognostic information which has been incorporated into CAD-RADS 2.0.
- In asymptomatic patients, currently, there is no evidence for the use of CCTA; however, ongoing trials aim to determine whether CCTA can provide additional prognostic information above those from coronary calcium scoring and clinical risk factors.

DISCLOSURE

M.C. Williams has given talks for Canon Medical Systems, Siemens Healthineers, and Novartis. The work of M.C. Williams is supported by the British Heart Foundation, United Kingdom (FS/ICRF/20/26002).

REFERENCES

1. Virani SS, Alonso A, Aparicio HJ, et al. Heart Disease and Stroke Statistics-2021 Update: A Report From the American Heart Association. Circulation 2021;143(8):e254–743.
2. Writing Committee M, Gulati M, Levy PD, et al. 2021 AHA/ACC/ASE/CHEST/SAEM/SCCT/SCMR Guideline for the Evaluation and Diagnosis of Chest Pain: A Report of the American College of Cardiology/American Heart Association Joint Committee on Clinical Practice Guidelines. J Cardiovasc Comput Tomogr 2022;16(1):54–122.
3. Gulati M, Levy PD, Mukherjee D, et al. 2021 AHA/ACC/ASE/CHEST/SAEM/SCCT/SCMR Guideline for the Evaluation and Diagnosis of Chest Pain: A Report of the American College of Cardiology/American Heart Association Joint Committee on Clinical Practice Guidelines. Circulation 2021;144(22):e368–454.
4. Litt HI, Gatsonis C, Snyder B, et al. CT angiography for safe discharge of patients with possible acute

coronary syndromes. N Engl J Med 2012;366(15): 1393–403.

5. Linde JJ, Hove JD, Sorgaard M, et al. Long-Term Clinical Impact of Coronary CT Angiography in Patients With Recent Acute-Onset Chest Pain: The Randomized Controlled CATCH Trial. JACC Cardiovasc Imaging 2015;8(12):1404–13.

6. Hoffmann U, Truong QA, Schoenfeld DA, et al. Coronary CT angiography versus standard evaluation in acute chest pain. N Engl J Med 2012;367(4): 299–308.

7. Hulten E, Pickett C, Bittencourt MS, et al. Outcomes after coronary computed tomography angiography in the emergency department: a systematic review and meta-analysis of randomized, controlled trials. J Am Coll Cardiol 2013;61(8):880–92.

8. D'Ascenzo F, Cerrato E, Biondi-Zoccai G, et al. Coronary computed tomographic angiography for detection of coronary artery disease in patients presenting to the emergency department with chest pain: a meta-analysis of randomized clinical trials. Eur Heart J Cardiovasc Imaging 2013;14(8):782–9.

9. Goldstein JA, Chinnaiyan KM, Abidov A, et al. The CT-STAT (Coronary Computed Tomographic Angiography for Systematic Triage of Acute Chest Pain Patients to Treatment) trial. J Am Coll Cardiol 2011; 58(14):1414–22.

10. Levsky JM, Spevack DM, Travin MI, et al. Coronary Computed Tomography Angiography Versus Radionuclide Myocardial Perfusion Imaging in Patients With Chest Pain Admitted to Telemetry: A Randomized Trial. Ann Intern Med 2015;163(3):174–83.

11. Hamilton-Craig C, Fifoot A, Hansen M, et al. Diagnostic performance and cost of CT angiography versus stress ECG–a randomized prospective study of suspected acute coronary syndrome chest pain in the emergency department (CT-COMPARE). Int J Cardiol 2014;177(3):867–73.

12. Levsky JM, Haramati LB, Spevack DM, et al. Coronary Computed Tomography Angiography Versus Stress Echocardiography in Acute Chest Pain: A Randomized Controlled Trial. JACC Cardiovasc Imaging 2018;11(9):1288–97.

13. Dedic A, Lubbers MM, Schaap J, et al. Coronary CT Angiography for Suspected ACS in the Era of High-Sensitivity Troponins: Randomized Multicenter Study. J Am Coll Cardiol 2016;67(1):16–26.

14. Aziz W, Morgan H, Demir OM, et al. Prospective RandOmised Trial of Emergency Cardiac Computerised Tomography (PROTECCT). Heart 2022;108(24): 1972–8.

15. Early computed tomography coronary angiography in patients with suspected acute coronary syndrome: randomised controlled trial. BMJ 2022;376: o438.

16. Linde JJ, Kelbaek H, Hansen TF, et al. Coronary CT Angiography in Patients With Non-ST-Segment Elevation Acute Coronary Syndrome. J Am Coll Cardiol 2020;75(5):453–63.

17. Ferencik M, Lu MT, Mayrhofer T, et al. Non-invasive fractional flow reserve derived from coronary computed tomography angiography in patients with acute chest pain: Subgroup analysis of the ROMICAT II trial. J Cardiovasc Comput Tomogr 2019; 13(4):196–202.

18. Chinnaiyan KM, Safian RD, Gallagher ML, et al. Clinical Use of CT-Derived Fractional Flow Reserve in the Emergency Department. JACC Cardiovasc Imaging 2020;13(2 Pt 1):452–61.

19. Nabi F, Chang SM, Pratt CM, et al. Coronary artery calcium scoring in the emergency department: identifying which patients with chest pain can be safely discharged home. Ann Emerg Med 2010;56(3): 220–9.

20. Chaikriangkrai K, Palamaner Subash Shantha G, Jhun HY, et al. Prognostic Value of Coronary Artery Calcium Score in Acute Chest Pain Patients Without Known Coronary Artery Disease: Systematic Review and Meta-analysis. Ann Emerg Med 2016;68(6): 659–70.

21. Grandhi GR, Mszar R, Cainzos-Achirica M, et al. Coronary Calcium to Rule Out Obstructive Coronary Artery Disease in Patients With Acute Chest Pain. JACC Cardiovasc Imaging 2022;15(2):271–80.

22. Douglas PS, Hoffmann U, Patel MR, et al. Outcomes of anatomical versus functional testing for coronary artery disease. N Engl J Med 2015;372(14):1291–300.

23. Stillman AE, Gatsonis C, Lima JAC, et al. Coronary Computed Tomography Angiography Compared With Single Photon Emission Computed Tomography Myocardial Perfusion Imaging as a Guide to Optimal Medical Therapy in Patients Presenting With Stable Angina: The RESCUE Trial. J Am Heart Assoc 2020;9(24):e017993.

24. Nielsen LH, Ortner N, Norgaard BL, et al. The diagnostic accuracy and outcomes after coronary computed tomography angiography vs. conventional functional testing in patients with stable angina pectoris: a systematic review and meta-analysis. Eur Heart J Cardiovasc Imaging 2014;15(9):961–71.

25. Foy AJ, Dhruva SS, Peterson B, et al. Coronary Computed Tomography Angiography vs Functional Stress Testing for Patients With Suspected Coronary Artery Disease: A Systematic Review and Meta-analysis. JAMA Intern Med 2017;177(11):1623–31.

26. Investigators S-H, Newby DE, Adamson PD, et al. Coronary CT Angiography and 5-Year Risk of Myocardial Infarction. N Engl J Med 2018;379(10): 924–33.

27. Group DT, Maurovich-Horvat P, Bosserdt M, et al. CT or Invasive Coronary Angiography in Stable Chest Pain. N Engl J Med 2022;386(17):1591–602.

28. Williams MC, Moss AJ, Dweck M, et al. Coronary Artery Plaque Characteristics Associated With Adverse

Outcomes in the SCOT-HEART Study. J Am Coll Cardiol 2019;73(3):291–301.

29. Dey D, Achenbach S, Schuhbaeck A, et al. Comparison of quantitative atherosclerotic plaque burden from coronary CT angiography in patients with first acute coronary syndrome and stable coronary artery disease. J Cardiovasc Comput Tomogr 2014;8(5):368–74.

30. Perez de Isla L, Alonso R, Gomez de Diego JJ, et al. Coronary plaque burden, plaque characterization and their prognostic implications in familial hypercholesterolemia: A computed tomographic angiography study. Atherosclerosis 2021;317:52–8.

31. Cury RC, Leipsic J, Abbara S, et al. CAD-RADS 2.0 - 2022 Coronary Artery Disease-Reporting and Data System: An Expert Consensus Document of the Society of Cardiovascular Computed Tomography (SCCT), the American College of Cardiology (ACC), the American College of Radiology (ACR), and the North America Society of Cardiovascular Imaging (NASCI). J Cardiovasc Comput Tomogr 2022;16(6):536–57.

32. Ferencik M, Mayrhofer T, Bittner DO, et al. Use of High-Risk Coronary Atherosclerotic Plaque Detection for Risk Stratification of Patients With Stable Chest Pain: A Secondary Analysis of the PROMISE Randomized Clinical Trial. JAMA Cardiol 2018;3(2):144–52.

33. Chang HJ, Lin FY, Lee SE, et al. Coronary Atherosclerotic Precursors of Acute Coronary Syndromes. J Am Coll Cardiol 2018;71(22):2511–22.

34. Lee JM, Choi KH, Koo BK, et al. Prognostic Implications of Plaque Characteristics and Stenosis Severity in Patients With Coronary Artery Disease. J Am Coll Cardiol 2019;73(19):2413–24.

35. Feuchtner GM, Barbieri F, Langer C, et al. Non obstructive high-risk plaque but not calcified by coronary CTA, and the G-score predict ischemia. J Cardiovasc Comput Tomogr 2019;13(6):305–14.

36. Otsuka K, Fukuda S, Tanaka A, et al. Napkin-ring sign on coronary CT angiography for the prediction of acute coronary syndrome. JACC Cardiovasc Imaging 2013;6(4):448–57.

37. Gaur S, Ovrehus KA, Dey D, et al. Coronary plaque quantification and fractional flow reserve by coronary computed tomography angiography identify ischaemia-causing lesions. Eur Heart J 2016;37(15):1220–7.

38. Williams MC, Kwiecinski J, Doris M, et al. Low-Attenuation Noncalcified Plaque on Coronary Computed Tomography Angiography Predicts Myocardial Infarction: Results From the Multicenter SCOT-HEART Trial (Scottish Computed Tomography of the HEART). Circulation 2020;141(18):1452–62.

39. Williams MC, Kwiecinski J, Doris M, et al. Sex-Specific Computed Tomography Coronary Plaque Characterization and Risk of Myocardial Infarction. JACC Cardiovasc Imaging 2021;14(9):1804–14.

40. Senoner T, Plank F, Barbieri F, et al. Added value of high-risk plaque criteria by coronary CTA for prediction of long-term outcomes. Atherosclerosis 2020;300:26–33.

41. Lopes PM, Ferreira AM, Albuquerque F, et al. Implications of three different testing strategies in the diagnostic approach to patients with stable chest pain and low pretest probability of obstructive coronary artery disease. J Cardiovasc Comput Tomogr 2023. https://doi.org/10.1016/j.jcct.2023.06.001.

42. Osborne-Grinter M, Kwiecinski J, Doris M, et al. Association of coronary artery calcium score with qualitatively and quantitatively assessed adverse plaque on coronary CT angiography in the SCOT-HEART trial. Eur Heart J Cardiovasc Imaging 2022;23(9):1210–21.

43. Nasir K, Cainzos-Achirica M, Valero-Elizondo J, et al. Coronary Atherosclerosis in an Asymptomatic U.S. Population: Miami Heart Study at Baptist Health South Florida. JACC Cardiovasc Imaging 2022;15(9):1604–18.

44. Di Cesare E, Patriarca L, Panebianco L, et al. Coronary computed tomography angiography in the evaluation of intermediate risk asymptomatic individuals. Radiol Med 2018;123(9):686–94.

45. Cho I, Chang HJ, Sung JM, et al. Coronary computed tomographic angiography and risk of all-cause mortality and nonfatal myocardial infarction in subjects without chest pain syndrome from the CONFIRM Registry (coronary CT angiography evaluation for clinical outcomes: an international multicenter registry). Circulation 2012;126(3):304–13.

46. Cho I, Al'Aref SJ, Berger A, et al. Prognostic value of coronary computed tomographic angiography findings in asymptomatic individuals: a 6-year follow-up from the prospective multicentre international CONFIRM study. Eur Heart J 2018;39(11):934–41.

47. Han D, Beecy A, Anchouche K, et al. Risk Reclassification With Coronary Computed Tomography Angiography-Visualized Nonobstructive Coronary Artery Disease According to 2018 American College of Cardiology/American Heart Association Cholesterol Guidelines (from the Coronary Computed Tomography Angiography Evaluation for Clinical Outcomes : An International Multicenter Registry [CONFIRM]). Am J Cardiol 2019;124(9):1397–405.

48. Muhlestein JB, Lappe DL, Lima JA, et al. Effect of screening for coronary artery disease using CT angiography on mortality and cardiac events in high-risk patients with diabetes: the FACTOR-64 randomized clinical trial. JAMA 2014;312(21):2234–43.

49. Available at: https://classic.clinicaltrials.gov/ct2/show/NCT03920176.

50. Detrano R, Guerci AD, Carr JJ, et al. Coronary calcium as a predictor of coronary events in four racial or ethnic groups. N Engl J Med 2008;358(13):1336–45.

51. Erbel R, Mohlenkamp S, Moebus S, et al. Coronary risk stratification, discrimination, and reclassification improvement based on quantification of subclinical coronary atherosclerosis: the Heinz Nixdorf Recall study. J Am Coll Cardiol 2010;56(17):1397–406.

52. Mohlenkamp S, Lehmann N, Greenland P, et al. Coronary artery calcium score improves cardiovascular risk prediction in persons without indication for statin therapy. Atherosclerosis 2011;215(1):229–36.

53. Hartaigh BO, Valenti V, Cho I, et al. 15-Year prognostic utility of coronary artery calcium scoring for all-cause mortality in the elderly. Atherosclerosis 2016;246:361–6.

54. Ahmadi N, Hajsadeghi F, Blumenthal RS, et al. Mortality in individuals without known coronary artery disease but with discordance between the Framingham risk score and coronary artery calcium. Am J Cardiol 2011;107(6):799–804.

55. Valenti V, B OH, Heo R, et al. A 15-Year Warranty Period for Asymptomatic Individuals Without Coronary Artery Calcium: A Prospective Follow-Up of 9,715 Individuals. JACC Cardiovasc Imaging 2015; 8(8):900–9.

56. Rozanski A, Gransar H, Shaw LJ, et al. Impact of coronary artery calcium scanning on coronary risk factors and downstream testing the EISNER (Early Identification of Subclinical Atherosclerosis by Noninvasive Imaging Research) prospective randomized trial. J Am Coll Cardiol 2011;57(15): 1622–32.

57. van der Aalst CM, Denissen S, Vonder M, et al. Screening for cardiovascular disease risk using traditional risk factor assessment or coronary artery calcium scoring: the ROBINSCA trial. Eur Heart J Cardiovasc Imaging 2020;21(11):1216–24.

58. Xie X, Zhao Y, de Bock GH, et al. Validation and prognosis of coronary artery calcium scoring in non-triggered thoracic computed tomography: systematic review and meta-analysis. Circ Cardiovasc Imaging 2013;6(4):514–21.

59. Fleisher LA, Fleischmann KE, Auerbach AD, et al. 2014 ACC/AHA guideline on perioperative cardiovascular evaluation and management of patients undergoing noncardiac surgery: a report of the American College of Cardiology/American Heart Association Task Force on Practice Guidelines. Circulation 2014;130(24):e278–333.

60. Kristensen SD, Knuuti J, Saraste A, et al. 2014 ESC/ ESA Guidelines on non-cardiac surgery: cardiovascular assessment and management: The Joint Task Force on non-cardiac surgery: cardiovascular assessment and management of the European Society of Cardiology (ESC) and the European Society of Anaesthesiology (ESA). Eur Heart J 2014;35(35): 2383–431.

61. Koshy AN, Ha FJ, Gow PJ, et al. Computed tomographic coronary angiography in risk stratification prior to non-cardiac surgery: a systematic review and meta-analysis. Heart 2019;105(17):1335–42.

62. Narula J, Chandrashekhar Y, Ahmadi A, et al. SCCT 2021 Expert Consensus Document on Coronary Computed Tomographic Angiography: A Report of the Society of Cardiovascular Computed Tomography. J Cardiovasc Comput Tomogr 2021;15(3):192–217.

63. Ren X, Liu K, Zhang H, et al. Coronary Evaluation Before Heart Valvular Surgery by Using Coronary Computed Tomographic Angiography Versus Invasive Coronary Angiography. J Am Heart Assoc 2021;10(15):e019531.

64. Norgaard BL, Leipsic J, Gaur S, et al. Diagnostic performance of noninvasive fractional flow reserve derived from coronary computed tomography angiography in suspected coronary artery disease: the NXT trial (Analysis of Coronary Blood Flow Using CT Angiography: Next Steps). J Am Coll Cardiol 2014;63(12):1145–55.

65. Lu MT, Ferencik M, Roberts RS, et al. Noninvasive FFR Derived From Coronary CT Angiography: Management and Outcomes in the PROMISE Trial. JACC Cardiovasc Imaging 2017;10(11):1350–8.

66. Min JK, Leipsic J, Pencina MJ, et al. Diagnostic accuracy of fractional flow reserve from anatomic CT angiography. JAMA 2012;308(12):1237–45.

67. Driessen RS, Danad I, Stuijfzand WJ, et al. Comparison of Coronary Computed Tomography Angiography, Fractional Flow Reserve, and Perfusion Imaging for Ischemia Diagnosis. J Am Coll Cardiol 2019;73(2):161–73.

68. Norgaard BL, Terkelsen CJ, Mathiassen ON, et al. Coronary CT Angiographic and Flow Reserve-Guided Management of Patients With Stable Ischemic Heart Disease. J Am Coll Cardiol 2018; 72(18):2123–34.

69. Patel MR, Norgaard BL, Fairbairn TA, et al. 1-Year Impact on Medical Practice and Clinical Outcomes of FFR(CT): The ADVANCE Registry. JACC Cardiovasc Imaging 2020;13(1 Pt 1):97–105.

70. Colleran R, Douglas PS, Hadamitzky M, et al. An FFR(CT) diagnostic strategy versus usual care in patients with suspected coronary artery disease planned for invasive coronary angiography at German sites: one-year results of a subgroup analysis of the PLATFORM (Prospective Longitudinal Trial of FFR(CT): Outcome and Resource Impacts) study. Open Heart 2017;4(1):e000526.

71. Becker LM, Peper J, Verhappen B, et al. Real world impact of added FFR-CT to coronary CT angiography on clinical decision-making and patient prognosis - IMPACT FFR study. Eur Radiol 2023;33(8):5465–75.

72. Curzen N, Nicholas Z, Stuart B, et al. Fractional flow reserve derived from computed tomography coronary angiography in the assessment and management of stable chest pain: the FORECAST randomized trial. Eur Heart J 2021;42(37):3844–52.

73. Hlatky MA, Wilding S, Stuart B, et al. Randomized comparison of chest pain evaluation with FFR(CT) or standard care: Factors determining US costs. J Cardiovasc Comput Tomogr 2023;17(1):52–9.

74. Mittal TK, Hothi SS, Venugopal V, et al. The Use and Efficacy of FFR-CT: Real-World Multicenter Audit of Clinical Data With Cost Analysis. JACC Cardiovasc Imaging 2023;16(8):1056–65.

75. Stuijfzand WJ, van Rosendael AR, Lin FY, et al. Stress Myocardial Perfusion Imaging vs Coronary Computed Tomographic Angiography for Diagnosis of Invasive Vessel-Specific Coronary Physiology: Predictive Modeling Results From the Computed Tomographic Evaluation of Atherosclerotic Determinants of Myocardial Ischemia (CREDENCE) Trial. JAMA Cardiol 2020;5(12):1338–48.

76. Hamilton MCK, Charters PFP, Lyen S, et al. Computed tomography-derived fractional flow reserve (FFR(CT)) has no additional clinical impact over the anatomical Coronary Artery Disease - Reporting and Data System (CAD-RADS) in real-world elective healthcare of coronary artery disease. Clin Radiol 2022;77(12):883–90.

77. Norgaard BL, Fairbairn TA, Safian RD, et al. Coronary CT Angiography-derived Fractional Flow Reserve Testing in Patients with Stable Coronary Artery Disease: Recommendations on Interpretation and Reporting. Radiol Cardiothorac Imaging 2019;1(5):e190050.

78. Pelgrim GJ, Dorrius M, Xie X, et al. The dream of a one-stop-shop: Meta-analysis on myocardial perfusion CT. Eur J Radiol 2015;84(12):2411–20.

79. Williams MC, Mirsadraee S, Dweck MR, et al. Computed tomography myocardial perfusion vs (15)O-water positron emission tomography and fractional flow reserve. Eur Radiol 2017;27(3): 1114–24.

80. Shu ZY, Cui SJ, Zhang YQ, et al. Predicting Chronic Myocardial Ischemia Using CCTA-Based Radiomics Machine Learning Nomogram. J Nucl Cardiol 2022; 29(1):262–74.

81. Michallek F, Nakamura S, Ota H, et al. Fractal analysis of 4D dynamic myocardial stress-CT perfusion imaging differentiates micro- and macrovascular ischemia in a multi-center proof-of-concept study. Sci Rep 2022;12(1):5085.

82. Yu M, Shen C, Dai X, et al. Clinical Outcomes of Dynamic Computed Tomography Myocardial Perfusion Imaging Combined With Coronary Computed Tomography Angiography Versus Coronary Computed Tomography Angiography-Guided Strategy. Circ Cardiovasc Imaging 2020;13(1):e009775.

83. Lubbers M, Coenen A, Kofflard M, et al. Comprehensive Cardiac CT With Myocardial Perfusion Imaging Versus Functional Testing in Suspected Coronary Artery Disease: The Multicenter, Randomized CRESCENT-II Trial. JACC Cardiovasc Imaging 2018;11(11):1625–36.

84. Jonas RA, Barkovich E, Choi AD, et al. The effect of scan and patient parameters on the diagnostic performance of AI for detecting coronary stenosis on coronary CT angiography. Clin Imaging 2022;84:149–58.

85. Muscogiuri G, Chiesa M, Trotta M, et al. Performance of a deep learning algorithm for the evaluation of CAD-RADS classification with CCTA. Atherosclerosis 2020;294:25–32.

86. Lin A, Manral N, McElhinney P, et al. Deep learning-enabled coronary CT angiography for plaque and stenosis quantification and cardiac risk prediction: an international multicentre study. Lancet Digit Health 2022;4(4):e256–65.

87. Kim Y, Choi AD, Telluri A, et al. Atherosclerosis Imaging Quantitative Computed Tomography (AI-QCT) to guide referral to invasive coronary angiography in the randomized controlled CONSERVE trial. Clin Cardiol 2023;46(5):477–83.

88. Antonopoulos AS, Sanna F, Sabharwal N, et al. Detecting human coronary inflammation by imaging perivascular fat. Sci Transl Med 2017;9:398.

89. Desai MY. Noninvasive detection of perivascular inflammation by coronary computed tomography in the CRISP-CT study and its implications for residual cardiovascular risk. Cardiovasc Res 2019;115(1): e3–4.

90. Oikonomou EK, Marwan M, Desai MY, et al. Noninvasive detection of coronary inflammation using computed tomography and prediction of residual cardiovascular risk (the CRISP CT study): a posthoc analysis of prospective outcome data. Lancet 2018;392(10151):929–39.

91. Tzolos E, Williams MC, McElhinney P, et al. Pericoronary Adipose Tissue Attenuation, Low-Attenuation Plaque Burden, and 5-Year Risk of Myocardial Infarction. JACC Cardiovasc Imaging 2022;15(6):1078–88.

92. Kim JN, Gomez-Perez L, Zimin VN, et al. Pericoronary Adipose Tissue Radiomics from Coronary Computed Tomography Angiography Identifies Vulnerable Plaques. Bioengineering (Basel) 2023;10(3). https://doi.org/10.3390/bioengineering10030360.

Cardiac Computed Tomography of Native Cardiac Valves

Jordi Broncano, MD[a],*, Kate Hanneman, MD, MPH, FRCPC[b],
Brian Ghoshhajra, MD, MBA[c], Prabhakar Shanta Rajiah, MD[d]

KEYWORDS

- Valvular heart disease • Cardiac computed tomography • Stenosis • Regurgitation
- Low-flow/low-gradient aortic stenosis • Valvular tumor • Infective endocarditis • Thrombus

KEY POINTS

- Cardiac computed tomography (CCT) may have a complementary role in certain specific situations when transthoracic echocardiography is inconclusive and plays a key role in planning for transcatheter valvular devices.
- Different gender thresholds for severe aortic calcification have been described helping to predict severe disease, excess of mortality, and providing incremental prognostic value beyond echocardiography.
- In patients with discordant echocardiographic Doppler severity of aortic stenosis (AS) or paradoxic low-flow/low-gradient with preserved LVEF, aortic valve calcification may be a useful marker for severe AS.
- Bicuspid aortic valve is the most frequent form of congenital aortic valvular heart disease (VHD), typically have commissural fusion and two unequally sized separated cusps and may be associated with AS, aortic regurgitation (AR), combined AS/AR, or no relevant functional VHD.
- Mitral regurgitation (MR) is the most common manifestation of VHD. Primary MR (degenerative) is produced by an anatomic abnormality or direct damage to the mitral valve or subvalvular apparatus, whereas secondary MR (functional) is produced by regional/global left ventricle dysfunction and/or dilatation leading to tethering and restriction of the mitral leaflets.

 Video content accompanies this article at http://www.radiologic.theclinics.com.

INTRODUCTION

Valvular heart disease (VHD) is a significant clinical problem with associated high morbidity and mortality. The prevalence in the United States is 2.5%, with over 20,000 VHD-related deaths in 2007, with aortic and mitral VHD the most common.[1–4] Up to 10% to 20% of surgical procedures in the United States are performed for treatment of VHD.[2] In developed countries, VHD is primarily

[a] Cardiothoracic Imaging Unit, Radiology Department, Hospital San Juan de Dios, HT Medica, Avenida El Brillante No 36, Córdoba 14012, Spain; [b] Department of Medical Imaging, Toronto General Hospital, Peter Munk Cardiac Center, University Health Network (UHN), University of Toronto, 1 PMB-298, 585 University Avenue, Toronto, Ontario M5G2N2, Canada; [c] Cardiovascular Imaging, Department of Radiology, Massachusetts General Hospital, Harvard Medical School, Charles River Plaza East, 165 Cambridge Street, Boston, MA 02114, USA; [d] Department of Radiology, Mayo Clinic, 201 West Center Street, Rochester, MN 55902, USA
* Corresponding author.
E-mail address: j.broncano.c@htime.org

Radiol Clin N Am 62 (2024) 399–417
https://doi.org/10.1016/j.rcl.2023.12.004
0033-8389/24/© 2024 Elsevier Inc. All rights reserved.

due to degenerative or inherited causes, depending on the patient's age. Post-rheumatic disease, the sequelae of acute systemic inflammatory reaction secondary to group A streptococcus infection, is the primary cause worldwide, with most severe involvement of the aortic valve (AV) and mitral valve (MV).[1,5] Other less frequent causes include infectious and noninfectious endocarditis, valvular neoplasms, or other valvular pseudomasses. Metastatic carcinoid tumor may involve right-sided cardiac valves through the secretion of vasoactive products.[6] Although not being the primary cardiac imaging modality, cardiac computed tomography (CCT) may help to exclude coronary artery disease (CAD) in patients with VHD undergoing surgery, evaluate the morphology and function of involved valves, grade its severity and proportionate important anatomic information when needed for percutaneous treatment planning.[7–9] The role of CCT for transcatheter device planning of cardiac valves has been the subject in detail of several recent reviews; hence, such topics are not included in this article.[10–17] In this review, the authors detail the current data available regarding the use of CCT in the evaluation of VHD in native valves, other than transcatheter device planning, imaging findings, and imaging hints for precisely determining the severity of VHD and assessing secondary cardiac remodeling.

ROLE OF IMAGING IN VALVULAR HEART DISEASE

Echocardiography is the primary imaging modality for the evaluation of VHD due to its widespread availability, noninvasiveness, and cost-effectiveness, providing in most cases adequate information for diagnosis, grading, risk stratification, and treatment planning.[18–20] Among its main limitations include interobserver variability, poor acoustic windows in patients with emphysema or large body habitus, low reliability in the evaluation of pulmonary valve (PV) and right heart function, and hemodynamic assumptions in some quantitative analysis. Although transesophageal echocardiography may be possible, it has several contraindications.[2]

Cardiac magnetic resonance (CMR) is a noninvasive imaging method that does not use ionizing radiation and is rapidly becoming the reference standard in VHD evaluation. Allowing qualitative and quantitative assessment of valvular and ventricular morphology and function, with high interstudy and interobserver reproducibility compared with echocardiography, excellent tissue characterization capabilities, and ability to visualize complex hemodynamic parameters.[1,21]

CCT may have a complementary role in certain specific situations when transthoracic echocardiography is inconclusive and plays a key role in planning for transcatheter valvular devices.[7] It allows for evaluation of CAD before surgical treatment in patients with VHD. Moreover, it may provide ancillary findings regarding cardiac chamber that may be important not only for diagnosis but also for percutaneous treatment planning. CT also allows for quantification of valvular calcification and morphology as well as characterization of valvular tumors, vegetations, and assessment of perivalvular complications.

CARDIAC COMPUTED TOMOGRAPHY PROTOCOL
Image Acquisition

Imaging of VHD requires high temporal and spatial resolution to reduce respiratory and cardiac motion artifacts. The current CT temporal resolution is approximately 60 to 180 millisecond and goes up to 83 millisecond with dual source technology.[1,7,22] Although the temporal resolution is still lower compared with CMR (25–50 millisecond) and echocardiography (5–60 millisecond), the spatial resolution and acquisition time of CT is superior.[4] Technological advances, such as multi-energy CT and photon-counting detector CT, have enabled tissue characterization with CT for detection of myocardial fibrosis and myocardial extracellular volume (ECV) quantification.[23]

Contrast-enhanced whole-heart retrospective ECG-gated acquisition is the preferred method for VHD. To avoid contrast material leaking into the right atrium (RA) and subsequent heterogeneous enhancement, the images should be acquired in mid-inspiration.[1] Although the radiation dose with retrospective ECG-gating (3–7 msV) was an issue in the past methods such as low-tube voltage scanning, iterative reconstruction, and ECG-based tube current modulation help to lower the dose.[24,25] If systolic phases are particularly important for valvular assessment, ECG-triggered radiation dose modulation may be used in diastole, lowering in up to 30% to 40% the final administered effective dose.[1] A 120-kV peak (kVp) is commonly used, although it may be reduced (100 kVp) in patients lower body mass index (<28–30).[7] Beam hardening artifact, seen in valvular prostheses, may be reduced by using high tube potential (up to 140 kVp) or high-energy virtual monoenergetic images from multi-energy CT. This artifact is more noticeable in retrospective rather than in prospective electrocardiogram (ECG) gating.

Unenhanced prospective ECG-gated acquisition may be useful for the assessment of aortic, coronary artery calcification, and valvular calcification, especially for severity grading in cases of low-flow/low-gradient aortic stenosis (AS). Other benefits of non-contrast imaging are identification of postsurgical changes, such as high attenuation pledgets, erroneously retained surgical objects or intramural hematomas in the aortic wall. In certain situation (infective endocarditis [IE]), adding a delayed CT acquisition may aid in the differentiation of vegetations from normal myocardium or thrombus as well as for the assessment of perivalvular findings and distant embolic events.[26,27]

Patient Preparation

Dependent on the inherent temporal resolution of the CT systems, oral or intravenous beta-blockers may be administered before scanning to reduce the heart rate and improve image quality if the patient does not have any conditions that prevent its administration. Contrast injection protocol should be tailored attending to the cardiac chamber under evaluation. Contrast media is infused commonly through and antecubital venous catheter (16–18 Gauge needle) and high flux (4–6 mL/s). Bolus tracking technique is the preferred method for real-time monitoring of the arrival of the contrast bolus to the target vascular structure.[2] A conventional triphasic contrast injection protocol (rapid infusion of contrast material followed by a mixture of contrast material and saline solution and a saline flush) is commonly used for the evaluation of left-sided valves (aortic and mitral). However, this approach may not be optimal for the opacification of right-sided cardiac valves. A modified triphasic contrast injection protocol (rapid infusion of contrast material followed by slower infusion of 100% contrast material and saline flush) may be used for better delineation of tricuspid and pulmonic valves.[1,2,7–9,22,24] Moreover, triggering the pulmonary artery (PA) during bolus tracking technique allow early initiation of the acquisition and proper opacification of the right-sided chambers (optimal enhancement: 400–450 HU).[28]

Image Reconstruction and Postprocessing

Currently, CT data sets may be reconstructed to obtain isotropic voxel resolution, with optimized reconstruction matrix and dedicated field of view. Artificial intelligence-based image reconstruction algorithms may improve the signal-to-noise and contrast-to-noise ratio as also low monoenergetic spectral imaging does in situations with unoptimized contrast enhancement. Both static and cine images can be obtained in different cardiac orientations.[1] Static images are created by using multiplanar reconstructions, thin-slab maximum intensity projections, or volume rendering for evaluating the cardiac valves in multiple motionless orthogonal cardiac planes.

Retrospective reconstruction of the entire cardiac cycle, every 5% to 10% of the entire R-R interval may be used for a dynamic valvular approach. In general, the number of reconstructed cardiac phases should be similar to the temporal resolution of the CT system used.[2] Dynamic 3D/4D cine evaluation of the valves is performed by obtaining conventional cardiac short-axis and long-axis views and a dedicated short-axis view exactly in the plane of the evaluated valve.[7] It may help to determine the phases of maximal opening and closure of native and prosthetic valves, planimetry of the valvular opening area (VOA) and regurgitant orifice area (ROA), leaflet thickening, and restricted motion. With current CCT technology, volumetric ventricular assessment is feasible, with high accuracy and reproducibility compared with CMR. This enables the calculation of regurgitant volume and fraction by indirect methods, which may be useful for grading isolated valvular insufficiency severity.[29,30] Although there are only scarce data, computational fluid dynamics (CFD) evaluation of CCT data sets may help to further dive in hemodynamic characteristics of certain VHD.[31]

NORMAL VALVULAR ANATOMY

Two semilunar valves (pulmonic and aortic) separate the right and left ventricles (LVs) form the PA and aorta, respectively. In the same manner, two atrioventricular valves (mitral and tricuspid) regulate the flow between left and right atria and ventricles, respectively. In both cases, pressure differences between chambers regulate the opening and closure of the valves, typically with unidirectional flow through them. In contrast to atrioventricular valves, AV and PV lack papillary muscles or chordae tendineae. Semilunar valve planimetry is better achieved on mid-systole (20%–30% of the RR interval or 50–100 millisecond for the R peak depending on the heart rate), whereas 0% to 5% of the RR interval are the best phase for atrioventricular valve ROA. Semilunar ROA planimetry and atrioventricular anatomic VOA are better depicted in mid-diastole (60%–75% RR interval).[32–34]

Aortic Valve

The AV complex is composed of an AV annulus, commissures, sinuses of Valsalva, coronary ostia, and sinotubular junction. The aortic annulus is a fibrous ring embedded in the endocardium and with structural continuity with the mitral annulus (intervalvular fibrosa). Commonly, the AV is composed of three cusps (right, left, and posterior), although it may range from 1 to 5 cusps.[2,35,36] At the nadir points of these cusps (hinge points), they anchor in the left ventricle outflow tract (LVOT) wall forming an oval crown-shaped virtual basal ring. Right and left cusps are inferior to the right and left coronary sinuses, where right and left coronary arteries arise, respectively.[1,2] No coronary artery arises from the posterior (noncoronary) cusp. Separating the three cusps, there are three commissures, roughly equally spaced around the AV annulus.[37] In systole, the LV pressure exceeds the aorta and causes aperture of the AV cusps producing a triangular-shaped orifice. In diastole, the LV pressure falls coapting the AV cusps. When AV closes, there is an overlap between the surfaces of each cusp as the closing edge is slightly proximal to the true anatomic edge of each cusp.[37] The normal AV area varies from 2.5 to 4 cm.[19,21,35]

Pulmonary Valve

The PV is a semilunar valve, commonly composed of three commissures and cusps (anterior, right, and left), and unlike AV, the PV lacks coronary ostia, and it is anatomically separate from the tricuspid valve (TV).[1] The left and right cusps are close to the left and coronary AV cusps, respectively. It also has a crown-shaped annulus inserted between the right ventricle outflow tract (RVOT) and the PA.[28] The PV leaflets are thinner than the AV leaflets as they supported lower blood pressures compared with left cardiac chambers.[28] The normal PV area is approximately 2 cm^2/m^2.

Mitral Valve

The MV is a bicuspid valve located between the left atrium (LA) and the LV, composed of five components (annulus, leaflets, commissures, papillary muscles, and chordae tendineae) synchronously actioned for its appropriate function. The annulus is a saddle-shaped fibrous ring embedded in the myocardium, anchoring the MV leaflets and in continuity with the AV annulus via the intervalvular fibrosa. MV have two leaflets (anterior and posterior mitral leaflets), each of them with three scallops (A1-A3 and P1-P3, respectively) of unequal size and shape.[10] Commissures are clefts that divide the leaflets from each other. Two papillary muscles connect the MV to the lateral wall of the LV, where they arise from.[37] Each of them comprises one to three muscular bundles.[10] The

chordae tendineae are fibrous tendons that arise from the tip of the papillary muscles and insert at the leaflets.[10,22,38,39] The MV area ranges 4 to 6 cm^2.[40]

Tricuspid Valve

TV is located between the RA and right ventricle (RV) and is composed of a fibrous annulus, leaflets, chordae tendineae, and papillary muscles.[1] The fibrous annulus is a D-shaped saddle-like, nonplanar structure with a larger posterolateral C-shaped segment and a straighter anteroseptal segment that changes its size dynamically through the cardiac cycle.[41] TV commonly has three leaflets (anterior, septal, and posterior) with variable size and mobility, although it may range from 2 to 4. The anterior leaflet is the largest one with the greatest motion, whereas the posterior is the smallest leaflet and the septal leaflet has the lowest mobility.[42] The anteroseptal commissure is near the noncoronary sinus of Valsalva, and the posterior-septal commissure is adjacent to the coronary sinus ostia.[41]

VALVULAR HEART DISEASE

A narrowing of the valvular orifice hindering antegrade blood flow is the hallmark of valvular stenosis. It can be due to valvular thickening or calcification, cusp or leaflet fusion, or congenital malformations. To compensate the increased afterload, the previous chamber rises its pressure, occasionally increasing its thickness (compensatory hypertrophy), to maintain cardiac output until it fails. Valvular insufficiency results from inadequate leaflet coaptation, allowing retrograde flow through the diseased valve and increasing the preload in the previous chamber. This increased volume overload produces irreversible ventricular remodeling, dilatation, and heart failure (HF).[1,7,22,37]

Aortic Valvular Heart Disease

Aortic stenosis

AS is defined as the obstruction of the forward blood flow through the LVOT at a valvular, supravalvular, or subvalvular level. Valvular stenosis is the most frequent type.[35,43,44] Although degenerative AS is the commonest cause in developed countries, rheumatic disease accounts for most of the cases worldwide. Moreover, age-related AS is associated with diffuse atherosclerotic disease.[1]

AS is characterized by a progressive decrease in VOA less than 2.5 cm^2, being hemodynamically significant when is less than 1 cm^2. Owing to its independence from hemodynamic factors, CCT-derived planimetric VOA measurement may be used to stratify AS severity with excellent correlation with echocardiography and mean transvalvular pressure gradient.[7,45,46] It has an excellent diagnostic accuracy for detecting moderate (100% of sensitivity, specificity, and accuracy, respectively) and severe (91%, 97%, 96% of sensitivity, specificity, and accuracy, respectively) AS.[45] For measuring the VOA, special care must be taken to position the plane precisely at the tips of the AV in systole. On cine imaging, limitation of the aortic cusps systolic excursion could be seen. Compensatory LV hypertrophy and ascending aorta dilatation may be present. The determination of increased myocardial ECV fraction on multi-energy CT in patients with AS has been described as an independent predictor of adverse outcomes (hazard ratio:1.25; $P < .001$) after valvular intervention.[23]

Although cusp thickening is a common feature among different etiologies, they differ on the pattern of calcification. In degenerative AS, the calcification, commonly heavy, begins at the annulus and progresses toward the cusps producing an asymmetric opening and closure of the valve. Fusion of adjacent cusps without commissural involvement may results in functional bicuspid valves (**Table 1**). Conversely, in rheumatic disease typically symmetric calcification, fusion of the three commissures occurs and reduction of its aperture occurs (**Table 2**).[37] Calcification not only correlates with severity of AS but also constitutes a subclinical indicator of atherosclerotic burden and coronary artery calcification severity.[7,45] Different gender thresholds for severe aortic calcification have been described ($\geq$1200 and $\geq$ 2000 Agatston units for severe AS in women and men, respectively) helping to predict severe disease, excess of mortality and providing incremental prognostic value beyond echocardiography (**Fig. 1**, Video 1).[47] Noticeably, in patients with discordant echocardiographic Doppler severity of AS or paradoxic low-flow/low-gradient with preserved left ventricle ejection fraction (LVEF), AV calcification may be a useful marker for severe AS.[48–51] Moreover, in cases where there is discordant information between echocardiography and CCT-derived VOA (VOA$\geq$1 cm^2), CCT CFD may be helpful for determining the hemodynamic severity.[31]

Aortic regurgitation

An incomplete coaptation of the valvular cusps with backflow of blood from the aorta to the LV is the hallmark for aortic regurgitation (AR) and can result from intrinsic valve disease, abnormal aortic root geometry, or both (**Box 1**).[1,7] Rheumatic disease constitutes the most common cause of AR in developing world, whereas bicuspid aortic valve (BAV) and aortic root ectasia are the most prevalent etiologies in developed world.[52]

Additional features depend on the chronicity of the AR onset. Acute AR due to endocarditis, trauma, or aortic dissection produces pulmonary congestion but with normal LV size as there has been no time for developing ventricular remodeling. Chronic AR may be secondary to valvular degeneration in older patients or congenital causes in younger individuals. Etiologies involving the aortic root and ascending aorta such as Stanford A aortic dissection, ascending aortic aneurysm, Marfan, or Ehlers Danlos disease can result in chronic AR. In chronic AR, the LV experiments an increased preload and ventricular filling pressure causing concentric or eccentric LV hypertrophy, dilatation, LA enlargement, and ultimately HF.[53] Nevertheless, up to 50% of patients with severe AR will develop HF in the following 10 years after the diagnosis.[32]

Shortened and thickened aortic cusps with or without aortic root ectasia may be seen on CCT in AR, with incomplete coaptation in mid-to-end diastole (70%–75%). Planimetric measurement of the ROA correlates with the severity of AR seen on echocardiography.[2] Different values based on ROA have been published in the literature (see **Table 2**). CCT may also calculate ventricular volumes and, therefore, derived aortic regurgitant volume (ARV = RV systolic volume–LV systolic volume) and fraction (ARF = ARV/LV systolic volume $\times$ 100) in the absence of other valvular regurgitation or shunts. Feutchner and colleagues observed good correlation between ARV and ARF compared with echocardiography. CT-derived ARV and ARF correctly classified 93% and 89% of severe AR, respectively (sensitivity and specificity of 98% and 90.3%). When ROA was added, the specificity improved to 97%.[54]

Congenital aortic valvular heart disease

BAV is the most frequent form of congenital aortic VHD, occurring in up to 1% to 2% of people. BAV typically have commissural fusion and two unequally sized separated cusps and may be associated with AS, AR, combined AS/AR, or no relevant functional VHD (see **Table 1**). Rarer anomalies of the AV include unicuspid, indeterminate, hypoplastic, or quadricuspid valves, which commonly present with AR.[37] Advanced cardiac imaging, either CCT or CMR, is recommended if any aortic segment could not be visualized on echocardiography, for ruling out coarctation or if any aortic segment measures $\geq$ 45 mm.[55] Three aspects

Table 1
Morphologic characteristics of aortic stenosis

	BAV	Degenerative	Rheumatic
Age	< 60 y	> 69 y	Variable
Epidemiology	Most common congenital VHD	Common in developed countries	Common worldwide
Opening	Asymmetric	Asymmetric	Symmetric
Cusps	Fusion of unequally sized cusps	Thickened Fusion without commissural involvement Functional bicuspid AV	Thickening Fusion three commissures
Calcification	Less severe Outline commissural edges and raphe	Heavy, asymmetric From the annulus toward cusps	Symmetric calcification

Abbreviations: AV, aortic valve; BAV, bicuspid aortic valve; VHD, valvular heart disease.

must be described in BAV: (1) the type, specific phenotype, and function; (2) the presence and characteristics of the raphe as well as the cusp size, shape, and symmetry; and (3) the presence and phenotype of BAV-related aortopathy and/or aortic coarctation (**Fig. 2**, Videos 2–4).[55] Contrarily to age-related or rheumatic AV calcification, BAV calcification is less severe, occurring predominantly at the commissural edges or outlining the raphe, when present.[37] For similar AS grades,

Table 2
Cardiac computed tomography findings on left-sided valvular heart disease

Cardiac Valve	Stenosis	Regurgitation
AV	Valvular findings • VOA ≤ 2.5 cm^2 (severe if ≤ 1 cm^2) • Limitation cusps excursion • Cusp thickening and fusion (functional bicuspid valves) • Leaflet calcification • Commissural fusion (rheumatic heart disease) Secondary findings • Compensatory LV hypertrophy • Ascending aorta dilatation • Increased ECV on DECT/spectral CT	Valvular findings • Shortening and thickening cusps • Malcoaptation (ROA quantification) Secondary findings • Concentric or eccentric LV hypertrophy • LV dilatation • LA enlargement • Aortic root ectasia • Heart failure
MV	Valvular findings • Leaflet thickening and calcification • "Funnel-shaped" appearance • Commissural fusion • Thickening and calcification chordae tendineae • VOA ≤ 2.5 cm^2 • Restricted leaflet motion Secondary findings • LA enlargement; LA appendage thrombus • Increased size pulmonary veins • Pulmonary edema; pulmonary hypertension • RV hypertrophy	Valvular findings • Leaflet thickening • Restricted leaflet motion and traction (tethering) • Apical displacement coaptation plane (tenting) • Malcoaptation (ROA quantification) • Systolic bowing ≥ 2 mm valvular plane • Flail leaflet motion Secondary findings • LV dilatation and eccentric remodeling • LA enlargement • Pulmonary edema • Heart failure

Abbreviations: AV, aortic valve; DECT, dual-energy computed tomography; ECV, extracellular volume; LA, left atrium; LV, left ventricle; MV, mitral valve; ROA, regurgitant orifice area; RV, right ventricle; VOA, valvular orifice area.

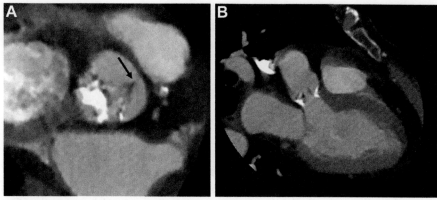

Fig. 1. A 82-year-old man with severe degenerative aortic stenosis. (*A*) Aortic view of CCT revealed a severely calcified (Agatston: 2600) tricuspid aortic valve, mainly in the noncoronary cusp, with partial fusion of the right and left coronary cusps (*black arrow*), irregularly thickened leaflets and VOA severely reduced (0.79 cm^2; indexed VOA: 0.5 cm^2/m^2). (*B*) CCT three-chamber view reveal a symmetric concentric hypertrophy (indexed mass: 102 g/m^2; relative wall thickness: 0.46) without ventricular dilatation and with normal LVEF (66%).

Box 1
Aortic regurgitation etiology

Intrinsic valve disease

- Age-related degeneration
- Rheumatic heart disease
- Infective endocarditis
- Bicuspid aortic valve

Dilated aortic root

- Systemic hypertension
- Aortic aneurysm
- Type A aortic dissection
- Thoracic trauma
- Syphilis
- Connective tissue diseases (Marfan, Ehlers-Danlos syndrome, and so forth).

Acute presentation

- Infectious endocarditis
- Type A aortic dissection
- Thoracic trauma

Chronic presentation

- Age-related degeneration
- Congenital (bicuspid aortic valve)
- Ascending aortic aneurysm
- Connective tissue diseases (Marfan, Ehlers-Danlos syndrome, and so forth)
- Syphilis

BAV have higher AV calcium scores compared with tricuspid AV.[7] In general, degenerative AS in patients with BAV occur earlier (<60 years) compared with TVs (>60 years).[2]

Mitral Valvular Heart Disease

Mitral stenosis

Rheumatic chronic inflammatory changes are the first cause worldwide of mitral stenosis (MS), followed by congenital abnormalities with parachute deformity, degenerative calcification, carcinoid syndrome, LA tumors or obstructive LA thrombus (**Box 2**).[1,7] CCT may be useful for the identification and quantification of MS, ascertain the underlying cause, and determine the suitability for surgical intervention and procedural planning.

On CCT, an adequate selection of the early-to-mid diastolic phase (60%–75% RR interval) for planimetry of the MV orifice by doing a double-oblique short axis plane through the tips of the MV is mandatory. In MS, an MV orifices ≤2.5 cm^2 with leaflet thickening, motion restriction on cine imaging, and funnel-shaped appearance may be seen. Calcification may be present and assessment of its morphology (focal or circumferential) and extension according to the Carpentier nomenclature is recommended. Rheumatic MS also produces calcification of the leaflets, commissural fusion, thickening, shortening, and calcification of chordae tendineae with a "dome-shape" appearance due to restricted motion of the leaflet tips.[37] Secondary signs of MS on CCT include LA enlargement with normal LV, increased size of pulmonary veins, pulmonary edema as well as pulmonary hypertension, RV hypertrophy, or LA appendage thrombus (see **Table 2**).[56]

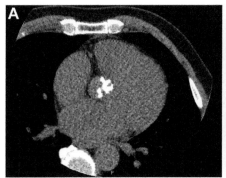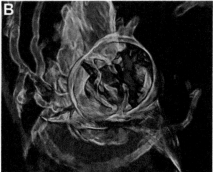

Fig. 2. A 61-year-old man. Triathlete with negative T waves on the lateral left ventricular wall on EKG and mild aortic stenosis on echocardiography. No significant coronary artery disease was detected on the CCT evaluation. (A) Non-contrast-enhanced ECG-gated CCT revealed mild calcium score results (Agatston: 80.4) but with moderate calcification of the aortic valve (Agatston AV: 1426). (B) 4D CCT revealed a bicuspid aortic valve due to fusion of noncoronary and right coronary cusps with raphe, with mild thickening of the leaflets border. Mild reduction of the VOA is present (1.7 cm^2).

Mitral regurgitation

Mitral regurgitation (MR) is the most common manifestation of VHD. Primary MR (degenerative) is produced by an anatomic abnormality or direct damage to the MV or subvalvular apparatus, such as rheumatic degeneration or MV prolapse (MVP). Secondary mitral valve regurgitation (MVR) (functional) is produced by regional/global LV dysfunction and/or dilatation leading to tethering and restriction of the mitral leaflets seen in ischemic heart disease, dilated cardiomyopathy, obstructive hypertrophic cardiomyopathy, papillary muscle rupture, or annular dilatation (**Box 3**).[10,57] Acute MR, seen on IE or papillary muscle rupture, results in LA sudden volume overload and enlargement with pulmonary edema without LV remodeling. In chronic MR, LV remodeling is patent with LV dilatation and eccentric remodeling, LA enlargement, and lately progression to HF.[1]

Rheumatic MR causes diffuse leaflet thickening without calcification and commissural fusion.[1] Adverse LV remodeling seen on secondary MR causes abnormal leaflet traction and motion restriction (tethering), which may be symmetric or asymmetric, apical displacement of the coaptation plane (tenting), with abnormal morphology of the anterior mitral leaflet.[58] CT-derived MV tenting area has been associated with MR severity.[38] Moreover, asymmetric tethering phenotype, seen on ischemic heart disease, has been related with severe MR.[59,60] ROA quantification by CCT has good correlation with echocardiography (see **Table 2**).[2] Estimation of MR volume (MRV) by CCT is feasible by calculating the difference between LV stroke volume (LVSV) and RV stroke volume, in the absence shunts or other valvular regurgitation. CCT MR fraction (MR fraction = MRV/LVSV

Box 2
Mitral stenosis etiology

Rheumatic heart disease

Congenital anomalies

Ager-related degenerative disease

Carcinoid syndrome

Connective tissue diseases

Left atrial tumor (ie, dynamic stenosis due to atrial myxoma)

Obstructive atrial thrombi

Box 3
Mitral regurgitation etiology

Primary (leaflet disorders)

- Rheumatic heart disease
- Mitral valve prolapse
- Connective tissue diseases
- Serotonergic drugs

Secondary (functional)

- Ruptured chordae tendineae
- Ruptured papillary muscle
- Papillary dysfunction
- Annular dilatation
- Hypertrophic cardiomyopathy left ventricle outflow tract obstruction (LVOTO)
- Dilated cardiomyopathy
- Ischemic heart disease

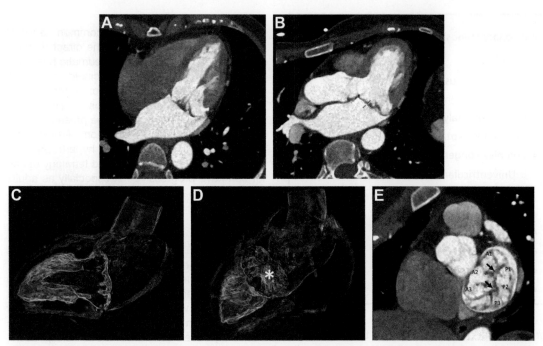

Fig. 3. A 56-year-old woman with rheumatic heart disease and mitral valve prolapse. (*A*) Four-chamber-oriented CCT. (*B*) Three-chamber-oriented CCT. (*C*) Two-chamber-oriented VR CCT. (*D*) 3D volume-rendering CCT focused on the mitral valve. A mitral valve prolapse of both leaflets is seen with mild thickening and billowing of anterior and posterior leaflets toward the left atrium of 6 mm (*). No mitral annular disjunction is present. (*E*) CCT oriented on the mitral valve closed, showing two valvular regurgitant orifices, one centered in A_1P_1 segment (0.06 cm^2) and the second one on A_2P_2 segment (0.11 cm^2). The total ROVA was 0.17 cm^2 (black arrows).

$\times$ 100) has good correlation with CMR.[10] Several parameters focusing on MV and LV remodeling have been associated with high rates of MR recurrence after surgical repair.[61]

Mitral prolapse

MVP is the most common cause of severe nonischemic MR, with a prevalence in general population of 1% to 2.5%.[62] Patients with MVP have higher risk for ventricular arrhythmias and sudden cardiac death.[63] Myxomatous valve disease is more frequent in older men with thickened and redundant valve leaflets. Barlow disease is a degenerative MV disease caused by enlarged, thickened and redundant MV leaflets, thickened chordae tendineae, and annular dilatation.[64] Secondary MVP prolapse may be present in connective tissue diseases or associated to congenital heart disease.[62]

CCT has high sensitivity (84.6%) and specificity (100%) for assessing MV abnormalities, being slightly less sensitive to echocardiography (92.3%), compared with intraoperative findings.[62] Assessment of the best cardiac phase to determine the location and extent of the MVP is mandatory. 4D CCT data sets in three-chamber view allows the evaluation dynamically of the MV coaptation line perpendicularly. A systolic bowing of the

MV above its annulus plane $\geq$ 2 mm toward the LA is diagnostic of MVP (**Fig. 3**). The prolapse scallop may be further classified as billowing leaflet (bowing of the leaflet body) or flail leaflet (free leaflet edge prolapse).[62] Flail leaflet motion occurs when chordae tendineae is ruptured requiring surgical treatment (see **Table 2**). Importantly, preoperative detection of aortic coarctation is mandatory in patients with MVP as if it is undetected, increases the mortality after MV repair due to elevated LVOT pressure.[65]

Pulmonary Valvular Heart Disease

Pulmonary stenosis

In 95% of cases pulmonary stenosis (PS) is due to congenital malformations, either isolated (atresia, bicuspid, or quadricuspid) or in the setting of other complex congenital heart diseases, such as tetralogy of Fallot.[19] Acquired PS is due to rheumatic disease and metastatic carcinoid syndrome (**Box 4**).[19,35,66]

CCT may be helpful not only to detect PS and evaluate its functional repercussion over the right heart but also for the evaluation of the pulmonary arteries, measurement of the RVOT, and evaluation of abnormal origin of coronary arteries for

---

Box 4
Pulmonary stenosis etiology

Congenital

- Unicuspid, bicuspid, dysplastic valve
- Hypoplastic right heart ventricle
- Ebstein anomaly
- Ventricular septal defect
- Complex congenital heart diseases
  - ○ Univentricular heart
  - ○ Tetralogy of Fallot
  - ○ Double outlet right ventricle

Acquired

- Rheumatic heart disease
- Carcinoid disease
- Cardiac tumors

---

preoperative planning.[28] In PS, thickening and fusion of the pulmonary leaflets, becoming easily visible on CCT, with reduced VOA and valve motion on cine imaging, is seen. Owing to a 90° angle orientation of the right PA, post-stenotic dilatation secondary to turbulent flow primarily involves the main and left PA. Secondary CCT findings include RV hypertrophy (free wall >4 mm) and dilatation, interventricular septal bowing and, in the late stages, HF (**Table 3**).[1,2,7,28]

Pulmonary regurgitation

Annular dilatation is the most common cause of pulmonary regurgitation (PR). The direct damage of PV leaflets can be seen in rheumatic heart disease, IE, or metastatic carcinoid syndrome (**Box 5**).[19] On CCT, malcoaptation of the PV leaflets and thickening of valve cusps, which become shortened and retracted, may be present.[67] Secondary findings include dilatation of pulmonary ring and PA, RV dilatation, and hypertrophy (see **Table 3**).[68] Patients with repaired tetralogy of Fallot can have progressive PR especially as adults post patch repair.

Tricuspid Valvular Heart Disease

Tricuspid stenosis

The most frequent cause of tricuspid stenosis (TS) is rheumatic heart disease, commonly associated, when present, with AV and MV involvement. Other less common etiologies include IE, more frequently seen on intravenous drug users, congenital tricuspid atresia, or metastatic carcinoid syndrome (**Box 6**).[1,2,56]

CCT findings include reduced VOA (≤ 3 cm^2), with shortened and thickened leaflets, commissural fusion and narrowed annulus. Associated findings include signs of RV HF, RA enlargement, dilated superior and inferior vena cava as well as hepatic veins, and signs of liver congestion (see **Table 3**).[56,69]

Table 3
Cardiac computed tomography findings on right-sided valvular heart disease

Cardiac Valve	Stenosis	Regurgitation
PV	Valvular findings • Leaflet thickening and fusion • Reduced VOA ≤ 3 cm^2; ≤ 2 cm^2/m^2 • Reduced leaflet motion Secondary findings • Post-stenotic dilatation (main and left PA) • RV hypertrophy (>4 mm) and dilatation • Interventricular septal bowing • Heart failure	Valvular findings • Thickening valve cusps • Leaflet shortening and retraction • Malcoaptation (ROA) Secondary findings • Dilatation pulmonary ring/ pulmonary artery • RV dilatation and/or hypertrophy
TV	Valvular findings • Leaflet thickening and shortening • Commissural fusion • Narrowed annulus • Reduced VOA (≤ 3 cm^2) Secondary findings • RV heart failure • RA enlargement • Dilated SVC and IVC • Dilated hepatic veins/signs liver congestion	Valvular findings • Cusp thickening • Leaflet retraction (tethering) • Leaflet reduced motion • Increased annular dilatation (tenting) • Leaflet malcoaptation (ROA) Secondary findings • RA and RV enlargement • Dilated IVC/hepatic veins • Other signs of underlying disease

Abbreviations: IVC, inferior vena cava; PA, pulmonary area; PV, pulmonary valve; RA, right atrium; ROA, regurgitant orifice area; RV, right ventricle; SVC, superior vena cava; TV, tricuspid valve; VOA, valvular orifice area.

Box 5
Pulmonary regurgitation etiology
Primary (direct leaflet damage)
• Congenital heart disease
• Prolapse leaflets
• Repaired tetralogy of Fallot
• Infective endocarditis
• Metastatic carcinoid syndrome
• Rheumatic disease
• Post-valvuloplasty
• Iatrogenic
Secondary (annular dilatation)
• Pulmonary artery hypertension
• Marfan syndrome

Box 7
Tricuspid regurgitation etiology
Primary (direct leaflet damage)
• Congenital (Ebstein anomaly)
• Rheumatic heart disease
• Infectious endocarditis
• Myxomatous degeneration
• Myocardial infarction
• Metastatic carcinoid syndrome
• Cardiothoracic trauma
• Marfan syndrome
Secondary (functional)
• Left-sided heart disease
• Pulmonary arterial hypertension
• RV enlargement/dysfunction (ischemia/infarction)
• Idiopathic tricuspid regurgitation

Tricuspid regurgitation

Primary tricuspid regurgitation (TR) due to anomalies in the TV may be secondary to congenital anomalies or acquired (rheumatic, IE or myxomatous degeneration).[41,70] Secondary (functional) TR is the most frequent cause (75%) and is produced by abnormalities in TV apparatus and RV remodeling. It could be seen also secondary to left heart diseases, PH, RV dysfunction, or idiopathic (Box 7).[71]

Mid-to-end systole short axis CCT views are used for the calculation of the ROA (20%–30% RR interval), whereas mid-to-end diastole two- and four-chamber views (60%–80% RR interval) are obtained for annular and leaflet coaptation evaluation. TR findings include cusp thickening with leaflet retraction and reduced motion on cine imaging. Increased annular dilatation (≥4 cm) with increased area and tenting height/area may be seen (**Fig. 4**).[41] TV annular dimensions and tenting height (≥7.2 mm) have been related with TR severity, prognosis, and recurrence after annuloplasty.[72,73] TR volume (RVSV-LVSV) and fraction (TRV/RVSV × 100) may be calculated by subtraction of RV and LV systolic volumes, with reduced accuracy of this approach if ventricular arrhythmias are present.[7,41] Secondary findings of TR include RA and RV enlargement, inferior vena cava, and hepatic veins congestion as well as other associated hallmarks related to the underlying cause of functional TR (see **Table 3**).

Role of cardiac computed tomography in multivalvular heart disease

Multiple VHD, defined by at least two moderate VHDs by the Euro Heart Survey, is present in up to 20% of patients with native VHD and 17% of those undergoing intervention, being associated with worse prognosis.[48,74,75] The most frequent associations were AS and AR, AS plus MR, and AR combined with MR. Multiple VHD is most often acquired, either post-rheumatic (51%) or degenerative (41%). Mixed aortic VHD is frequently congenital or degenerative in industrialized countries, being IE (1%) and post-rheumatic less frequent (9%–13%). Mixed mitral VHD mainly results from rheumatic and degenerative processes.[48]

When significant MR is present in cases of AS plus MR, there is a risk of AS underestimation due to low forward flow through the AV. These low-flow/low-gradient AS coexist with reduced (classical form) or normal (paradoxic form) LVEF.[76] Combination of AS plus MS is less frequent, poorly tolerated, and may also lead to

Box 6
Tricuspid stenosis etiology
Rheumatic heart disease
Congenital tricuspid atresia
Ebstein anomaly
Infective endocarditis (intravenous drug users)
Metastatic carcinoid syndrome
Right atrial tumors

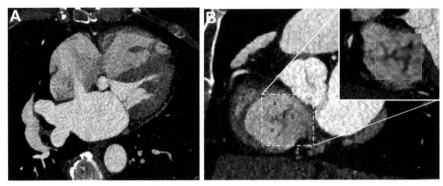

Fig. 4. A 65-year-old woman with type 1 ostium secundum atrial septal defect (ASD). (*A*) 4D chamber-oriented CCT with left-to-right shunt of contrast media secondary to ASD (area 1.7 cm^2). Associated right ventricle and right atrial enlargement was seen (RV/LV ratio: 1.4). (*B*) Tricuspid valve-oriented CCT revealing a tricuspid mal-coaptation of leaflets secondary to annular dilatation (43 mm; normal if < 40 mm) with a regurgitant orifice area of 0.16 cm^2.

underestimation of AS due to reduced LV cardiac output.[48] In both cases, calculation of AV calcium load with CCT may help to adequately evaluate AS severity.[76] Opposing loading conditions may be seen in combination of AR and MS. In those cases, calculation of MR by continuity equation may be invalid due to significant AR. This could be solved by direct quantification of mitral ROA either with echocardiography or with CCT, when suboptimal ultrasound imaging.[48]

Infective endocarditis

IE is a life-threatening infectious condition involving native valve endocarditis (NVE) or pros-thetic valve endocarditis (PVE), endocardium, or implantable cardiac devices. Its global incidence is 3 to 10 cases per 10^5 people/year, being higher in older people, and patients with comorbidities, with a slight male predominance. Although CCT is not the first imaging modality, it is recommended for establishing the diagnosis and in situations where echocardiography is inconclusive or non-diagnostic in NVE or PVE (class IB), as well as for evaluation perivalvular involvement or other noncardiac embolic phenomena (class IB).[77]

Vegetations are variable-sized, low-to-interme-diate attenuation and mobile lesions attached to the endocardial surface or prosthetic valve. They are commonly located at the low-pressure side of the cardiac valve. A delayed portal venous phase (60–70 seconds) may improve detection. Large (>10 mm) and mobile vegetations have higher risk of embolization and constitute an indi-cation of urgent surgery (**Table 4**).[78,79] Inflamma-tion of the valve may lead to destruction and regurgitation, but also stenosis. Right heart vege-tations are more common among intravenous drug users or people PV and, occasionally, may produce secondary pulmonary embolisms (**Fig. 5**). Other valvular signs of IE include leaflet perforation or pseudoaneurysm.[24]

Perivalvular extension in IE has been described in up to 35% of cases, being more frequent in PVE rather than in NVE.[79] If new or changing con-duction abnormalities are noted, CCT should be considered to rule out perivalvular extension. Peri-valvular aneurysm is seen as contrast-filled (200–400 HU) saccular or fusiform perivalvular cavity, with narrow neck and variable size, which commu-nicates with the aortic root or cardiac chamber. Perivalvular abscess are distinguished by a low (20–50 HU) or heterogeneous fluid collection of variable size with occasionally peripheral rim enhancement ("capsule") more prominently evident in delayed phases. Adjacent signs of inflammation, such as pericardial fat stranding, pericardial effusion, or loss of normal periaortic fatty tissue (1–30 HU) may also be present.[24,80] A perivalvular fistula, which is an abnormal connec-tion between two neighboring cavities, may form in rare cases and is typically linked with an ab-scess or a pseudoaneurysm.[77]

Valvular Cardiac Masses

Thrombus

Constitutes the most common cardiac mass, appearing generally in slow-flowing locations (atrial appendage or hypo-akinetic myocardial segments), but also have been described along valves in hypercoagulable states.[81] A low-attenuated (<200 HU; <145 HU cutoff) non-enhancing filling defects may be seen, often lobular but also laminar or linear in chronic stages (see **Table 4**).[82] CT may provide prognostic infor-mation about treatment response because low-density (<90 HU) thrombi are more likely to

Table 4
Clinical features, imaging findings, and treatment of valvular lesions

	Clinical Background	Valve Location	Morphology	Treatment
Vegetation	Fever and nonspecific symptoms Embolic phenomena (30%) 10% culture: negative IE	All (left-side > right-side valves) Low-pressure side	Soft-tissue and mobile lesions Large (>10 mm) and mobile lesions have higher tendency to embolization	Medical therapy Surgery when high risk of embolization (large and mobile)
PFE	Second most common primary valvular tumor 75% of valvular neoplasms Frequently incidentally discovered	Left-sided (AV > MV) more frequent than right-sided (TV > PV) High- pressure side	Highly mobile soft-tissue lesions attached with a stalk to the valve, away from the leaflet free edge	Surgery is indicated
Thrombi	Most common cardiac mass Slow-flowing locations (atrial appendage; hypo- akinetic segments) Hypercoagulable states (valves)	Along valves	Low attenuated (<200 HU; <145 HU cutoff) non-enhancing filling defects Lobular Laminar/linear in chronic stages	Medical treatment
Lambl's excrescences	Incidentally discovered	Left-sided cardiac valves Low-pressure side	Thin, hypermobile, soft-tissue bands located in the cusps boundary at the low-pressure side. Occasionally associated with embolic events	N/A
NBTE	No signs of infection Association with malignancy and autoimmune disorders Valvular dysfunction Heart failure Embolic systemic phenomena	Mainly in left-sided valves Low-pressure side	Small (<1 cm), irregular, and broad-based Valve destruction is infrequent Small, irregular, and broad based soft-tissue density lesions	Depending on the underlying condition
CNMA	Symptomatic clinical presentation	Mitral annulus Centered on the annulus	Well-demarcated, homogeneous Highly attenuated mitral annular mass (calcification). No enhancement after contrast-media Central hypodensity due to liquefaction	N/A

(continued on next page)

Table 4 (continued)				
	Clinical Background	**Valve Location**	**Morphology**	**Treatment**
Mitral blood cyst	Frequently seen on infants (50% in infants <2 months) Rarity in the adulthood	Mitral leaflets or subvalvular apparatus	Well-defined cystic lesion with contrast filling	Only require surgery if symptomatic

Abbreviations: AV, aortic valve; CNMA, caseous necrosis of the mitral annulus; MV, mitral valve; NBTE, non-bacterial thrombotic endocarditis; PFE, papillary fibroelastoma; PV, pulmonary valve; TV, tricuspid valve.

completely lysed than those between 90 and 145 HU.[24,82]

Papillary fibroelastoma

Papillary fibroelastoma (PFE) is the most common primary cardiac tumor and accounts for 75% of all valvular neoplasms. Aortic and MVs are more commonly involved rather than right-sided valves.[81] PFE is low-attenuated and highly mobile, "frond-like" and stalked lesions attached along the valve's downstream surface and distant from the leaflet border (**Fig. 6**, see **Table 4**). CCT has excellent capabilities for characterizing these lesions due to its inherent high spatial resolution.[83]

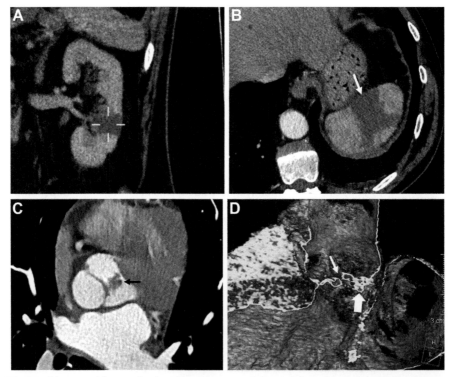

Fig. 5. A 55-year-old man with constitutional symptoms and fever. (*A*) Coronal abdominal CT in portal phase revealing a subsegmental and well-defined hypodense area in the lower pole of the left ventricle in keeping with renal infarction (*yellow cross*). (*B*) Axial abdominal CT in portal phase showing a well-defined hypodense area in the upper pole of the spleen, compatible with splenic infarction (*white arrow*). (*C*) CCT axially oriented at the level of the aortic valve showing a soft-tissue mass anchored in the ventricular side of the left coronary cusp, with mild leaflet thickening due to infective endocarditis vegetation (*black arrow*). (*D*) 3D volume-rendering CCT focused on the aortic valve revealing the vegetation located at the ventricular side of the left coronary aortic cusp (*thick white arrow*). Please note the absence of complete coaptation of the aortic leaflets suggesting secondary aortic regurgitation (*thin white arrow*).

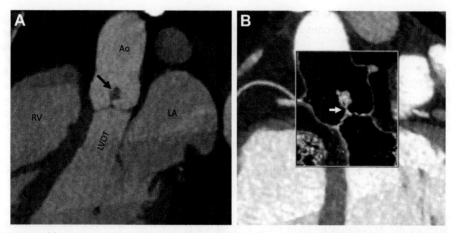

Fig. 6. A 47-year-old woman with incidentally discovered aortic valve lesion on transthoracic echocardiography. (*A*) Three-chamber-oriented CCT. A frond-like, hypermobile, and pediculated soft-tissue lesion (*black arrow*) attached to the downstream side of the aortic valve is depicted, in keeping with papillary fibroelastoma. (*B*) Detailed 3D volume-rendering CCT of the aortic valve lesion demonstrating the pedicular nature of the focal aortic valve lesion as well as its attachment through a thin (2 mm) and well-defined stalk (*white arrow*) to the high-pressure side of the left coronary cusp of the aortic valve.

Cardiac Pseudomasses

Lambl's excrescences

Lambl's excrescences are incidentally found valvular and hypermobile fronds arising from endothelial wear and tear. They appear as thin, soft-tissue CCT bands located in the valvular cusps' boundary, primarily on the low-pressure side (see **Table 4**). They are more common in left-sided cardiac valves and occasionally may be associated with embolic events.[84]

Noninfective valvular endocarditis

Noninfective valvular endocarditis is characterized as a sterile/aseptic soft-tissue CCT density vegetation that is small (<10 mm) and irregular, and broadly based. It is more frequently found in left-sided cardiac valves and is linked with malignancy or other autoimmune disorders (Libman–Sacks endocarditis) (see **Table 4**). It may manifest with systemic embolic events that mirror left-sided IE symptoms.[85,86]

Caseous necrosis of the mitral valve

Caseous necrosis of the MV is a rare and benign process (<0.6% of mitral annular calcifications), more frequently seen in women and characteristically asymptomatic. Caseous calcification is made up of basophilic areas surrounded with fibrous tissue. CCT reveals a high-attenuated, well-defined oval or crescent-shaped mass with peripheral calcification. Commonly, it is located along the

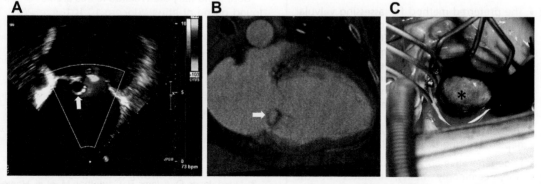

Fig. 7. A 61-year-old man with atrial fibrillation, dyspnea, and previous history of infective endocarditis. (*A*) Transthoracic echocardiography revealing an anechoic round and well-defined valvular lesion attached at the atrial side of the mitral valve (*white arrow*). (*B*) Two-chamber-oriented CCT shows a well-defined cystic lesion attached to the atrial side of the mitral valve filled with contrast (*white arrow*). (*C*) Intraoperative view of the atrial side of the mitral valve revealing a well-defined bluish mass compatible with mitral blood cyst (*).

posterior mitral annulus and does not show enhancement after iodinated-contrast media administration (see **Table 4**).[87–89]

Mitral blood cysts

Mitral blood cysts constitute congenital benign valvular lesions more frequently seen on infants (<6 months) produced by invagination of the endothelium located in the cusps or subvalvular apparatus of auriculoventricular valves. They have been described in up to 50% of children less than 2 months and are a rarity in the adulthood. Blood cysts can also be seen in adults postsurgery. A well-defined cystic lesion filled with iodinated contrast material attached to the valvular leaflet or subvalvular apparatus is seen (**Fig. 7**, see **Table 4**). These lesions only require surgery when symptomatic.[90,91]

SUMMARY

CCT constitutes a useful and valuable imaging modality for the evaluation of VHD in native valves, refining and giving important information not only for its diagnosis but also for treatment planning, risk stratification, and prognosis. CCT helps to assess other less frequent forms of valvular diseases, such as neoplasms, IE, nonbacterial infectious endocarditis, or pseudomasses, and may help to refine the severity gradation in cases of multiple VHD. Although there are scarce data, some new developments in tissue characterization (myocardial ECV) and advanced hemodynamic parameters (CFD) may help to further dive in the pathophysiology, risk stratification, and prognosis in VHD.

CLINICS CARE POINTS

- The preferred method for assessing valvular heart disease (VHD) is contrast-enhanced whole-heart retrospective ECG-gated acquisition. Semilunar valve planimetry is optimally achieved during mid-systole, while 0-5% of the RR interval proves most effective for measuring atrioventricular valve regurgitant orifice area. In contrast, semilunar regurgitant orifice area planimetry and atrioventricular anatomic valve opening area are best depicted during mid-diastole.

- In degenerative aortic stenosis (AS), calcification, commonly heavy, initiates at the annulus and progresses towards the cusp, resulting in asymmetric opening and closure. Conversely, rheumatic disease typically exhibits symmetric calcification, commissural fusion, and reduced aperture.

- Calcification not only correlates with AS severity but also serves as a subclinical surrogate marker for atherosclerotic burden and coronary artery calcification. Gender – specific thresholds for severe aortic calcification aid in predicting disease severity, mortality excess, and offer incremental prognostic value, particularly in patients with discordant echocardiographic Doppler severity of AS or paradoxical low flow-low gradient with preserved LVEF.

- Bicuspid aortic valve (BAV) respresents the most frequent form of congenital aortic VHD, characterized by commissural fusion and two unequally – sized cusps. BAV may be associated with AS, AR, combined AS/AR or no relevant functional VHD. Each case should detail (1) the type, specific phenotype, and function; (2) the presence and characteristics of the raphe, as well as the cusp size, shape, and symmetry; and (3) the presence and phenotype of BAV-related aortopathy and/or aortic coarctation.

- Mitral regurgitation (MR) is the most common manifestation of VHD, classified as primary or secondary. Primary MR results from anatomic abnormalities or direct damage to the mitral valve or subvalvular apparatus, while secondary MR is associated with regional/global left ventricular dysfunction and/or dilatation. leading to tethering and restriction of the mitral leaflets. Computed tomography - derived MV tenting area has been linked to the severity of MR.

DISCLOSURE

The authors do not have any relevant disclosures.

SUPPLEMENTARY DATA

Supplementary data related to this article can be found online at https://doi.org/10.1016/j.rcl.2023.12.004.

REFERENCES

1. Chen JJ, Manning MA, Frazier AA, et al. CT angiography of the cardiac valves: normal, diseased, and postoperative appearances. Radiographics 2009; 29(5):1393–412.
2. Ketelsen D, Fishman EK, Claussen CD, et al. Computed tomography evaluation of cardiac valves: a review. Radiol Clin North Am 2010;48(4):783–97.
3. Lloyd-Jones D, Adams R, Carnethon M, et al. Heart disease and stroke statistics–2009 update: a report from the American Heart Association Statistics Committee and Stroke Statistics Subcommittee. Circulation 2009;119(3):480–6.

4. Vogel-Claussen J, Pannu H, Spevak PJ, et al. Cardiac valve assessment with MR imaging and 64-section multi-detector row CT. Radiographics 2006; 26(6):1769–84.

5. Rowe JC, Bland EF, Sprague HB, et al. The course of mitral stenosis without surgery: ten- and twenty-year perspectives. Ann Intern Med 1960;52:741–9.

6. Fox DJ, Khattar RS. Carcinoid heart disease: presentation, diagnosis, and management. Heart 2004;90(10):1224–8.

7. Litmanovich DE, Kirsch J. Computed tomography of cardiac valves: review. Radiol Clin North Am 2019; 57(1):141–64.

8. Gaztanaga J, Pizarro G, Sanz J. Evaluation of cardiac valves using multidetector CT. Cardiol Clin 2009;27(4):633–44.

9. Patel KP, Vandermolen S, Herrey AS, et al. Cardiac computed tomography: application in valvular heart disease. Front Cardiovasc Med 2022;9:849540.

10. Weir-McCall JR, Blanke P, Naoum C, et al. Mitral valve imaging with CT: relationship with transcatheter mitral valve interventions. Radiology 2018;288(3):638–55.

11. Godoy M, Mugharbil A, Anastasius M, et al. Cardiac computed tomography (CT) evaluation of valvular heart disease in transcatheter interventions. Curr Cardiol Rep 2019;21(12):154.

12. Boutsikou M, Tzifa A. Noninvasive imaging prior to percutaneous pulmonary valve implantation. Hellenic J Cardiol 2022;67:59–65.

13. Francone M, Budde RPJ, Bremerich J, et al. CT and MR imaging prior to transcatheter aortic valve implantation: standardisation of scanning protocols, measurements and reporting-a consensus document by the European Society of Cardiovascular Radiology (ESCR). Eur Radiol 2020;30(5):2627–50.

14. Layoun H, Schoenhagen P, Wang TKM, et al. Roles of cardiac computed tomography in guiding transcatheter tricuspid valve interventions. Curr Cardiol Rep 2021;23(9):114.

15. Lopes BBC, Hashimoto G, Bapat VN, et al. Cardiac computed tomography and magnetic resonance imaging of the tricuspid valve: preprocedural planning and postprocedural follow-up. Interv Cardiol Clin 2022;11(1):27–40.

16. Maggiore P, Anastasius M, Huang AL, et al. Transcatheter mitral valve repair and replacement: current evidence for intervention and the role of ct in preprocedural planning-a review for radiologists and cardiologists alike. Radiol Cardiothorac Imaging 2020; 2(1):e190106.

17. Yucel-Finn A, Nicol E, Leipsic JA, et al. CT in planning transcatheter aortic valve implantation procedures and risk assessment. Clin Radiol 2021;76(1):73.e1–19.

18. Bolger AF, Eigler NL, Maurer G. Quantifying valvular regurgitation. Limitations and inherent assumptions of Doppler techniques. Circulation 1988;78(5 Pt 1): 1316–8.

19. Manghat NE, Rachapalli V, Van Lingen R, et al. Imaging the heart valves using ECG-gated 64-detector row cardiac CT. Br J Radiol 2008;81(964):275–90.

20. Simpson IA, Sahn DJ. Quantification of valvular regurgitation by Doppler echocardiography. Circulation 1991;84(3 Suppl):I188–92.

21. Grothues F, Smith GC, Moon JCC, et al. Comparison of interstudy reproducibility of cardiovascular magnetic resonance with two-dimensional echocardiography in normal subjects and in patients with heart failure or left ventricular hypertrophy. Am J Cardiol 2002;90(1):29–34.

22. Ko SM, Song MG, Hwang HK. Evaluation of the aortic and mitral valves with cardiac computed tomography and cardiac magnetic resonance imaging. Int J Cardiovasc Imag 2012;28(Suppl 2):109–27.

23. Suzuki M, Toba T, Izawa Y, et al. Prognostic Impact of Myocardial Extracellular Volume Fraction Assessment Using Dual-Energy Computed Tomography in Patients Treated With Aortic Valve Replacement for Severe Aortic Stenosis. J Am Heart Assoc 2021; 10(18):e020655.

24. Saeedan MB, Wang TKM, Cremer P, et al. Role of cardiac CT in infective endocarditis: current evidence, opportunities, and challenges. Radiol Cardiothorac Imaging 2021;3(1):e200378.

25. Hermann F, Martinoff S, Meyer T, et al. Reduction of radiation dose estimates in cardiac 64-slice CT angiography in patients after coronary artery bypass graft surgery. Invest Radiol 2008;43(4):253–60.

26. Grob A, Thuny F, Villacampa C, et al. Cardiac multidetector computed tomography in infective endocarditis: a pictorial essay. Insights Imaging 2014;5(5):559–70.

27. Faure ME, Swart LE, Dijkshoorn ML, et al. Advanced CT acquisition protocol with a third-generation dual-source CT scanner and iterative reconstruction technique for comprehensive prosthetic heart valve assessment. Eur Radiol 2018;28(5):2159–68.

28. Costantini P, Perone F, Siani A, et al. Multimodality imaging of the neglected valve: role of echocardiography, cardiac magnetic resonance and cardiac computed tomography in pulmonary stenosis and regurgitation. J Imaging 2022;8(10):278.

29. Raman SV, Shah M, McCarthy B, et al. Multi-detector row cardiac computed tomography accurately quantifies right and left ventricular size and function compared with cardiac magnetic resonance. Am Heart J 2006;151(3):736–44.

30. Lembcke A, Borges AC, Dushe S, et al. Assessment of mitral valve regurgitation at electron-beam CT: comparison with Doppler echocardiography. Radiology 2005;236(1):47–55.

31. Mittal TK, Reichmuth L, Bhattacharyya S, et al. Inconsistency in aortic stenosis severity between CT and echocardiography: prevalence and insights into mechanistic differences using computational fluid dynamics. Open Heart 2019;6(2):e001044.

32. LaBounty TM, Sundaram B, Agarwal P, et al. Aortic valve area on 64-MDCT correlates with transesophageal echocardiography in aortic stenosis. AJR Am J Roentgenol 2008;191(6):1652–8.

33. Feuchtner GM, Dichtl W, Müller S, et al. 64-MDCT for diagnosis of aortic regurgitation in patients referred to CT coronary angiography. AJR Am J Roentgenol 2008;191(1):W1–7.

34. Lembcke A, Durmus T, Westermann Y, et al. Assessment of mitral valve stenosis by helical MDCT: comparison with transthoracic Doppler echocardiography and cardiac catheterization. AJR Am J Roentgenol 2011;197(3):614–22.

35. Brickner ME, Hillis LD, Lange RA. Congenital heart disease in adults. First of two parts. N Engl J Med 2000;342(4):256–63.

36. Meng Y, Zhang L, Zhang Z, et al. Cardiovascular magnetic resonance of quinticuspid aortic valve with aortic regurgitation and dilated ascending aorta. J Cardiovasc Magn Reson 2009;11(1):28.

37. Chheda SV, Srichai MB, Donnino R, et al. Evaluation of the mitral and aortic valves with cardiac CT angiography. J Thorac Imag 2010;25(1):76–85.

38. Delgado V, Tops LF, Schuijf JD, et al. Assessment of mitral valve anatomy and geometry with multislice computed tomography. JACC Cardiovasc Imaging 2009;2(5):556–65.

39. Garbi M, Monaghan MJ. Quantitative mitral valve anatomy and pathology. Echo Res Pract 2015;2(3):R63–72.

40. Ranganathan N, Lam JH, Wigle ED, et al. Morphology of the human mitral valve. II. The value leaflets. Circulation 1970;41(3):459–67.

41. Ahn Y, Koo HJ, Kang JW, et al. Tricuspid valve imaging and right ventricular function analysis using cardiac CT and MRI. Korean J Radiol 2021;22(12):1946–63.

42. Saremi F, Hassani C, Millan-Nunez V, et al. Imaging evaluation of tricuspid valve: analysis of morphology and function With CT and MRI. AJR Am J Roentgenol 2015;204(5):W531–42.

43. Maganti K, Rigolin VH, Sarano ME, et al. Valvular heart disease: diagnosis and management. Mayo Clin Proc 2010;85(5):483–500.

44. Nkomo VT, Gardin JM, Skelton TN, et al. Burden of valvular heart diseases: a population-based study. Lancet 2006;368(9540):1005–11.

45. Pouleur AC, le Polain de Waroux JB, Pasquet A, et al. Aortic valve area assessment: multidetector CT compared with cine MR imaging and transthoracic and transesophageal echocardiography. Radiology 2007;244(3):745–54.

46. Nasir K, Katz R, Al-Mallah M, et al. Relationship of aortic valve calcification with coronary artery calcium severity: the Multi-Ethnic Study of Atherosclerosis (MESA). J Cardiovasc Comput Tomogr 2010;4(1):41–6.

47. Clavel MA, Pibarot P, Messika-Zeitoun D, et al. Impact of aortic valve calcification, as measured by MDCT, on survival in patients with aortic stenosis: results of an international registry study. J Am Coll Cardiol 2014;64(12):1202–13.

48. Unger P, Pibarot P, Tribouilloy C, et al. Multiple and mixed valvular heart diseases. Circ Cardiovasc Imaging 2018;11(8):e007862.

49. Pawade T, Clavel MA, Tribouilloy C, et al. Computed tomography aortic valve calcium scoring in patients with aortic stenosis. Circ Cardiovasc Imaging 2018; 11(3):e007146.

50. Falk V, Baumgartner H, Bax JJ, et al. 2017 ESC/EACTS Guidelines for the management of valvular heart disease. Eur J Cardio Thorac Surg 2017; 52(4):616–64.

51. Clavel MA, Messika-Zeitoun D, Pibarot P, et al. The complex nature of discordant severe calcified aortic valve disease grading: new insights from combined Doppler echocardiographic and computed tomographic study. J Am Coll Cardiol 2013;62(24):2329–38.

52. Enriquez-Sarano M, Tajik AJ. Clinical practice. aortic regurgitation. N Engl J Med 2004;351(15):1539–46.

53. Carlsson E, Gross R, Holt RG. The radiological diagnosis of cardiac valvar insufficiencies. Circulation 1977;55(6):921–33.

54. Feuchtner GM, Spoeck A, Lessick J, et al. Quantification of aortic regurgitant fraction and volume with multi-detector computed tomography comparison with echocardiography. Acad Radiol 2011;18(3):334–42.

55. Michelena HI, Corte AD, Evangelista A, et al. International consensus statement on nomenclature and classification of the congenital bicuspid aortic valve and its aortopathy, for clinical, surgical, interventional and research purposes. Radiol Cardiothorac Imaging 2021;3(4):e200496.

56. Rajani R, Khattar R, Chiribiri A, et al. Multimodality imaging of heart valve disease. Arq Bras Cardiol 2014;103(3):251–63.

57. Hickey AJ, Wilcken DE, Wright JS, et al. Primary (spontaneous) chordal rupture: relation to myxomatous valve disease and mitral valve prolapse. J Am Coll Cardiol 1985;5(6):1341–6.

58. Piérard LA, Carabello BA. Ischaemic mitral regurgitation: pathophysiology, outcomes and the conundrum of treatment. Eur Heart J 2010;31(24):2996–3005.

59. Dudzinski DM, Hung J. Echocardiographic assessment of ischemic mitral regurgitation. Cardiovasc Ultrasound 2014;12:46.

60. Enriquez-Sarano M, Akins CW, Vahanian A. Mitral regurgitation. Lancet 2009;373(9672):1382–94.

61. Lancellotti P, Tribouilloy C, Hagendorff A, et al. Recommendations for the echocardiographic assessment of native valvular regurgitation: an executive summary from the European Association of Cardiovascular Imaging. Eur Heart J Cardiovasc Imaging 2013;14(7):611–44.

62. Koo HJ, Yang DH, Oh SY, et al. Demonstration of mitral valve prolapse with CT for planning of mitral valve repair. Radiographics 2014;34(6):1537–52.

63. Hayek E, Gring CN, Griffin BP. Mitral valve prolapse. Lancet 2005;365(9458):507–18.

64. Anyanwu AC, Adams DH. Etiologic classification of degenerative mitral valve disease: Barlow's disease and fibroelastic deficiency. Semin Thorac Cardiovasc Surg 2007;19(2):90–6.

65. Ludman P, Yacoub M, Dancy M. Mitral valve prolapse and occult aortic coarctation. Postgrad Med 1990;66(780):834–7.

66. Sandmann H, Pakkal M, Steeds R. Cardiovascular magnetic resonance imaging in the assessment of carcinoid heart disease. Clin Radiol 2009;64(8): 761–6.

67. Saremi F, Gera A, Ho SY, et al. CT and MR imaging of the pulmonary valve. Radiographics 2014;34(1): 51–71.

68. Bennett CJ, Maleszewski JJ, Araoz PA. CT and MR imaging of the aortic valve: radiologic-pathologic correlation. Radiographics 2012;32(5):1399–420.

69. Naoum C, Blanke P, Cavalcante JL, et al. Cardiac computed tomography and magnetic resonance imaging in the evaluation of mitral and tricuspid valve disease: implications for transcatheter interventions. Circ Cardiovasc Imaging 2017;10(3):e005331.

70. Dahou A, Levin D, Reisman M, et al. Anatomy and physiology of the tricuspid valve. JACC Cardiovasc Imaging 2019;12(3):458–68.

71. Dreyfus GD, Martin RP, Chan KMJ, et al. Functional tricuspid regurgitation: a need to revise our understanding. J Am Coll Cardiol 2015;65(21):2331–6.

72. Kabasawa M, Kohno H, Ishizaka T, et al. Assessment of functional tricuspid regurgitation using 320-detector-row multislice computed tomography: risk factor analysis for recurrent regurgitation after tricuspid annuloplasty. J Thorac Cardiovasc Surg 2014;147(1):312–20.

73. Kim H, Kim IC, Yoon HJ, et al. Prognostic usefulness of tricuspid annular diameter for cardiovascular events in patients with tricuspid regurgitation of moderate to severe degree. Am J Cardiol 2018; 121(11):1343–50.

74. Abramowitz Y, Kazuno Y, Chakravarty T, et al. Concomitant mitral annular calcification and severe aortic stenosis: prevalence, characteristics and outcome following transcatheter aortic valve replacement. Eur Heart J 2017;38(16):1194–203.

75. Iung B, Baron G, Butchart EG, et al. A prospective survey of patients with valvular heart disease in Europe: The Euro Heart Survey on Valvular Heart Disease. Eur Heart J 2003;24(13):1231–43.

76. Leong DP, Pizzale S, Haroun MJ, et al. Factors associated with low flow in aortic valve stenosis. J Am Soc Echocardiogr 2016;29(2):158–65.

77. Delgado V, Ajmone Marsan N, de Waha S, et al. 2023 ESC Guidelines for the management of endocarditis. Eur Heart J 2023;ehad193. https://doi.org/10.1093/eurheartj/ehad193.

78. Vilacosta I, Graupner C, San Román JA, et al. Risk of embolization after institution of antibiotic therapy for infective endocarditis. J Am Coll Cardiol 2002;39(9): 1489–95.

79. Prendergast BD, Tornos P. Surgery for infective endocarditis: who and when? Circulation 2010;121(9): 1141–52.

80. Khalique OK, Veillet-Chowdhury M, Choi AD, et al. Cardiac computed tomography in the contemporary evaluation of infective endocarditis. J Cardiovasc Comput Tomogr 2021;15(4):304–12.

81. Young PM, Foley TA, Araoz PA, et al. Computed tomography imaging of cardiac masses. Radiol Clin North Am 2019;57(1):75–84.

82. Rajiah P, Moore A, Saboo S, et al. Multimodality imaging of complications of cardiac valve surgeries. Radiographics 2019;39(4):932–56.

83. Tamin SS, Maleszewski JJ, Scott CG, et al. Prognostic and bioepidemiologic implications of papillary fibroelastomas. J Am Coll Cardiol 2015;65(22): 2420–9.

84. Ammannaya GKK. Lambl's excrescences: current diagnosis and management. Cardiol Res 2019; 10(4):207–10.

85. Asopa S, Patel A, Khan OA, et al. Non-bacterial thrombotic endocarditis. Eur J Cardio Thorac Surg 2007;32(5):696–701.

86. Hurrell H, Roberts-Thomson R, Prendergast BD. Non-infective endocarditis. Heart 2020;106(13): 1023–9.

87. Elgendy IY, Conti CR. Caseous calcification of the mitral annulus: a review. Clin Cardiol 2013;36(10): E27–31.

88. Parato VM, Nocco S, Alunni G, et al. Imaging of cardiac masses: an updated overview. J Cardiovasc Echogr 2022;32(2):65–75.

89. Srivatsa SS, Taylor MD, Hor K, et al. Liquefaction necrosis of mitral annular calcification (LNMAC): review of pathology, prevalence, imaging and management: proposed diagnostic imaging criteria with detailed multi-modality and MRI image characterization. Int J Cardiovasc Imag 2012;28(5): 1161–71.

90. Romano S, Krishnasamy K, Jariwala N, et al. Giant mitral blood cyst: Cardiovascular magnetic resonance imaging features. Int J Cardiol 2016;203: 17–8.

91. Cianciulli TF, Ventrici JF, Marturano MP, et al. Blood cyst of the mitral valve: echocardiographic and magnetic resonance imaging diagnosis. Circ Cardiovasc Imaging 2015;8(2):e002729.

Pretranscatheter and Posttranscatheter Valve Planning with Computed Tomography

Thomas Clifford, MBChB[a,1], Vitaliy Androshchuk, MBChB[b,1],
Ronak Rajani, DM, MD, FRCP, FESC, FSCCT, FRCR[c,2],
Jonathan R. Weir-McCall, MBChB, PhD[d,*,2]

KEYWORDS

- Cardiac computed tomography • Transcatheter heart valve
- Transcatheter aortic valve replacement • Transcatheter mitral valve replacement
- Transcatheter tricuspid valve replacement • Transcatheter pulmonary valve replacement

KEY POINTS

- The range of indications for transcatheter heart valve intervention is increasing
- Computed tomography provides detailed anatomic assessment for device selection and procedure planning
- Risk factors for procedural complications can be identified to better guide patients' decisions and adjust the procedure where required to mitigate risk

INTRODUCTION

There are few areas in medicine in which there has been such rapid progression from proof of concept to clinical practice as with transcatheter heart valves (THVs). Since the first insertion of a stented valve into a pulmonary conduit in 2000,[1] the field has evolved with improvements in stent design, deployment systems, and adaptation of design to meet the unique anatomic demands of each of the heart valves.

Cardiac computed tomography (CT) has played a central role in the expansion of the use of THVs. Due to its high spatial resolution, rapidity, and ability for simultaneous valve and vascular access assessment, CT has become the preferred modality for procedural planning in THV workup.[2] The utility of CT is not limited to preprocedural planning. It can also be used as an adjunct to echocardiography in patients who develop valve-related complications.

This review provides an overview of CT in the preprocedural planning of THVs in the aortic, mitral, tricuspid and pulmonary valves. This will include optimizing scan protocols for each of the valves, key anatomic measures and predictors of procedural risk requiring highlighting, and post-THV imaging.

[a] Department of Radiology, Royal Papworth Hospital, Cambridge, UK; [b] Department of Cardiology, Guy's and St Thomas' Hospital, London, UK; [c] School of Biomedical Engineering and Imaging Sciences, King's College London, London, UK; [d] Department of Radiology, School of Clinical Medicine, University of Cambridge, Box 219, Level 5, Cambridge Biomedical Campus, Cambridge CB2 0QQ, UK
[1] Joint first authors with equal contribution.
[2] Joint senior authors with equal contribution
* Corresponding author. Department of Radiology, Box 218 Cambridge Biomedical Campus, Cambridge CB2 0QQ
E-mail address: Jw2079@cam.ac.uk
Twitter: @jweirmccall (J.R.W.-M.)

Radiol Clin N Am 62 (2024) 419–434
https://doi.org/10.1016/j.rcl.2024.01.007

AORTIC VALVE
Indications for Transcatheter Aortic Valve Replacement

Aortic stenosis (AS) is increasing in prevalence, largely due to an aging population with a dramatic increase in almost every country in the world over the last 2 decades.[3] The evidence for TAVR has rapidly expanded, with randomized controlled trials supporting its consideration even in low-risk patients with symptomatic severe AS.[4] In patients aged 65 to 80 years, the choice of surgery versus TAVR has shifted to a joint decision-making process with the patient based on both their surgical risk and anatomic suitability for TAVR.[5] In those aged older than 80 years or with less than 10 years of remaining life expectancy, transfemoral TAVR is the recommended approach.[5]

Preprocedural Transcatheter Aortic Valve Replacement Planning Computed Tomography

Scan protocols are summarized in **Table 1**. Specific TAVR considerations are as follows.

Noncontrast cardiac computed tomography
This is not an essential component of the TAVR workup; however, the aortic valve calcium score can provide further information on stenosis severity in the 30% of patients whose echocardiographic parameters are nonconcordant.[6] The images can also be used to plan the subsequent contrast-enhanced cardiac CT.

Contrast-enhanced cardiac computed tomography
Imaging of the heart in at least the systolic phase is essential.[7] In practice, the whole cardiac cycle is recommended. This provides additional data for analysis if the systolic phase is degraded by artifact.

Transcatheter Aortic Valve Replacement Reporting Considerations

Valve morphology and calcification
The valve calcium score should exclude left ventricular outflow tract (LVOT) and aortic wall calcification. An Agatston score of greater than 2063 in men and greater than 1377 in women in indicative of severe AS.[8]

Approximately 6% of patients presenting for TAVI have bicuspid valves.[9] Where a bicuspid valve is detected, the presence or absence of a raphe should be reported, as well as whether the raphe is calcified. The presence of both severe leaflet calcification and a raphe portends higher risk of post-TAVR morbidity and mortality.[10]

Device sizing
The aortic valve annulus is typically largest in early to mid-systole.[11] However, images of the root should be reviewed in all phases to ensure this is the case.[12] The annular 2-plane diameter, perimeter, and area are to be reported.

Device landing zone
The LVOT forms part of the TAVR landing zone. Calcium here increases risk of paravalvular regurgitation, conduction system injury and root rupture.[13,14] Location in relation to the valve cusps, and degree of protrusion into the LVOT should also be provided. A qualitative assessment should be reported as none, mild (single, nonprotruding, <5 mm), moderate or severe (multiple, protruding, or >10 mm).

Root assessment
Coronary occlusion is a rare (0.66%) complication with a 40% 30 day mortality.[15] The risk is increased with a coronary height less than 11 mm, and sinus less than 30 mm, particularly when occurring together (**Fig. 1**).[15] Where the software allows, modeling a virtual TAVR in situ may improve risk prediction, with a distance from the virtual valve to the coronary ostium of less than 4 mm indicative of an increased risk of occlusion.[15]

Membranous septal length
Shorter membranous septal lengths are an independent predictor for postprocedural PPM implantation. Membranous septum measurement is performed in the coronal plane, from the annulus to the muscular septum. Lengths greater than 7 mm are at low risk, while less than 3 mm is at high risk.[16]

C-arm angulation
A fluoroscopic view perpendicular to the annulus is required during TAVI to ensure optimal prosthesis deployment and should be included in the report.

Vascular access
Minimum iliofemoral diameter should be quoted bilaterally. The minimum required diameter is in part dependant on the device and access sheath to be used, with a sheath to vessel ratio of 1.12 or greater considered at high risk.[17] Circumferential calcification restricts vessel expansion and can lead to rupture in borderline narrow vessels. Calcification of the anterior common femoral artery can prevent vessel puncture and hinder postprocedure closure devices. Tortuosity is an independent risk factor for periprocedural access and bleeding complications especially if associated with calcification.[18]

Table 1
Scanning considerations and protocols in the workup of structural heart disease for transcatheter intervention

	TAVR	TMVR/r	TTVR/r	TPVR
Scanner requirements	≥64-detector row scanner. Higher temporal resolution and greater number of detector rows provide greater cranio-caudal coverage and faster acquisition, reducing the likelihood of motion and misregistration artifact			
Patient preparation: • General	Intravenous cannulation, preferably in the antecubital vein should be performed for the administration of iodinated contrast			
Patient preparation: • Specific considerations	BB + GTN relatively contraindicated	BB if HR ≥ 100 ±GTN if coronary assessment required	BB if HR ≥ 100 ±GTN if coronary assessment required	BB if HR ≥ 100 ±GTN if coronary assessment required
Noncontrast CT	Optional Acquire using same parameters as for coronary artery calcium scoring	Not required	Not required	Not required
Contrast-enhanced CT: • General	Collimation: ≤0.625 mm Scan range: From the tracheal bifurcation to below the apex Reconstruction: Ideally use of an iterative algorithm with slice thickness of <1 mm (preferably 0.5–0.625 mm). The entire cardiac cycle should be reconstructed at 5%–10% of the R–R interval, or 50–100 ms kV and mAs modulated based on patient size			
Contrast-enhanced CT: • Specific considerations	Minimum = systolic acquisition Preferred = Whole cycle Gated may cover whole chest, or just aortic root and heart Bolus triggering in the ascending aorta	Whole cardiac cycle Bolus triggering in the left ventricle	Whole cardiac cycle Bolus tracking in the proximal descending aorta	Whole cardiac cycle Imaging coverage should be from the top of the aortic arch to the diaphragm to cover the heart and central pulmonary arteries
Vascular access	Arterial phase from skull base to lesser trochanter	Not routinely required Venous phase abdomen and pelvis if prior DVT/ prior long term femoral line/known venous stenosis	Nongated scan of neck, chest, abdomen, and pelvis from the external auditory canal to lesser trochanter at 60–90 s may be acquired	Not routinely required For evaluation of the inferior and superior vena cava a delayed nongated scan at 60–90 s should be acquired

(continued on next page)

Table 1
(continued)

	TAVR	TMVR/r	TTVR/r	TPVR
Contrast	4–6 mL/s, using a bolus of 50–100 mL (100 mL required in larger patients, or in older generation scanners with smaller z-axis coverage) In CKD slower injection rates (3 mL/s) with lower kVp (80–90 kVp) scanning can be considered to reduce contrast volume	4–5 mL/s If a transseptal approach is being considered, a triphasic injection to ensure right heart opacification and adequate delineation of the interatrial septum is required: 40 mL contrast at 5 mL/s, followed by 20 mL contrast with 20 mL saline, then by 40 mL of saline	Triphasic protocol to enable adequate visualization of the RCA, the right ventricle, and the inferior and superior vena cava: 50 mL of neat contrast at 5 mL/s followed by 100 mL of a contrast saline mix in a 50% mix ratio at 5 mL/s and thereafter 50 mL of a saline flush at the same flow rate	Triphasic protocol to enable adequate visualization of the RCA, the right ventricle, and the inferior and superior vena cava: 50 mL of neat contrast at 5 mL/s followed by 100 mL of a contrast saline mix in a 50% mix ratio at 5 mL/s and thereafter 50 mL of a saline flush at the same flow rate

Abbreviations: BB, beta-blocker; CKD, chronic kidney disease (eGFR<30); CT, computed tomography; GTN, Glyceryl trinitrate; TAVR, transcatheter aortic valve replacement; TMVR/r, transcatheter mitral valve replacement/repair; TPVR, transcatheter pulmonary valve replacement; TTVR/r, transcatheter tricuspid valve replacement/repair.

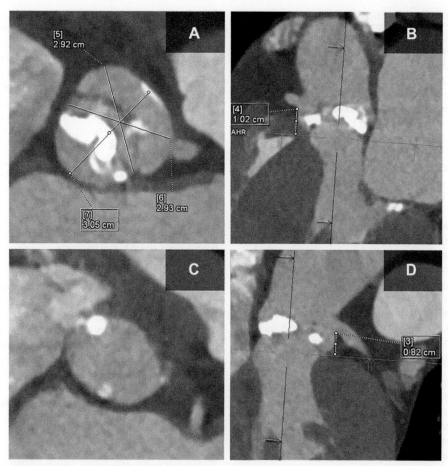

Fig. 1. Bicuspid valve with a small sinus (*A*) and low left and right coronary heights (*B, D*), and severe LVOT calcification (*B*). This constellation of high-risk features guided this patient to choose surgical valve replacement.

Where transfemoral access is not feasible, axillary/subclavian and carotid access should be reviewed and reported according to the same parameters as the iliofemoral vessels.

Coronary assessment

With retrospective acquisition and 10% reconstructions, the coronary arteries are imaged in multiple phases. This allows for the exclusion of prognostically significant proximal/mid coronary artery disease with high accuracy despite a high burden of coronary calcification and arrythmia in this cohort.[19]

MITRAL VALVE
Indications for Transcatheter Mitral Valve Replacement

Unlike the aortic valve where replacement is the only option, transcatheter mitral valve repair (TMVr) and replacement (TMVR) are both possible. Currently, the principal indication for intervention is symptomatically severe mitral regurgitation (MR) with high/prohibitive surgical risk. This constitutes a significant group, with clinical registries data showing that up to 50% of symptomatic patients with severe MR have a prohibitive risk for surgery.[20]

Transesophageal echocardiography is the initial imaging technique of choice in patients with MR. It provides information on underlying mechanism and severity and allows accurate assessment of whether TMVr is feasible.[21] Not all patients are suitable for TMVr, with large coaptation gap (>10 mm), calcification at the potential grasping sites, and immobile or restricted leaflets all associated with lower likelihood of success. In these instances, CT is used to assess for suitability for TMVR.

Preprocedural TMVR Planning Computed Tomography

Scan protocols are summarized in **Table 1**.

TMVR Reporting Considerations

Annulus assessment

Mitral annular dimensions are dynamic and should therefore be analyzed in both systolic and diastolic phases. Dedicated software, allowing for the contouring of the entire annulus including LVOT provides for the most detailed assessment. A manual technique can also be undertaken, which follows a similar technique as for the aortic valve, with the 3 cusp hingepoints replaced instead by the medial and lateral trigone, and ventricular insertion point of the posterior mitral valve leaflet.[22] The annulus report should include area, perimeter, intertrigonal, intercommissural and septolateral distances, mitral annular calcification (MAC), leaflet length, distance between papillary muscles, and the course of the coronary sinus and circumflex artery relative to the annular plane. Valve-in-valve or valve-in ring TMVR's are an emerging option for patients considered high risk for reoperation. If the model and size of the surgical device is unknown, short axis CT images can be used to calculate the inner diameter and guide TMVR sizing.

Annulus assessment in mitral annular calcification

MAC provides a rigid landing zone for anchoring of TMVR devices, allowing for the use of Sapien aortic valves in the mitral position. The circumferential extent, radial thickness, longitudinal depth, and whether it involves the trigones and anterior mitral valve leaflet should all be commented upon. There is an increased risk of embolization if involvement is less than 270°, the trigones are not involved, and the thickness/depth of the calcification is less than 10 mm.[23] The same measures should be obtained as for a native annulus, but using the inner aspect of the mitral calcification as the perimeter (**Fig. 2**).

Left ventricular outflow tract obstruction

Left ventricular outflow tract obstruction (LVOTO) is one of the most serious complications of

TMVR and is defined as an increase in LVOT gradient of greater than 10 mm Hg compared with baseline.[24] The likelihood of its occurrence can be predicted using CT, through the implantation of a virtual valve (the sizing of which is based on the annular area) from which the neo-LVOT area can then be calculated. Current recommendations are for measurement in the mid to end systolic phase (using an open aortic valve to define systole).[24] An area of 1.7 to 1.9 cm^2 is considered the lower cutoff, below which severe LVOTO is likely (**Fig. 3**).[25] Those perceived to be at an increased risk of LVOTO are not necessarily precluded from undergoing TMVR. Preprocedural catheter-guided alcohol septal ablation can be performed to increase the LVOT area in patients with a thickened basal septum.

Percutaneous access planning

Access for TMVr is performed via the transapical or transseptal route. Planning of access site for the transapical approach is achieved by virtually extending the trajectory of the deployment device to the chest wall. This method allows identification of the optimal intercostal space and degree of laterality for puncture. Peripheral venous imaging is not required for TMVr and not routinely required for TMVR as venous stenosis is rare as is venous tortuosity/calcification.

TRICUSPID VALVE
Indications for Tricuspid Valve Replacement/ Repair

The burden of significant tricuspid regurgitation (TR) is relatively high, with prevalence of 0.55% in the entire population, which increases to 4% in patients over 75 years of age.[26]

Surgical repair or replacement is recommended for

- Severe TR if undergoing surgery for left-sided valve disease
- Primary TR in the presence of symptoms and/ or evidence of right ventricular (RV) dilatation

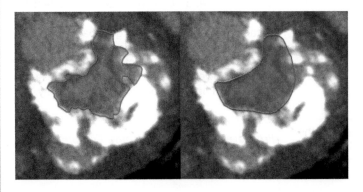

Fig. 2. Severe MAC in TMVR. Contouring the MAC precisely leads to a distorted assessment of the annular dimensions, and changes the epicenter. The smoother contour on the right better represents the native D-shaped annulus for modeling the TMVR. The 340° coverage, including the trigones and anterior mitral valve leaflet as well as the thickness of greater than 10 mm all indicate low risk of embolization.

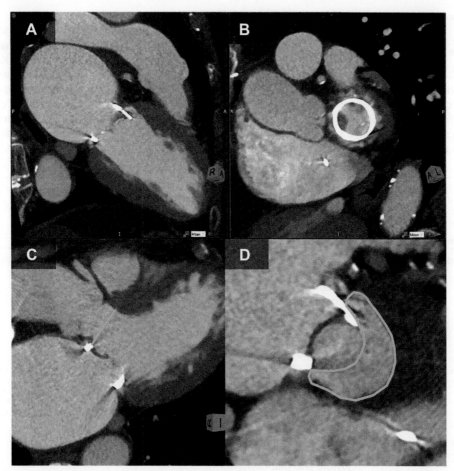

Fig. 3. 79M with degenerate mitral valve replacement as evidenced by leaflet thickening and calcification (*A, B*). The annulus to interventricular distance was 24 mm (*C*) while the neo-LVOT was 3.9 cm^2 (*D*), both in keeping with a low risk of LVOT obstruction. Patient underwent successful TMVR with a Sapien 3 valve.

- Secondary TR with no significant pulmonary hypertension or RV dysfunction, in the presence of symptoms or RV dilatation.

Where patients are not suitable candidates for surgery, they may be considered for transcatheter intervention.[2,5]

As with mitral intervention, both transcatheter tricuspid valve repair (TTVr) and replacement (TTVR) are options. Several anatomic features are associated with a poor result with TTVr, favoring TTVR as an alternative option, with these the same as for TMVr (discussed earlier).[27] Currently available TTVR devices may be categorized as orthotopic or heterotopic. Orthotopic valves (Cardiovalve, NaviGate, Evoque, Trisol, LUX-Valve, Intrepid, Tricares) are deployed at the tricuspid valve annulus, whereas heterotopic valves (Sapien, TricValve Tricento) are placed in one or both vena cavae to reduce the extracardiac hemodynamic impact of TR.[28]

COMPUTED TOMOGRAPHY IN TTVR
Tricuspid Valve Anatomy

The annulus exhibits a dynamic change in size of almost 30% through the cardiac cycle and is largest in late diastole following atrial contraction.[29] Relevant adjacent anatomy includes the right coronary artery (RCA), and the triangle of Koch, which contains the atrioventricular node—located at the ostium of the coronary sinus at the base of the septal leaflet. Both the RCA and atrioventricular node may be susceptible to damage during TTVR.

Computed Tomography Requirements for TTVR Evaluation

Echocardiography remains the gold standard for evaluation of TR severity and etiology. CT nevertheless provides complementary information that permits a better understanding of the anatomy of the right heart in relation to its adjacent structures.

Scan protocols are summarized in **Table 1**.

Objectives of Computed Tomography in TTVR Planning

CT provides comprehensive evaluation of anatomy, which helps with patient-specific selection for an appropriate TTVR device.[30] Systematic image analysis can assist with a number of different stages of procedure planning (**Table 2**).

TTVR device sizing

Assessment of anulus dimensions, including maximal antero-posterior and septo-lateral diameters, perimeter, and area. Given the dynamic change in annular size, measurements should be performed in both end-systole and mid-diastole (**Figs. 4** and **5**).[30] Measuring the dimensions of vena cavae at the right atrio-caval junction and distance to the first hepatic vein is key for heterotropic caval valve sizing and avoidance of hepatic vein obstruction.[30]

Table 2
Morphologic analysis for transcatheter tricuspid valve repair and replacement computed tomography report

Anatomic Structure	Measurements	Orientation
Tricuspid valve anulus	• Area, perimeter, and antero-posterior and septo-lateral diameter measured in end systole and mid-diastole • Distance from the tricuspid annulus to the apex of the right ventricle • Presence of annular calcification	• Short axis view at the level of the annulus • 4-chamber view
Subvalvular anatomy	• Presence of prominent trabeculae and the moderator band	• 4-chamber and 2-chamber views • Double oblique view
RCA	• Assess the sub, trans, or supra-annular course of the RCA relative to the tricuspid annulus • Distance from the RCA to anterior and posterior leaflets in end systole and mid-diastole	• Short axis of the tricuspid valve • 4-chamber and 2-chamber views
Tricuspid valve leaflet tethering	• Height, area, and angle of leaflet tenting between annular plane and coaptation point of anterior and septal leaflets	• 4-chamber and 2-chamber views
Right atrium	• Area, width, and length	• 4 and 2 RV chamber views

Vena cavae	• Maximum and minimum SVC dimensions at the level of
	  a. Brachiocephalic vein convergence
	  b. Pulmonary artery
	  c. Right atrial junction
	• Maximum and minimum IVC dimensions at the level of
	  a. Right atrial junction
	  b. First hepatic vein
	  c. 5 cm below IVC-right atrial junction
	Distance between first hepatic vein and IVC-right trial junction
		• Double-oblique transverse view
		• Single oblique sagittal view

Additional	• Coaxial implantation angle • Coaptation defect assessment • Fluoroscopic simulation of device implantation • Delivery sheath simulation for optimal access to the landing zone	

Abbreviations: IVC, inferior vena cava; SCS, superior vena cava.

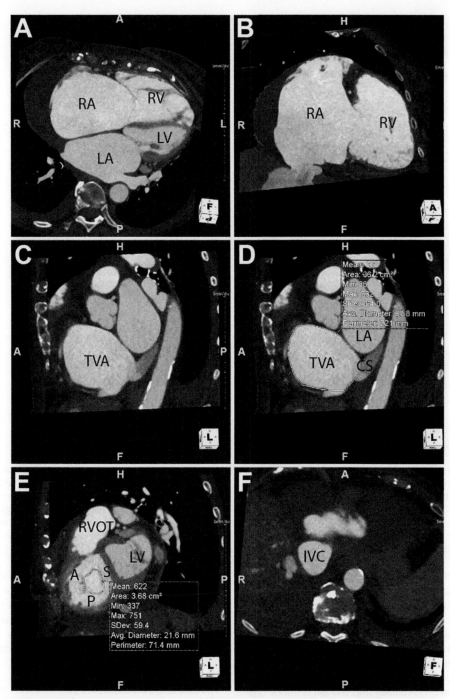

Fig. 4. 77F with severe functional TR. (*A, B*) A severely dilated RA and RV in the 4-chamber and right ventricular inflow view. (*C, D*) The D-shaped tricuspid annulus and the measurement of its size (*D*). (*E*) The tricuspid valve leaflets in end-systole with a large coaptation defect measuring 3.7 cm². (*F*) The size of the IVC at its entry point into the RA. A, anterior tricuspid valve leaflet; CS, coronary sinus; IVC, inferior vena cava; LA, left atrium; P, posterior tricuspid valve leaflet; RA, right atrium; RV, right ventricle; RVOT, right ventricular outflow tract; S, septal tricuspid valve leaflet; TVA, tricuspid valve annulus.

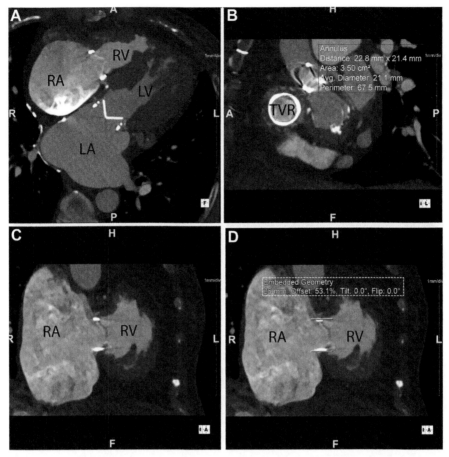

Fig. 5. Valve-in-valve tricuspid planning in a 52F with previous mechanical aortic and mitral valve replacement and re-do mitral valve replacement and tissue tricuspid valve replacement. (*A*) The 4-chamber view with a bioprosthetic tricuspid valve with calcified leaflets. (*B*) The measurement of the sewing ring of the bioprosthetic valve and (*C*) the RV inflow view of the valve. (*D*) A simulated implant of a Sapien 3 valve inside the bioprosthetic tricuspid valve. A, anterior tricuspid valve leaflet; CS, coronary sinus; IVC, inferior vena cava; LA, left atrium; P, posterior tricuspid valve leaflet; RA, right atrium; RV, right ventricle; RVOT, right ventricular outflow tract; S, septal tricuspid valve leaflet; TVA, tricuspid valve annulus; TVR, tricuspid valve replacement.

Device landing zone assessment

Target anchoring sites for TTVR implants around the tricuspid valve anulus, the right atrium, and the vena cavae are required. The optimal fluoroscopic projections for coplanar device implantation with the tricuspid anulus should be defined: the right anterior oblique view—obtained tangentially to the annulus—allows the evaluation of the implant trajectory and co-axiality and the left anterior oblique caudal view provides the surgical "en face" view from the RV.[31] Simulating device implantation using embedded geometry can also help to assess implantation depth, optimize device positioning and anticipate paravalvular regurgitation.

Evaluation of adjacent structures and risk of possible impediment

Assessing the course of the RCA and the distance at each point from the annulus is required to avoid the risk of coronary injury. Large papillary muscles or trabeculations can interfere with device navigation or cause entanglement. The degree of prosthesis protrusion may be assessed by measuring the distance between the annular plane and the moderator band and prominent trabeculae.

Vascular access route

The size and patency of the inferior vena cava (IVC) at the junction with the right atrium and at the level of the first hepatic vein are important measures when assessing the suitability of transfemoral venous or alternative access strategies (jugular, subclavian, and axillary). Measuring the angulation between the IVC and annulus helps to assess the feasibility of achieving coaxial alignment, while the distance between the ostium of the IVC and the tricuspid valve anulus determines whether the delivery system has enough length to deliver the device.

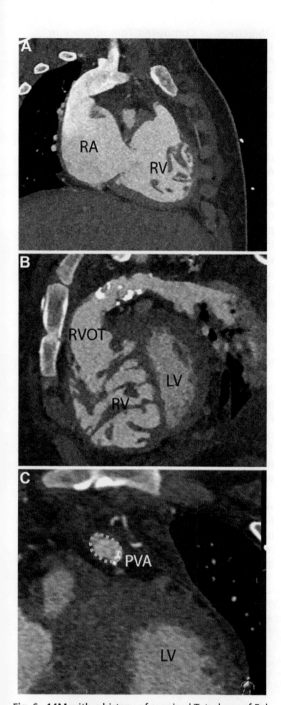

Fig. 6. 14M with a history of repaired Tetralogy of Fallot and pulmonary atresia repair with an RV to PA homograft. (*A*) The RV inflow view and (*B*) the RV outflow view with pulmonary homograft calcification and stenosis. (*C*) The measurement of the pulmonary valve annulus in preparation for a TPVR with a Venus P-valve. A, anterior tricuspid valve leaflet; CS, coronary sinus; IVC, inferior vena cava; LA, left atrium; P, posterior tricuspid valve leaflet; RA, right atrium; RV, right ventricle; RVOT, right ventricular outflow tract; S, septal tricuspid valve leaflet; TVA, tricuspid valve annulus.

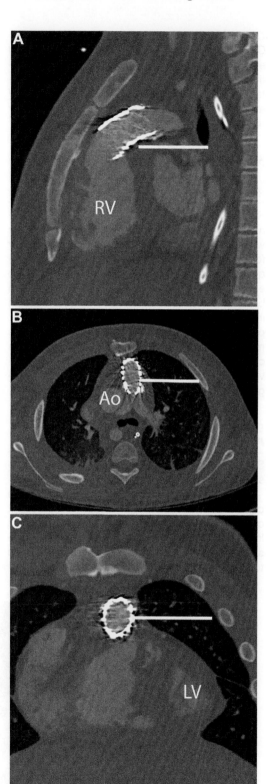

Fig. 7. Electrocardiogram-gated cardiac CT in a patient who successfully underwent deployment of a Venus P valve (*solid line*) for pulmonary homograft stenosis in the sagittal view (*A*), axial view (*B*), and the coronal view (*C*). Ao, Aorta; LV, left ventricle; RV, right ventricle.

Other considerations

CT can accurately measure RV end-diastolic and end-systolic volume to assess RV ejection fraction, assisting with patient selection. This is important as an acute increase in afterload on the RV after TTVR may not be tolerated, resulting in higher risk of acute right heart failure postprocedurally.[32]

PULMONARY VALVE
Indications for Transcatheter Pulmonary Valve Replacement

Right ventricular outflow tract (RVOT) and pulmonary valve dysfunction are common in patients with congenital heart disease, after surgical repair for congenital abnormalities and as a consequence of acquired conditions such as infective endocarditis.[33] Repeat surgical interventions can be technically challenging and associated with increased morbidity and mortality.[34] Transcatheter pulmonary valve replacement (TPVR) is one of the most common procedures in patients with congenital heart disease, permitting earlier intervention and reducing the need for multiple surgeries over a lifetime.

Computed Tomography in Transcatheter Pulmonary Valve Replacement

Scan protocols are summarized in **Table 1**. TPVR-specific considerations are as follows:

Given the younger age of this cohort in the context of congenital heart disease, an important consideration is to keep the radiation dose as low as reasonably achievable. Appropriate acquisition length, using the lowest possible kVp and tube current modulation is essential.

Objectives of Computed Tomography in Transcatheter Pulmonary Valve Replacement Planning

Systematic evaluation using CT is key to assessing the suitability of different TPVR devices, with several important objectives.

Transcatheter pulmonary valve replacement device sizing

Accurate device sizing is essential for preventing complications such as device embolization and paravalvular regurgitation. At present, there is no consensus on which standardized measurements provide the most reliable information for TPVR sizing. In practice, CT is used to identify patients with measurements beyond the limits for a particular device, with ultimate TPVR implant sizing ultimately determined via catheter balloon-sizing during the procedure. The size of the native pulmonary valve annulus, RVOT and main pulmonary artery, the dimensions of the surgical conduit, and the length of the main pulmonary artery until bifurcation are important determinants for the use of TPVR devices (**Fig. 6**).

Assessment of right ventricular outflow tract morphology

Five different types of RVOT have been described, with the shape being an important determinant of TPVR outcome. Type 1 (pyramidal) morphology is associated with a high risk of device embolization, while the other types are usually suitable for TPVR.[35]

Access route assessment

Measurement of minimum vessel diameters can be used to plan optimal percutaneous access route, which can include transfemoral, transjugular, and subclavian.

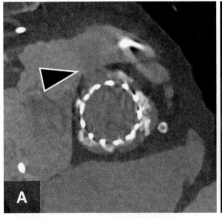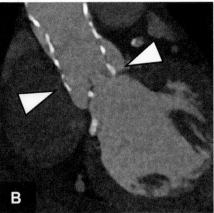

Fig. 8. Post-THV complications. (*A*) Post-TAVR VSD communicating with the RV (*black arrow*). (*B*) The Evolut valve has migrated superiorly with one part of the stent frame above the aortic cusp while the other is just below it (*white arrows*). This was associated with moderate aortic regurgitation.

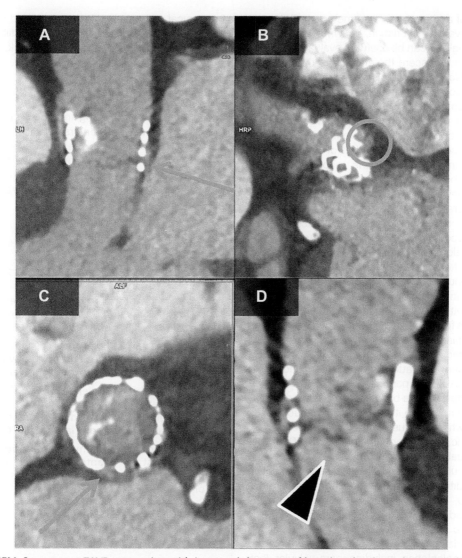

Fig. 9. 85M, 8 years post-TAVR, presenting with increased shortness of breath. Echo showed severe paravalvular regurgitation. CT shows a small leak between the left and noncoronary cusps (*arrows* and *circle* in *A–C*). It also revealed a flail leaflet (*black arrow* in *D*) in keeping with the main regurgitation being transvalvular. Patient underwent valve-in-valve with almost complete resolution of the aortic regurgitation.

Coronary artery anatomy

Measuring the distance from coronary arteries to the RVOT or conduit is important for avoiding coronary compression during TPVR. The main indicator of risk is close proximity (<2 mm) and should be assessed in systole and diastole since the position changes with the cardiac phase.[36]

Conduit assessment

Right ventricular-pulmonary conduits can become calcified and stenotic over time, which affects their distensibility. CT can identify patients who may require conduit rehabilitation before TPVR (**Fig. 7**). Small caliber conduits may require preprocedure covered stent to create a uniform landing zone for

TPVR,[37] whereas larger conduits may require placement of an RVOT reducer.[38]

Simulation and three-dimensional fusion imaging

In patients with complex anatomy, CT can be used to create patient-specific three-dimensional printed models, which improves the understanding of anatomy and can be used to simulate procedures.[39]

POSTPROCEDURAL IMAGING IN TRANSCATHETER HEART VALVES

Echocardiography remains the imaging modality of choice for post-THV follow-up, providing both functional and anatomic parameters. In the presence of valve dysfunction, or when images are suboptimal, CT can be useful to evaluate the valve as well as to discern the etiology of the dysfunction.[2,40] Cardiac CT is also a valuable adjunct to echocardiogram in patients who are suspected to have complications such as patient prosthesis mismatch, valve thrombosis, infective endocarditis, or structural valve degeneration (**Fig. 8**).[41]

Scan acquisition follows that of preprocedural assessment for each of the respective valves. Higher tube voltages (120 kVp) can be used to reduce device-related streak artifact. Peripheral vasculature does not need to be imaged unless there is consideration of a transcatheter valve-in-valve procedure or suspected access site complications.

Hypoattenuated leaflet thickening (HALT) and hypoattenuation affecting motion (HAM) are common findings in both surgical and transcatheter valves, with their presence suggestive of leaflet thrombus formation.[42] Location, length, and extent of thickening should be described.[12] HAM should be reported as present or absent. A key consideration when hypoattenuation is identified is to discern HALT from pannus formation. HALT is typically centered in the base of the leaflet and is usually asymmetrical in its involvement of each of the cusps, while pannus tends to be subvalvular, concentric, and uniform in its ingrowth. The presence of calcification is indicative of chronic structural valvular degeneration. In cases of infective endocarditis, the hypoattenuating vegetation is lobulated, with the presence and extent of any associated abscess commented upon.

Cardiac CT is helpful in the identification and characterization of several other issues related to device implantation including para-valvular leak (PVL; **Fig. 9**) and access site complications.

PVL is one of the more common post-THV complications and is associated with increased mortality.[43] On CT, PVLs appear as contrast opacified channels running alongside the valve. Size, length, and location should be reported as well as predicted gantry angle for potential closure. Evaluation for both PVLs and the THV leaflet position is important as transvalvular and paravalvular regurgitation can coexist, and due to the acoustic shadowing from the THV stent frame, these can occasionally be mistaken for one another on echocardiography (see **Fig. 9**). Access site complications are common and range from self-limiting hematomas to large pseudoaneurysms and retroperitoneal hemorrhages requiring intervention. CT is an ideal modality for assessment with a triple-phase protocol being adopted for the assessment of active hemorrhage. Left ventricular pseudoaneurysm is a rare transapical or transseptal access-related complication.[44] These appear as focal contrast filled outpouchings from the LV with a narrow neck.

SUMMARY

The range of transcatheter solutions to valve disease is increasing, bringing treatment options to those in whom surgery confers significant risk. As the range of devices and their indications grow, so too will the demand for procedural planning. CT will continue to enable this growth through the provision of accurate device sizing and procedural risk assessment.

CLINICS CARE POINTS

- THVs are transforming clinical care, enabled by high-quality preprocedural planning with CT.
- Accurate sizing and assessment of the landing zone reduces the incidence of paravalvular leak, device embolization, and annular injury.
- It is important to understand how the THV will sit in the native anatomy to be able to assess for the risk of complications beyond the annulus such as coronary or LVOTO.
- Percutaneous vascular image acquisition protocols must be adapted according to the planned procedural approach (transarterial or transvenous).

DISCLOSURE

J.R. Weir-McCall is supported by the NIHR Cambridge Biomedical Research Centre (BRC-1215–20,014). The views expressed are those of the authors and not necessarily those of the NIHR or the Department of Health and Social Care.

REFERENCES

1. Bonhoeffer P, Boudjemline Y, Saliba Z, et al. Percutaneous replacement of pulmonary valve in a right-ventricle to pulmonary-artery prosthetic conduit with valve dysfunction. Lancet 2000;356(9239): 1403–5.
2. Vahanian A, Beyersdorf F, Praz F, et al. 2021 ESC/EACTS Guidelines for the management of valvular heart disease. Eur J Cardio Thorac Surg 2021; 60(4):727–800.
3. Coffey S, Roberts-Thomson R, Brown A, et al. Global epidemiology of valvular heart disease. Nat Rev

Cardiol 2021. https://doi.org/10.1038/s41569-021-00570-z. 0123456789.

4. Mack MJ, Leon MB, Thourani VH, et al. Transcatheter Aortic-Valve Replacement with a Balloon-Expandable Valve in Low-Risk Patients. N Engl J Med 2019. https://doi.org/10.1056/NEJMoa1814052. NEJMoa1814052.

5. Otto CM, Nishimura RA, Bonow RO, et al. 2020 ACC/AHA Guideline for the Management of Patients With Valvular Heart Disease: A Report of the American College of Cardiology/American Heart Association Joint Committee on Clinical Practice Guidelines. Circulation 2021;143(5):e72–227.

6. Clavel MA, Messika-Zeitoun D, Pibarot P, et al. The complex nature of discordant severe calcified aortic valve disease grading: New insights from combined Doppler echocardiographic and computed tomographic study. J Am Coll Cardiol 2013;62(24):2329–38.

7. Steffen J, Beckmann M, Haum M, et al. Systolic or diastolic CT image acquisition for transcatheter aortic valve replacement – An outcome analysis. Journal of Cardiovascular Computed Tomography 2022;16(5):423–30.

8. Pawade T, Clavel M-A, Tribouilloy C, et al. Computed Tomography Aortic Valve Calcium Scoring in Patients With Aortic Stenosis. Circulation: Cardiovascular Imaging 2018;11(3):e007146.

9. Yoon S-H, Bleiziffer S, De Backer O, et al. Outcomes in Transcatheter Aortic Valve Replacement for Bicuspid Versus Tricuspid Aortic Valve Stenosis. J Am Coll Cardiol 2017;69(21):2579–89.

10. Yoon SH, Kim WK, Dhoble A, et al. Bicuspid Aortic Valve Morphology and Outcomes After Transcatheter Aortic Valve Replacement. J Am Coll Cardiol 2020;76(9):1018–30.

11. Suchá D, Tuncay V, Prakken NHJ, et al. Does the aortic annulus undergo conformational change throughout the cardiac cycle? A systematic review. European Heart Journal Cardiovascular Imaging 2015;16(12):1307–17.

12. Blanke P, Weir-McCall JR , Achenbach S, et al. Computed tomography imaging in the context of transcatheter aortic valve implantation (TAVI)/transcatheter aortic valve replacement (TAVR): An expert consensus document of the Society of Cardiovascular Computed Tomography. Journal of Cardiovascular Computed Tomography 2019;13(1):1–20.

13. Hansson NC, Nørgaard BL, Barbanti M, et al. The impact of calcium volume and distribution in aortic root injury related to balloon-expandable transcatheter aortic valve replacement. Journal of Cardiovascular Computed Tomography 2015;9(5):382–92.

14. Hansson NC, Leipsic J, Pugliese F, et al. Aortic valve and left ventricular outflow tract calcium volume and distribution in transcatheter aortic valve replacement: Influence on the risk of significant paravalvular

regurgitation. Journal of Cardiovascular Computed Tomography 2018;12(4):290–7.

15. Khan JM, Kamioka N, Lisko JC, et al. Coronary Obstruction From TAVR in Native Aortic Stenosis: Development and Validation of Multivariate Prediction Model. JACC Cardiovasc Interv 2023;16(4):415–25.

16. Hamdan A, Guetta V, Klempfner R, et al. Inverse Relationship between Membranous Septal Length and the Risk of Atrioventricular Block in Patients Undergoing Transcatheter Aortic Valve Implantation. JACC Cardiovasc Interv 2015;8(9):1218–28.

17. Okuyama K, Jilaihawi H, Kashif M, et al. Transfemoral access assessment for transcatheter aortic valve replacement: Evidence-based application of computed tomography over invasive angiography. Circulation: Cardiovascular Imaging 2014;8(1). https://doi.org/10.1161/CIRCIMAGING.114.001995.

18. Mach M, Poschner T, Hasan W, et al. The Iliofemoral tortuosity score predicts access and bleeding complications during transfemoral transcatheter aortic valve replacement: Data from the VIenna Cardio Thoracic aOrtic valve registrY (VICTORY). Eur J Clin Invest 2021;51(6):e13491.

19. van den Boogert TPW, Claessen BEPM, Opolski MP, et al. DEtection of ProxImal Coronary stenosis in the work-up for Transcatheter aortic valve implantation using CTA (from the DEPICT CTA collaboration). Eur Radiol 2022;32(1):143–51.

20. Mirabel M, Iung B, Baron G, et al. What are the characteristics of patients with severe, symptomatic, mitral regurgitation who are denied surgery? Eur Heart J 2007;28(11):1358–65.

21. Hashimoto G, Lopes BBC, Sato H, et al. Computed Tomography Planning for Transcatheter Mitral Valve Replacement. Structural Heart 2022;6(1):100012.

22. Weir-McCall JR , Blanke P, Naoum C, et al. Mitral Valve Imaging with CT: Relationship with Transcatheter Mitral Valve Interventions. Radiology 2018;288(3):638–55.

23. Guerrero M, Wang DD, Pursnani A, et al. A Cardiac Computed Tomography–Based Score to Categorize Mitral Annular Calcification Severity and Predict Valve Embolization. JACC (J Am Coll Cardiol): Cardiovascular Imaging 2020;13(9):1945–57.

24. Reid A, Ben Zekry S, Turaga M, et al. Neo-LVOT and Transcatheter Mitral Valve Replacement: Expert Recommendations. JACC (J Am Coll Cardiol): Cardiovascular Imaging 2021;14(4):854–66.

25. Yoon S-H, Bleiziffer S, Latib A, et al. Predictors of Left Ventricular Outflow Tract Obstruction After Transcatheter Mitral Valve Replacement. JACC Cardiovasc Interv 2019;12(2):182–93.

26. Topilsky Y, Maltais S, Medina Inojosa J, et al. Burden of Tricuspid Regurgitation in Patients Diagnosed in the Community Setting. JACC Cardiovasc Imaging 2019;12(3):433–42.

27. Condello F, Gitto M, Stefanini GG. Etiology, epidemiology, pathophysiology and management of tricuspid regurgitation: an overview. RCM (Rapid Commun Mass Spectrom) 2021;22(4):1115–42.

28. Goldberg YH, Ho E, Chau M, et al. Update on Transcatheter Tricuspid Valve Replacement Therapies. Front Cardiovasc Med 2021;8:619558.

29. Fukuda S, Saracino G, Matsumura Y, et al. Three-dimensional geometry of the tricuspid annulus in healthy subjects and in patients with functional tricuspid regurgitation: a real-time, 3-dimensional echocardiographic study. Circulation 2006;114(1 Suppl):I492–8.

30. van Rosendael PJ, Kamperidis V, Kong WKF, et al. Computed tomography for planning transcatheter tricuspid valve therapy. Eur Heart J 2017;38(9):665–74.

31. Asmarats L, Puri R, Latib A, et al. Transcatheter Tricuspid Valve Interventions: Landscape, Challenges, and Future Directions. J Am Coll Cardiol 2018;71(25):2935–56.

32. Preda A, Melillo F, Liberale L, et al. Right ventricle dysfunction assessment for transcatheter tricuspid valve repair: A matter of debate. Eur J Clin Invest 2021;51(12):e13653.

33. Driesen BW, Warmerdam EG, Sieswerda G-J, et al. Percutaneous Pulmonary Valve Implantation: Current Status and Future Perspectives. Curr Cardiol Rev 2019;15(4):262–73.

34. Verheugt CL, Uiterwaal CSPM, Grobbee DE, et al. Long-term prognosis of congenital heart defects: a systematic review. Int J Cardiol 2008;131(1):25–32.

35. Pugliese L, Ricci F, Luciano A, et al. Role of computed tomography in transcatheter replacement of "other valves": a comprehensive review of preprocedural imaging. J Cardiovasc Med 2022;23(9):575–88.

36. Malone L, Fonseca B, Fagan T, et al. Preprocedural Risk Assessment Prior to PPVI with CMR and Cardiac CT. Pediatr Cardiol 2017;38(4):746–53.

37. Zahn EM. Self-Expanding Pulmonary Valves for Large Diameter Right Ventricular Outflow Tracts. Interv Cardiol Clin 2019;8(1):73–80.

38. Boudjemline Y, Agnoletti G, Bonnet D, et al. Percutaneous pulmonary valve replacement in a large right ventricular outflow tract: an experimental study. J Am Coll Cardiol 2004;43(6):1082–7.

39. Byrne N, Velasco Forte M, Tandon A, et al. A systematic review of image segmentation methodology, used in the additive manufacture of patient-specific 3D printed models of the cardiovascular system. JRSM Cardiovasc Dis 2016;5. https://doi.org/10.1177/2048004016645467. 2048004016645467.

40. Dvir D, Bourguignon T, Otto CM, et al. Standardized Definition of Structural Valve Degeneration for Surgical and Transcatheter Bioprosthetic Aortic Valves. Circulation 2018;137(4):388–99.

41. Nishimura RA, Otto CM, Bonow RO, et al. 2017 AHA/ACC Focused Update of the 2014 AHA/ACC Guideline for the Management of Patients With Valvular Heart Disease: A Report of the American College of Cardiology/American Heart Association Task Force on Clinical Practice Guidelines. Circulation 2017;135(25):e1159–95.

42. Yanagisawa R, Hayashida K, Yamada Y, et al. Incidence, Predictors, and Mid-Term Outcomes of Possible Leaflet Thrombosis After TAVR. JACC (J Am Coll Cardiol): Cardiovascular Imaging 2017; 10(1):1–11.

43. Hwang HY, Choi J-W, Kim H-K, et al. Paravalvular Leak After Mitral Valve Replacement: 20-Year Follow-Up. Ann Thorac Surg 2015;100(4):1347–52.

44. Sawlani N, Berry N, Sobieszczyk P, et al. Percutaneous Closure of a Delayed Left Ventricular Pseudoaneurysm After Transseptal Transcatheter Mitral Valve Replacement. JACC Cardiovasc Interv 2017; 10(14):1464–5.

Cardiac Computed Tomography in Congenital Heart Disease

Evan J. Zucker, MD[a],*

KEYWORDS

- Cardiac • Congenital heart disease • Adult congenital heart disease • Computed tomography
- Computed tomography angiography • Coronary artery • Single ventricle • Tetralogy of Fallot

KEY POINTS

- Computed tomography (CT) has become an essential imaging modality in the preoperative and postoperative congenital heart disease (CHD) patient, supplementing echocardiography and MR imaging and often obviating the need for invasive angiography.
- CT is most adept for assessing the systemic and pulmonary veins, pulmonary and coronary arteries, and aorta, along with the lungs and airways, but can also elucidate intracardiac anatomy and cardiac chamber size and function.
- CT is particularly useful in the adult CHD population due to the presence of stents and other postsurgical materials that limit routine surveillance and assessment of complications by other imaging modalities.
- With ongoing CT advances such as dual-source and multispectral technology, the applications of CT in CHD continue to grow with decreasing radiation, iodinated contrast, and breath-holding/sedation requirements.

INTRODUCTION

Congenital heart disease (CHD) comprises a broad spectrum of pathology defined by structural anomalies of the heart or intrathoracic great vessels with variable physiologic consequences.[1] Despite the rarity of individual malformations, CHD is in fact collectively common, occurring in up to nearly 1% of births.[2] With continued advances in CHD treatment, most patients now survive into adulthood but are at risk for late postoperative complications along with acquired systemic and cardiovascular abnormalities.[2,3]

Given the vast nature of potential anomalies and need for lifelong monitoring, imaging plays a central role in the preoperative and postoperative management of CHD. Echocardiography remains the first-line modality but often suboptimally depicts the extracardiac vasculature and complex malformations and may be limited by poor acoustic windows particularly in larger or postoperative patients. Once the reference standard cardiac catheterization, due to its invasive nature, is now reserved when possible for cases in which concurrent intervention is planned. Finally, cardiac MR imaging can offer much comprehensive information but may be unfeasible due to traditionally long scans and need for specialized expertise and regardless may provide inadequate anatomic detail or suffer from artifacts.[4]

In recent years, computed tomography (CT) has solidified its role as an essential imaging adjunct in the evaluation of CHD patients. Rapidly and effectively, CT enables delineation of intricate preoperative and postoperative cardiovascular malformations and any complicating features with continually decreasing technical requirements and drawbacks. In this article, the ever-

[a] Department of Radiology, Divisions of Pediatric and Cardiovascular Imaging, Massachusetts General Hospital, 55 Fruit Street, Boston, MA 02114, USA
* Corresponding author.
E-mail address: ezucker@mgh.harvard.edu

Radiol Clin N Am 62 (2024) 435–452
https://doi.org/10.1016/j.rcl.2023.12.015
0033-8389/24/© 2024 Elsevier Inc. All rights reserved.

expanding role of CT in CHD is reviewed. Current imaging approaches are emphasized, whereas major clinical applications are highlighted.

NORMAL ANATOMY

Although the myriad potential malformations in CHD can be daunting, the sequential segmental approach provides a structured framework to ensure systematic anatomic reporting that can be readily applied to any imaging modality including CT. Assessment should include determination of situs (based on atrial appendage morphology and bronchial configuration), identification of the major cardiovascular segments (systemic and pulmonary venous drainage, atria, ventricles, great vessels, and coronary arteries), and documentation of intersegmental connections (venoatrial, atrioventricular, and ventriculoarterial), noting any anomalies (eg, shunts) or combinations of anomalies (eg, tetralogy of Fallot [TOF]) where present.[5] The segmental anatomy may be summarized using a three-letter shorthand system corresponding to the visceroatrial situs, ventricular loop (direction of cardiac "bending" determined in development), and relative position of the great vessels (aorta and main pulmonary artery [PA]).[6]

It is also incumbent on the cardiac imager to gain familiarity with the range of potential surgeries that may be pursued in CHD. In turn, this knowledge can help ensure prompt recognition of postoperative complications. While too expansive to enumerate in detail, the CHD surgeries and procedures more commonly encountered by CT are highlighted through selected case examples later in this text.[7,8]

IMAGING TECHNIQUE

Modern multidetector CT (MDCT) with angiographic technique (CTA) facilitates a quick and comprehensive anatomic CHD assessment of the heart, great vessels, and relevant extracardiac structures such as the lungs and airways, generally with a single acquisition.[4] Non-contrast imaging may be considered to distinguish calcifications, stents, and other hyperattenuating surgical/implanted material, especially if these structures might be mistaken for active arterial extravasation in the setting of acute decompensation. Delayed venous phase imaging may also be required to optimize assessment of the system veins or to achieve diagnostic opacification in the context of altered cardiovascular physiology (eg, total cavopulmonary connection/Fontan).[9] Concomitant scanning of the abdomen and pelvis in arterial and/or venous phases can also be performed if clinically appropriate, such as

to assess the access vasculature in preparation for percutaneous valve placement.[10]

Adequate preparation is crucial in any cardiac CT for CHD, particularly in young children who may require immobilization or sedation to mitigate patient motion. To optimize coronary imaging, administration of nitroglycerine (to dilate the coronaries) and beta-blockers (to decrease the heart rate) may be considered, the latter less essential in newer scanners with higher temporal resolution; these medications are more commonly given in adults.[4,11] Non-electrocardiographic (ECG)-synchronized scanning is generally sufficient for evaluating the extracardiac thoracic vasculature, lungs, and airways. It may also be adequate for assessing the intracardiac structures when using newer generation, high temporal resolution dual-source scanners with high-pitch modes that help to mitigate respiratory and cardiac motion even in free-breathing infants with sub-second acquisitions; high-pitch scan modes can also be ECG-synchronized.[9,11]

Prospective ECG-triggered axial sequential or retrospective ECG-gated spiral/helical scanning should be used when reliable coronary and detailed intracardiac imaging is needed, along with functional information if desired. Although prospective compared with retrospective mode generally results in less radiation exposure (although greater than in high-pitch helical mode), it is also more prone to stair-step artifacts at the interface between acquisition slabs. Both prospective and retrospective scanning may require breath-holding, which can be prohibitive in young children or otherwise incooperative patients.[4,11]

In general, radiation risks remain the chief drawback of cardiac CT, meriting special concern in the CHD population prone to repeated follow-up into adulthood. However, newer technology (eg, 320-MDCT) combined with dose-saving measures (eg, low kilovoltage [kV] potential [kVp] settings, iterative or artificial intelligence-based reconstruction of noisier images) has helped facilitate very low, even sub-millisievert effective doses. Another downside is the need for iodinated intravenous (IV) contrast, which may precipitate allergic reactions or nephrotoxicity in select patients. However, current nonionic, low-osmolality contrasts have lower allergy rates compared with older agents.[4] Moreover, recent data have cast doubt on the actual risk of contrast-induced nephropathy, which may be negligible even in patients with chronic renal disease.[12]

Advanced Scanning Techniques

A variety of newer scanning techniques have expanded the role of cardiac CT in CHD. Myocardial delayed enhancement assessment can be achieved with CT through a prospectively triggered or retrospectively ECG-gated acquisition obtained 5 to 15 minutes after IV contrast administration. Rivaling late gadolinium enhancement imaging, delayed enhancement CT is a viable alternative for patients in whom MR imaging is contraindicated or unfeasible. Another useful technique is four-dimensional (4D) CT, acquired throughout the respiratory cycle and thereby allowing dynamic cardiovascular and airway evaluation.[11]

In addition, there has been much interest in dual-energy/multispectral CT that uses both high and low tube potentials to allow greater material decomposition. As a result, this approach facilitates generation of virtual non-contrast images (potentially obviating the need for a true non-contrast acquisition), production of virtual monoenergetic reconstructions (which may salvage a poor contrast bolus at lower simulated kV near the k-edge of iodine or decrease metallic beam hardening artifacts at higher simulated kV), and creation of iodine/perfused blood volume maps (which can serve as a surrogate for lung perfusion).[13] However, dual-energy mode must be preselected at the time of acquisition and does not allow simultaneous high-pitch imaging that is often preferred in unsedated children.

More recently, photon-counting detector (PCD) CT, in which incident photons are directly converted into electric signal, has recently become clinically available, offering substantial noise reduction along with enhanced spatial and contrast resolution and in turn lower radiation and contrast media dose requirements.[14] Moreover, in PCD CT (unlike dual-energy CT), spectral information is always available without the need for preselection of a specific scan mode or compromise of temporal or spatial resolution.[15] The applications of this nascent technology in CHD are just emerging and will continue to evolve with time.

Advanced Postprocessing Tools

In addition to newer scan modes, a variety of novel postprocessing tools are now available to expand the utility of CT data in the CHD patient. Multiplanar reformatting, minimum and maximum intensity projections, and three-dimensional (3D) volume rendering capabilities have long been available.[4] Multispectral CT processing can occur at the scanner console or offline through a variety of software packages. Cinematic rendering improves on traditional volume rendering through the simulation of light rays, producing more realistic surgical depiction of relevant anatomy.[16] Augmented reality systems involving the overlay of manipulable

digital holograms on a real-life scene (such as 3D CT data in the operating room) may help improve surgical technique.[17] Finally, 3D printing of CT data after segmentation has gained increasing traction for CHD patients. Such models can be used not only for preoperative planning but also virtual simulated surgery on the printed physical specimens.[18]

In addition to enhancing anatomic rendering, postprocessing tools can also be used to generate novel physiologic information from existing cardiac CT data sets. For example, fractional flow reserve derived from coronary CTA (CT-FFR), based on computational fluid dynamics modeling (approved by the US Food and Drug Administration) or machine learning approaches (experimental), is now in routine use for interrogating the hemodynamic significance of coronary artery stenoses analogous to invasive FFR. In the CHD context, CT-FFR seems promising for evaluating the physiologic consequences of anomalous coronary arteries although is not currently approved for this indication.[19] Another typical limitation of CT in CHD is the lack of flow information, which is usually derived noninvasively from echocardiography and phase contrast MR imaging. Recently, 4D flow CT was described, simulating flow measurements from cardiac CT data with close correlation to 4D phase contrast MR imaging measurements.[20] Although this technique is thus promising for a "one-stop shop" CHD CT combining anatomy, function, and flow in one examination, it still remains in investigational stages.

IMAGING PROTOCOLS

CT protocols in CHD optimally require individualized tailoring to best address the specific clinical questions of interest for a given patient's unique anatomy and physiology.[11] Nonetheless, for surgically corrected adult CHD (ACHD), a similar protocol can suffice in most cases if more intensive physician oversight is not possible. For thoracic indications, a sample protocol (after scout topograms) consists first of a non-contrast ECG-triggered/gated calcium scoring scan spanning from approximately 1 cm below to the carina through the apex of the heart. The field-of-view can be extended through the aortic arch to cover all relevant segmental anatomy.[10] Alternatively, the non-contrast acquisition can be omitted in younger patients for whom radiation concerns outweigh the likelihood of coronary artery disease, and assessment of calcifications and hyperattenuating surgical material is not necessary.

Next, an ECG-triggered/gated arterial phase acquisition extending from above the aortic arch through the heart is performed. This is typically accomplished with a bolus-tracking technique, placing a region of interest (ROI) in the ascending thoracic aorta after acquiring a monitoring slice and automatically scanning 4 to 5 seconds after a threshold Hounsfield unit (HU) attenuation (eg, 100–150 HU) is reached. Alternatively, some institutions may prefer a test bolus technique in which a small amount of contrast is first injected before to monitor the attenuation in the ROI with time and then select the optimal delay for peak vascular enhancement in the diagnostic acquisition; while more controlled, this method adds to contrast dose and time.[10,21] The descending aorta may be preferred for placement of the ROI given that it is more likely to be identified with altered anatomy (eg, right aortic arch) and visible on a range of potential monitoring slice selections.[10] If cardiac function analysis is desired, radiation pulsing should be sufficient throughout the cardiac cycle to visualize the ventricles in end-systole and end-diastole for postprocessing purposes (including "padding" if in prospective mode to extend the acquisition window).[11]

Finally, a non-gated delayed venous scan covering the same anatomy can be performed for better assessment of the systemic veins and other venous structures. Although usually optional unless otherwise clinically warranted, such an acquisition, typically performed 75 to 90 seconds after contrast injection, is critical in the setting of single ventricle physiology post-Fontan in whom there will be heterogeneous opacification of the superior and inferior cavopulmonary anastomosis pathways in the arterial phase in the absence of simultaneous upper and lower extremity IV injection. On the other hand, the Fontan circuit will appear homogeneous on delayed imaging, allowing confirmation of patency or identification of thrombi.[9]

CHD contrast injection protocols should similarly be tailored when possible. However, in general, for corrected ACHD, a typical biphasic injection protocol would consist of 60 to 100 mL of contrast administered at rate of at least 4 to 5 mL/second, followed by a saline flush of 30 to 40 mL, sufficing for most indications.[10] A triphasic injection protocol may alternatively be considered, administering a mix of iodine and saline in the added second phase (eg, 20% and 80%, respectively), between the pure contrast and saline flush phases, to provide differential opacification of the left and right heart, which can be useful for quantification purposes.[21]

On the other hand, achieving optimal contrast opacification in neonates and young children with uncorrected CHD can be especially challenging and merits special consideration. In general, suggested total contrast and fluid (contrast plus saline) limits for a diagnostic CT are 2 mL/kg and 10 mL/kg, respectively. The goal is to achieve injection duration (typically 15–25 seconds) sufficient for all steps of the scan (monitoring, moving the CT table, breath-hold if needed, diagnostic acquisition). Thus, although contrast (2 mL/kg up to 100–150 mL) followed by a saline chaser (generally 1 mL/kg up to 40 mL) is administered as in adults, the rate of administration is decreased (eg, to as low as 0.8–1 mL/second) or the contrast diluted (eg, 50% contrast/50% saline) via the power injector to achieve the desired injection duration, rather than working from a predetermined injection rate (eg, 4–5 mL/second).[22] Moreover, unlike in adults, a foot rather than arm IV is often preferred especially in children under 5 kg. This can help mitigate otherwise common superior vena cava (SVC) streak artifact, which in turn can obscure adjacent small structures (such as right PA branches).[9,22]

In addition, if feasible, for young pediatric patients, manual scan triggering (rather than automated triggering after reaching a threshold HU) during bolus tracking with real-time physician oversight may be preferred due to anatomic complexity and more variable enhancement pattern depending on the CHD lesion. There is also greater potential for misplacement of the ROI by an inexperienced operator or premature automated triggering due to ROI translation off the structure of interest in the setting of rapid cardiorespiratory rates and propensity for patient motion. Placement of a mid-cardiac monitoring slice allowing qualitative visualization of enhancement over time in the cardiac chambers and descending aorta is an appropriate starting place for most CHD lesions.[11]

IMAGING FINDINGS: UNREPAIRED CONGENITAL HEART DISEASE

The major strengths of cardiac CT in unrepaired CHD center on the assessment of the extracardiac vasculature. Although the intracardiac anatomy is usually adequately characterized by echocardiography, particularly in neonates and young children with more optimal acoustic windows, a systematic approach using segmental analysis is nonetheless recommended to ensure all findings are appreciated.[22] Herein, the examples of unrepaired CHD involving the aorta, pulmonary arteries, systemic and pulmonary veins, coronary arteries, valves, and pericardium are presented.

Aortic Anomalies

Coarctation

Aortic coarctation is characterized by an obstructive, fibromuscular shelf-like narrowing near the region of the ductus arteriosus (either preductal or postductal) and/or tubular arch hypoplasia (**Fig. 1**). It is thought to result from disordered aortic arch development along with altered blood flow.[23,24] Coarctation is among the most common CHD, accounting for 6% to 8% of all lesions, and may be associated with other defects, most commonly bicuspid aortic valve. With severe obstruction, patients may present with symptoms of marked systemic hypoperfusion after physiologic closure of the ductus arteriosus, whereas mild disease may remain undetected into adulthood or manifest late with hypertension.[23] Rarely, there may be complete lack of continuity between the aortic arch and descending aorta, a condition known as interrupted aortic arch, which can be considered on the spectrum of extreme coarctation.[22] CT is effective for diagnosing and characterizing the coarctation for pretreatment planning purposes, demonstrating the extent of any collaterals, providing accurate aortic measurements, and identifying associated anomalies.[23]

Aortic arch anomalies and vascular rings
A wide variety of aortic arch anomalies may arise secondary to abnormal formation or involution of branchial arches during the development. These may occur in isolation or in association with other CHD or chromosomal abnormalities and can be asymptomatic or present with difficulty breathing or swallowing depending on the lesion.[24–26] The normal aortic arch is left-sided, giving rise to the brachiocephalic, left common carotid, and left subclavian arteries. Normal variants include a common origin of the brachiocephalic and left common carotid arteries or a direct origin of the left vertebral artery off the arch. The most common

left aortic arch anomaly is an aberrant right subclavian artery, which may or may not arise from a dilated origin known as a diverticulum of Kommerell (**Fig. 2**). Other rarer left arch anomalies include an isolated subclavian artery with no connection to the arch and a left circumflex aorta in which the descending aorta crosses midline. A right-sided aortic arch occurs in approximately one in 1000 individuals with subtypes including mirror image branching (symmetric to the normal left arch but on the opposite side), aberrant left subclavian artery (ALSA) that may or may not arise from a diverticulum of Kommerell, isolated subclavian artery, and right circumflex aorta (where the descending aorta crosses to the left). Additional arch variants include a double aortic arch with or without partial or complete atresia of either arch and the rare persistent fifth (double lumen) aortic arch.[24–26]

In evaluating aortic arch anomalies, it is important to recognize the presence of a vascular ring in which vessels (or their atretic remnants) encircle the trachea and esophagus, causing compression of the airways and/or esophagus.[26] The most common complete vascular rings are the right aortic arch with ALSA and left ligamentum arteriosum and the double aortic arch, accounting for 90% of cases.[22,24] CT well depicts any arch anomalies and any associated mass effect on surrounding structures and can also provide accurate size measurements. Of note, however, atretic portions of vessels along with the ductus arteriosus/ligamentum arteriosum, which contribute to the complete of vascular rings, may not opacify or be visible on CT (or other imaging), and thus their presence can only be inferred by the arch pattern and relationship to nearby anatomy (**Fig. 3**).[26]

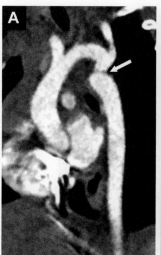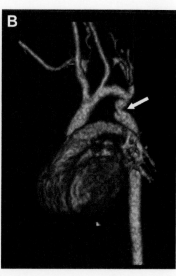

Fig. 1. Aortic coarctation in a 7-month-old boy. (*A*) Oblique sagittal and (*B*) 3D reformatted images from a CT angiogram of the chest show a focal shelf-like narrowing (*arrows*) of the juxtaductal thoracic aorta, consistent with coarctation.

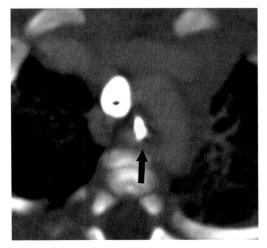

Fig. 2. Left aortic arch with aberrant right subclavian artery in a 29-day-old girl. Oblique axial MIP-reformatted image from a CT angiogram of the chest shows the aberrant right subclavian artery (*arrow*) coursing posterior to the esophagus, which contains a hyperattenuating enteric tube. There is no associated diverticulum of Kommerell.

Patent ductus arteriosus

Patent ductus arteriosus (PDA) refers to a persistent communication between the descending thoracic aorta and PA secondary to lack of normal closure of the fetal ductus arteriosus. It is a relatively common CHD, accounting for 5% to 10% of cases. PDA may be isolated or occur in association with other cardiac anomalies, in which case it is essential remain open to allow the mixing of oxygenated with deoxygenated blood.[22] CT can be helpful for delineating a complex PDA with tortuosity, particularly in preparation for PDA closure or stent placement to preserve patency (**Fig. 4**).[24]

Pulmonary Artery Anomalies

Congenital PA anomalies result from abnormal PA development, most commonly in association with CHD or syndromes such as Williams and Alagille (**Fig. 5**).[24,27] PA stenosis most often occurs at the level of pulmonary valve related to abnormal bulbus cordis formation during the fifth week of gestation but may occur above or below the valve or involve peripheral PA branches. Idiopathic PA dilation also may rarely occur, possibly in association with connective tissue disease.[27]

Conotruncal malformations

The CHD most commonly associated with PA anomalies is the class of disorders known as the conotruncal malformations, characterized by abnormal ventriculo-arterial alignments and connections. Of these, the prototype conotruncal malformation is TOF consisting of four main components: pulmonary outflow tract obstruction, right ventricular (RV) hypertrophy, malaligned subaortic ventricular septal defect (VSD), and overriding aorta.[28] TOF is thought to be caused embryologically by an abnormal relationship of the conal septum relative to the ventricular endocardial cushion. It is relatively common, comprising 5% to 10% of all CHD, and is the most common etiology of cyanotic CHD. PA stenosis is a fundamental component of the disorder and may be valvular, subvalvular, or supravalvular or involve peripheral PA branches (**Fig. 6**).[24,27,28]

In actuality, TOF has a heterogeneous phenotype including two distinct subtypes beyond the conventional form: TOF with absent pulmonary valve (TOF/APV) and TOF with pulmonary atresia (TOF/PA). In TOF/APV, a malformed or completely

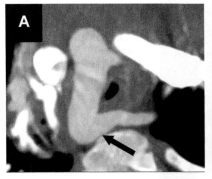

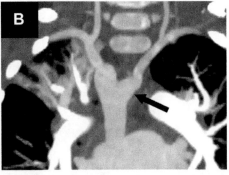

Fig. 3. Right aortic arch with aberrant left subclavian artery arising from a diverticulum of Kommerell in a 1-year-old boy. (*A*) Oblique axial and (*B*) oblique coronal maximum intensity projection (MIP)-reformatted images from an ECG-synchronized, high-pitch helical CT angiogram of the chest show a right aortic with aberrant left subclavian artery arising from a diverticulum of Kommerell (*arrows*), with associated effacement of the esophagus and mild tracheal narrowing. This loose vascular ring is completed by a left ligamentum arteriosum, which is not visible by CT.

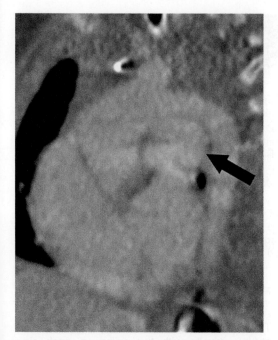

Fig. 4. Patent ductus arteriosus (PDA) in a 54-day-old boy. Oblique sagittal reformatted image from a routine contrast-enhanced chest CT shows a large, tortuous PDA (*arrow*) arising from the descending aorta.

APV results in severe pulmonic regurgitation (PR) with resultant marked PA dilation and secondary tracheobronchial compression (**Fig. 7**). In TOF/PA, the pulmonary valve is atretic, and major aortopulmonary collaterals (MAPCAs) and/or a PDA supply the PAs[22,27,28] (**Fig. 8**). CT is well-equipped in characterizing these complex anomalies and other rarer conotruncal malformations such as truncus arteriosus (abnormal division of the aorta and PAs), transposition of the great arteries (TGA) (main PA and aorta arising from the left and right ventricles, respectively), and double outlet right ventricle (both main PA and aorta arising from the right ventricle by 50% or more circumference).[22,27]

Pulmonary sling

Left PA sling is a rare anomaly characterized by an aberrant left PA origin from the right PA, attributed to abnormal development of the sixth pulmonary arch (**Fig. 9**). The anomalous left PA courses between the trachea and esophagus with associated compression, resulting in symptoms such as stridor usually in the first year of life. Concomitant abnormal tracheal bronchial branching occurs in most cases, usually with a low-set carina, distal tracheal stenosis, and bridging bronchus straddling the mediastinum from its left main bronchus origin and supplying the right middle and lower lobes. The right upper lobe bronchus may be absent or atretic, or there may be an accessory right upper lobe tracheal bronchus. CT is adept at characterizing these vascular and airway anomalies along with any associated CHD that occurs nearly one-third of patients.[24,27]

Systemic Veins

Left superior vena cava

A left SVC is the most frequent congenital thoracic venous anomaly. It is observed in up to 0.5% of normal individuals but in up to 10% of CHD patients and in up to 70% of cases of heterotaxy syndrome (ambiguous situs of the chest and abdomen).[22,24] Usually, the left SVC drains to the coronary sinus without clinical consequence. Uncommonly, it may drain directly to the left atrium, causing a left-to-right shunt that remains, however, generally physiologically insignificant (**Fig. 10**). A normal right-sided SVC typically is still present, with a bridging vein between the SVCs in 25% to 35% of cases.[22] Although a left SVC may be incidental, it is well-demonstrated by CT and should

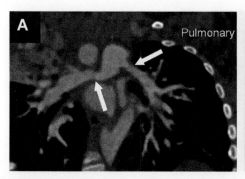
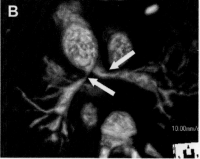

Fig. 5. Pulmonary artery stenosis in a 22-month-old boy with Alagille syndrome. (*A*) Curved planar and (*B*) 3D (posterior perspective) reformatted images from a high-pitch helical CT angiogram of the chest show bilateral proximal pulmonary arterial stenoses (*arrows*).

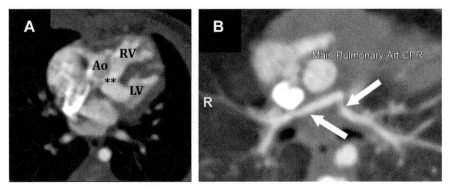

Fig. 6. Tetralogy of Fallot (conventional) in a 4-day-old boy. (A) Axial image from a high-pitch helical CT angiogram of the chest shows a dilated and hypertrophied right ventricle (RV), communicating with the left ventricle (LV) via a malalignment ventricular septal defect (*asterisks*) with an overriding aorta (Ao). (B) Curved planar reformatted image shows diffusely hypoplastic central pulmonary arteries (*arrows*), which remained in communication with the right ventricular outflow tract, augmented by a patent ductus arteriosus (not shown).

be noted particularly in preparation for any future cardiothoracic intervention (eg, pacemaker, superior cavopulmonary anastomosis).[22,24]

Interrupted inferior vena cava

Interrupted inferior vena cava (IVC) is an infrequent developmental anomaly in which the IVC terminates at the level of the hepatic veins due to focal agenesis or fusion between the hepatic and prerenal IVC segments in embryogenesis.[29] The infrahepatic IVC often continues as the azygos vein or another tributary such as the hemiazygos (**Fig. 11**). Although the anomaly may be isolated, it occurs in up to 2% of patients with CHD and a majority (>80%) of patients with left atrial isomerism (bilateral left-sided heterotaxy pattern). Like a left-sided SVC, interrupted IVC is generally incidental but can present procedural challenges (eg, during right heart catheterization, IVC filter placement, and Fontan creation) and thus should be reported on CT, where it is effectively depicted.[24,29]

Pulmonary Veins

Anomalous pulmonary venous return

The pulmonary veins normally drain to the left atrium, usually with two veins on each side, although there is substantial normal variation.[30] In partial anomalous pulmonary venous return (PAPVR), one or more (but not all) pulmonary veins drain to a location other than the left atrium, usually the right atrium or SVC, and often in association with a sinus venous atrial septal defect (**Fig. 12**). Although a single isolated PAPVR is usually asymptomatic and clinically insignificant, patients with greater numbers of anomalous pulmonary veins may develop cardiomegaly and exercise intolerance.[24,30] Scimitar syndrome is a type of PAPVR in which all pulmonary veins from one lung (generally the right) drain to the IVC near the diaphragm, in association with a hypoplastic right PA and lung and often a right lung sequestration with aortic arterial supply.[30] Finally, in rare total anomalous pulmonary venous return (TAPVR), all pulmonary veins drain to a location other than

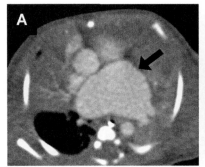
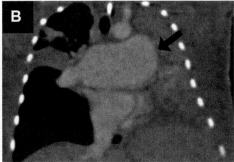

Fig. 7. Tetralogy of Fallot with absent pulmonary valve in a 2-day-old girl. (A) Axial and (B) coronal-reformatted images from a CT angiogram of the chest shows marked dilation of the central pulmonary arteries (*arrows*) with resultant airway compression and downstream atelectasis in the lungs.

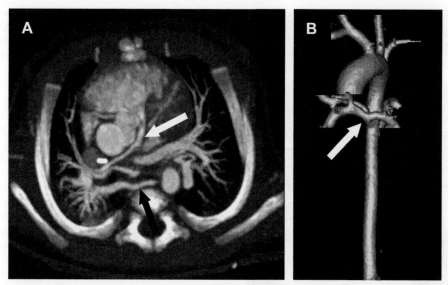

Fig. 8. Tetralogy of Fallot with pulmonary atresia and major aortopulmonary collaterals (MAPCAs) in a 33-day-old girl. (A) Oblique axial maximum intensity projection (MIP)-reformatted image from a high-pitch helical CT angiogram of the chest shows confluent but hypoplastic central pulmonary arteries (*white arrow*). There are multiple MAPCAs (*black arrow*—example), arising from the descending aorta. (B) 3D reformatted image better displays the multiple descending aortic MAPCAs (*arrow*).

the left atrium with three types: supracardiac (SVC or innominate veins), cardiac (right atrium or coronary sinus), or infracardiac (hepatic or portal veins). The severity of TAPVR depends on the site of anomalous drainage and the degree of venous obstruction.[22]

CT is an excellent modality for demonstrating aberrant pulmonary venous drainage, the presence and extent of any pulmonary venous stenosis and occlusion, and associated anomalies.[24,30]

Moreover, normal anatomic variants may also be relevant before intervention. In particular, pulmonary venous CT mapping is commonly obtained before radiofrequency ablation for atrial fibrillation.[30]

Coronary Arteries

Coronary anomalies
Coronary anomalies are anatomic variants in which one or more coronaries arise from an unusual

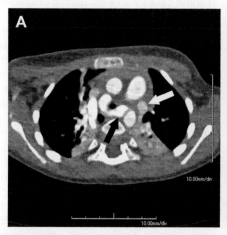
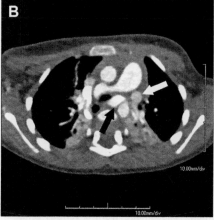

Fig. 9. Pulmonary sling in a 13-month-old girl. Contiguous axial high-pitch helical chest CT angiogram images from (A) cranial to (B) caudal show the left pulmonary artery (*black arrows*) arising from the right pulmonary artery and coursing between the trachea and esophagus, consistent with a left pulmonary artery sling. A left superior vena cava (*white arrows*) is incidentally also present.

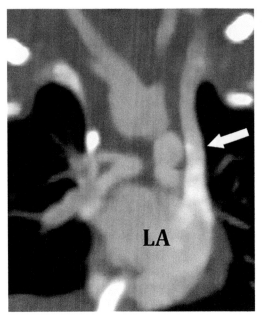

Fig. 10. Left superior vena cava (SVC) with left atrial connection in a 12-day-old girl. Oblique coronal MIP-reformatted image from a high-pitch helical CT angiogram of the chest shows the left SVC (*arrow*) draining directly to the left atrium (LA).

location, either from an atypical sinus of Valsalva or outside the aorta. While occurring in less than 1% of the general population, they arise in up to 5% to 10% of CHD patients.[22,24] Anomalous coronaries arising from the aorta may have an interarterial, pre-pulmonic, retroaortic, or transseptal (subpulmonic) course.[22,31] Unlike other variants in this group that in general lack hemodynamic significance (benign),

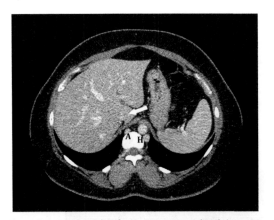

Fig. 11. Interrupted inferior vena cava (IVC) in a 38-year-old woman. Axial image from a venous phase CT of the chest and abdomen shows absence of the IVC in expected location (*arrow*) below the level of the hepatic veins. The azygos (A) and hemiazygos (H) veins are prominent.

an interarterial (malignant) course (between the aorta and main PA) poses an increased risk of sudden cardiac especially when high-risk features (slit-like ostium, acute takeoff angle, intramural segment in the aortic wall) are present (**Fig. 13**).[31] The rare anomalous origin of the left coronary artery from the PA or Bland–White–Garland syndrome, accounting for less than 0.5% of CHD, usually presents in infancy with acute myocardial ischemia and heart failure.[22,24]

Cardiac CT is in general the most reliable noninvasive modality for evaluating coronary anomalies, including their origin, course, and termination and any associated collateralization. Moreover, even normal variants may be of clinical significance in anticipation of surgery or other intervention.[24] For example, retroaortic and prepulmonic coronaries are at risk to be injured during aortic valve intervention and median sternotomy, respectively, without appropriate planning.[22]

Cardiac Valves

Congenital cardiac valve anomalies, caused by abnormal semilunar (aortic/pulmonic) or atrioventricular (mitral/tricuspid) valve development, are relatively common and found in more than half of patients with CHD.[32,33] *Bicuspid aortic valve*, resulting from variable coronary cusp fusion (right/left > right/noncoronary > left/noncoronary), is in fact the most frequent form of CHD, occurring up to 2% of the general population and associated with premature aortic valve disease and aortopathy (**Fig. 14**).[33] *Mitral valve prolapse*, characterized by abnormal displacement of a thickened mitral valve leaflet into the left atrium during systolic, occurs in up to 3% of individuals, in some cases with a congenital or syndromic (eg, Marfan) component; sequelae may include valvular regurgitation, congestive heart failure, and arrhythmia.[32] Congenital valvular *pulmonic stenosis*, occurring in 1 per 2000 live births, is usually an isolated defect but also often arises in conotruncal malformations; although it can be relatively asymptomatic, it may lead to such complications as right atrial and ventricular enlargement, RV hypertrophy, and PA dilation.[33] *Ebstein anomaly* is a rare but unique malformation arising in approximately 1 in 20,000 live births and characterized by dysplasia and downward displacement of the septal and posterior tricuspid valve leaflets into the RV cavity with resultant tricuspid regurgitation. Its severity is correlated with the degree of leaflet displacement, which causes much of the right ventricle to become contiguous with a dilated right atrium with a so-called "atrialized" appearance (**Fig. 15**).[4,33]

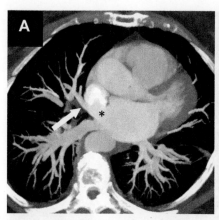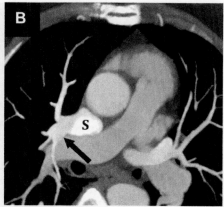

Fig. 12. Partial anomalous pulmonary venous return (PAPVR) and sinus venosus atrial septal defect in a 69-year-old woman. (*A*) Oblique axial maximum intensity projection (MIP)-reformatted image from a high-pitch helical, ECG-synchronized CT angiogram of the chest demonstrates anomalous drainage of the right middle pulmonary vein (*arrow*) to the level of a sinus venosus defect (*asterisk*). (*B*) More cranial axial MIP-reformatted chest CT angiogram shows that the right upper lobe pulmonary vein (*arrow*) also drains anomalously to the superior vena cava (S).

The noninvasive quantitative assessment of valvular stenosis and regurgitation is most directly performed with echocardiography or cardiac MR imaging. Nonetheless, cardiac CT is a useful adjunct in characterizing valve morphology, including the presence of calcification or implanted material and secondary manifestations of congenital valve lesions such as aortic or pulmonary arterial enlargement.[4,32,33] In addition, valvular stenosis and regurgitation may be indirectly evaluated, respectively, through systolic planimetric measurement of valve area and calculation of stroke volume difference based on quantified ventricular volumes (assuming only a single significantly regurgitant valve and absent shunts).[4,28,34] Moreover, CT has become standard of care before transcatheter valve interventions.[34] Further information on CT for imaging cardiac valves and planning for transcatheter procedures is detailed separately in this Special Issue.

Pericardium

Congenital absence of the pericardium
Congenital absence of the pericardium (CAP) is caused by failure of growth and fusion of the lateral pleuropericardial folds, most often on the left. It is a rare disease, with an incidence of less than one in 10,000, associated with other cardiac or lung anomalies in up to 50% of patients. Although most cases are discovered incidentally and asymptomatic, CAP may present with nonspecific symptoms such as non-exertional chest pain and poses increased risk of atrioventricular strangulation and coronary compression in partial defects.[35,36] The lack of visualization of the pericardium on cross-sectional imaging is not reliable for diagnosing CAP.[36] Nonetheless, CT is adept at demonstrating the characteristics indirect findings of the disorder. For left-sided lesions, these include lung tissue interposed between the ascending aorta and main PA and between the heart and diaphragm and displacement of the heart to the left with horizontal elongation of the cardiac chambers and posterior orientation of the left ventricular apex (**Fig. 16**).[35,36] Features of right-sided defects include lung interposed between the SVC and ascending aorta or ascending aorta and right PA and lateral bulging of the right heart border.[36] Any associated cardiopulmonary complications and anomalies may also be readily assessed.[35,36]

Fig. 13. Anomalous right coronary artery (RCA) in a 57-year-old woman. Oblique axial-reformatted image from a retrospectively ECG-gated cardiac CT angiogram shows an anomalous RCA (*arrow*) arising from the left coronary cusp with an interarterial course between the aorta and main pulmonary artery. High-risk features are present with a slight-like orifice, acute takeoff angle, and narrowing of the interarterial segment.

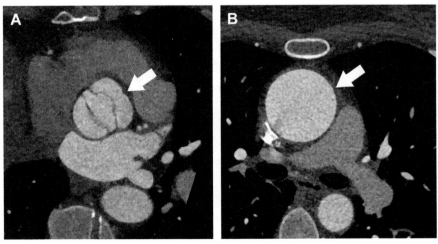

Fig. 14. Bicuspid aortic valve with secondary aortopathy in a 44-year-old woman. (*A*) Short-axis reformatted image from a prospectively ECG-triggered cardiac CT angiogram in systole demonstrates fusion between the left and right coronary cusps (*arrow*). (*B*) Axial image at the level of the main pulmonary artery shows an associated ascending aortic aneurysm (*arrow*).

IMAGING FINDINGS: REPAIRED CONGENITAL HEART DISEASE

Although the workup of clinically significant unrepaired CHD is often limited to specialized centers, even the general radiologist is likely to encounter repaired CHD on CT given increasing patient survival rates.[9,37,38] The potential indications for cardiac CT in repaired CHD are multifold including routine surveillance, assessment of postoperative complications, and planning for repeat intervention. In this section, examples in each of these categories for the more commonly encountered CHD at CT (TOF, TGA, and single ventricle disease) are presented after an overview of general considerations.

Repaired Congenital Heart Disease: General Considerations

Early postoperative complications

Infection and bleeding are among the early postoperative complications common to many types of CHD repair. The latter may manifest as a mediastinal hematoma or active arterial extravasation and the former as a rim-enhancing collection or pseudoaneurysm (**Fig. 17**).[28,38] Injury to the coronary arteries or other structures intentionally or iatrogenically manipulated (eg, aortic cannulation sites) is also possible.[38] CT is an excellent modality for expediently and confidently detecting such abnormalities to guide further management.[28]

Implanted material

Foreign material and devices are frequently implanted in CHD patients, including vascular shunts (typically from aorta or branch to PA), conduits (rerouting extracardiac blood flow), baffles (rerouting intracardiac blood flow), and stents.[22,24,28] All of these may be subject to frank thrombosis, stenosis, dystrophic/degenerative wall calcification, infection, or nearby seroma or hematoma formation (**Fig. 18**).[24] CT is especially well-suited for assessing the integrity of these materials,

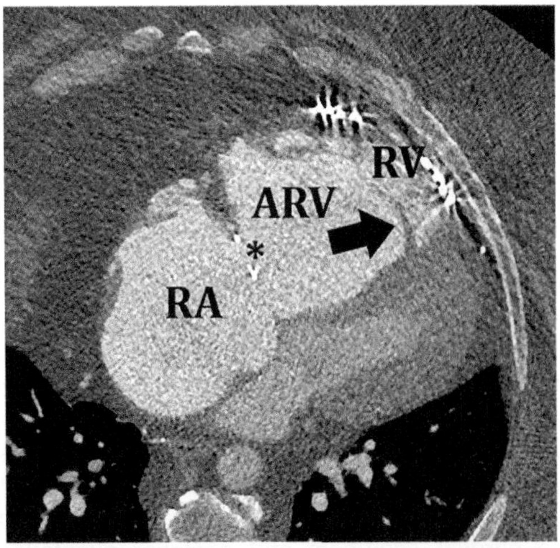

Fig. 15. Ebstein anomaly in a 48-year-old man. Axial image from a prospectively ECG-triggered cardiac CT angiogram shows marked apical displacement of the septal tricuspid valve leaflets (*arrow*) with dilation of the right atrium (RA) and atrialized right ventricle (ARV). The true right ventricle (RV) is small. Partially imaged postsurgical changes of prior tricuspid annuloplasty are present (*asterisk*).

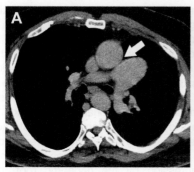
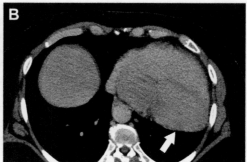

Fig. 16. Congenital absence of the pericardium in a 60-year-old man. (*A*) Axial contrast-enhanced chest CT image shows lung (*arrow*) interposed between the ascending aorta and main pulmonary artery. (*B*) More caudal axial image shows displacement of the heart into the left chest, horizontal elongation of the cardiac chambers, and posterior orientation of the left ventricular apex (*arrow*).

especially stents, which are prone to extensive ferromagnetic artifacts on MR imaging.[24,28]

Repaired Congenital Heart Disease: Selected Entities

Tetralogy of Fallot

TOF is among the most common repaired CHD encountered at cross-sectional imaging. Patients require regular monitoring post-repair to gauge RV size and function and the degree of PR to help determine when pulmonic valve replacement is necessary in combination with other clinical data. MR imaging is, in general, the preferred modality for such surveillance. However, ECG-gated cardiac CT provides a ready substitute when MR imaging is contraindicated (eg, incompatible pacemaker), suboptimal, or otherwise unfeasible,

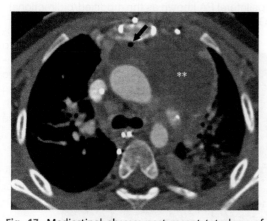

Fig. 17. Mediastinal abscess post recent tetralogy of Fallot repair in a 4-year-old girl with fever and concern for infection. Axial image from a contrast-enhanced chest CT shows a large, partially rim-enhancing mediastinal fluid collection (*asterisks*) located deep to the median sternotomy and containing a focus of gas (*arrows*), compatible with abscess.

allowing analogous postprocessing of a functional series in end-diastole and end-systole to quantify ventricular volumes, function, and myocardial mass if desired; this method is widely applicable and not limited to repaired TOF (**Fig. 19**). Although PR cannot be directly measured, it can be estimated as the stroke volume difference divided by RV stroke volume in the absence of other significant valvular regurgitation or shunts and may be qualitatively observed as incomplete coaptation of valve leaflets in diastole. If pulmonic valve replacement is indicated, CT can also be used for preprocedural planning for either a transcatheter approach or redo sternotomy.[28,37,38]

Other non-immediate sequelae post-TOF repair may include residual or recurrent PA stenosis, VSD patch leak, and gradually increasing aortic dilation. The older, transannular patch approach to relieve RV outflow tract (RVOT) obstruction is more likely to result in RVOT dyskinesia and aneurysm/pseudoaneurysm formation, whereas the newer valve-sparing technique is associated with less PR but greater likelihood of residual RVOT obstruction. In TOF/PA, valved RV-PA conduits are commonly placed but undergo calcific degeneration with subsequent stenosis over time. On the other hand, TOF/APV patients may develop residual or recurrent PA aneurysms that require reduction plasty.[28,37,38] All of these complicating features can be readily evaluated at CT.

Transposition of the great arteries

Dextro-TGA (d-TGA) is characterized by atrioventricular concordance (right and left atria aligned with right and left ventricular, respectively) but ventriculoarterial discordance (right and left ventricles arising from aorta and main PA, respectively). There are two main approaches to repair: atrial switch and arterial switch. In the atrial switch operation, an intra-atrial baffle is used to direct SVC and IVC

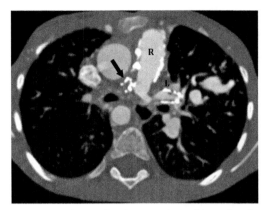

Fig. 18. Stent complications post-tetralogy of Fallot repair in a 9-year-old boy. Axial imaged from a high-pitch helical CT angiogram of the chest shows occlusion of a right pulmonary artery (RPA) stent (*arrow*) and the downstream RPA. Peripheral calcifications and nonocclusive thrombus/intimal hyperplasia are also noted in the patient's right ventricular to pulmonary artery conduit (R) and left pulmonary artery stent (L).

flow to the left ventricle and pulmonary venous flow to the right, using either prosthetic material (Mustard procedure) or atrial septal tissue (Senning procedure) (**Fig. 20**). In the arterial switch operation (Jatene procedure), the aortic and PA root are transected at a supravalvular level and connected, respectively, to the distal main PA and aorta, to become the neopulmonic and neoaortic root, with accompanying coronary artery reimplantation. This is usually accompanied by a LeCompte maneuver consisting of translocation of the PAs anterior to the neoaortic root/transected pulmonic trunk (**Fig. 21**). Although the arterial switch is now preferred to the atrial switch due to better long-

term survival rates, there are many patients still living post-atrial switch who will thus be encountered at imaging.[37–39]

Complications of atrial switch include RV enlargement and dysfunction due to volume and pressure overload, baffle stenosis, baffle leakage, and systemic and pulmonary venous obstruction. Complications of arterial switch include left ventricular dysfunction, stenosis at anastomotic sites (most commonly at the neopulmonic root-distal PA attachment), PA stenosis secondary to compression by the neoaortic root, neoaortic root dilation, supravalvular aortic stenosis, and coronary ostial stenosis.[37,38] All of these abnormalities can be readily observed at CT. Moreover, as in TOF, if MR imaging is not possible, an ECG-gated acquisition can be used to facilitate quantification of ventricular volumetry, mass, and function and indirect interrogation of valvular regurgitation (most commonly neoaortic).[28,39]

Single ventricle palliation

Single ventricle disease connotes a broad spectrum of disorders in which effectively only one ventricle has adequate size and function to pump blood to the body, and biventricular physiology cannot be achieved.[40] The final common pathway to (palliative) repair in these patients is creation of a total cavopulmonary connection/Fontan circuit to redirect systemic venous blood directly to the lungs, allowing the monoventricle to pump oxygenated pulmonary venous blood to the systemic circulation. This is achieved in two major steps. First, SVC flow is redirected to the PA, usually with an end to side anastomosis between the transected distal SVC and undivided ipsilateral PA known as the modified/bidirectional Glenn procedure. Second, IVC flow is redirected

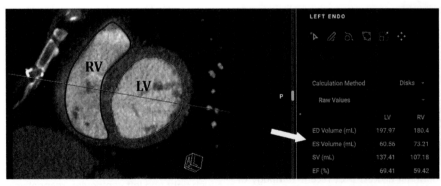

Fig. 19. Quantification of ventricular volumetry by cardiac CT in a 57-year-old woman with repaired complex congenital heart disease (atrioventricular septal defect) who could not tolerate cardiac MR imaging. Sample end-diastolic short-axis reformatted image from a retrospectively ECG-gated cardiac CT angiogram shows endocardial contours drawn for the right ventricle (RV) and left ventricle (LV). After tracing end-diastolic and end-systolic endocardial contours for all slices covering the ventricles, the software can calculate ventricular volume and function data (*arrow*).

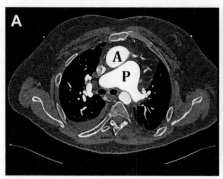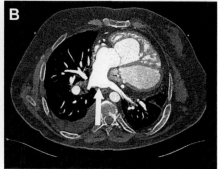

Fig. 20. Dextro-transposition of the great arteries (d-TGA) post-atrial switch in a 45-year-old man. (*A*) Axial image from a retrospectively ECG-gated cardiac CT angiogram shows the ascending aorta (A) abnormally located anterior and to the right of the main pulmonary artery (P), consistent with d-TGA. (*B*) More caudal axial image shows patent pulmonary veins baffled to the right-sided atrium (*arrow*).

to the PA, either via a lateral/intra-atrial tunnel within the right atrium (lateral tunnel/intracardiac Fontan) or extracardiac conduit (extracardiac Fontan) (**Fig. 22**).[37,38,40]

Complications of post-total cavopulmonary connection may include thrombosis, occlusion, stenosis, dilation, or leak of the Fontan circuit, pulmonary arterial stenosis or thromboembolism, atrial dilation, and ventricular dysfunction, all of which may be readily assessed at cardiac CT (**Fig. 23**).[37,38,40] As previously noted, with a sole upper or lower extremity IV injection, apparent filling defects in the Fontan circulation should not be mistaken for clot on arterial phase CT due to incomplete upper and lower systemic venous mixing if not confirmed on delayed imaging.[9] Patients are also prone to developing venovenous collaterals

secondary to systemic venous hypertension and aortopulmonary collaterals due to chronic hypoxia.[37,38] Although the total collateral burden is not numerically quantifiable by CT (unlike on MR imaging), large collaterals can be coil embolized and thus should be noted.[40]

Pulmonary arteriovenous malformations (PAVMs) are also common in Fontan patients and attributed to IVC blood bypassing the liver before reaching the lungs. The portions of the lung that are subsequently not bathed in "hepatic factors" tend to develop PAVMs. In addition, extra-cardiovascular complications of the Fontan circulation are frequent secondary to lymphatic and hepatic congestion and may include lymphatic dilation, pleural and

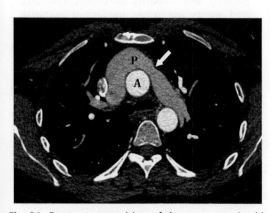

Fig. 21. Dextro-transposition of the great arteries (d-TGA) post-arterial switch with LeCompte maneuver in a 36-year-old woman. Axial image from a prospective ECG-triggered cardiac CT angiogram shows the pulmonary arteries (P) draped anterior to the ascending aorta (A), consistent with the LeCompte maneuver. There is mild narrowing of the left pulmonary artery origin (*arrow*).

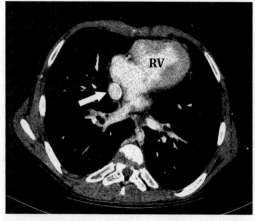

Fig. 22. Hypoplastic left heart syndrome post-Fontan in a 14-year-old man. Axial image from a dual-energy CT angiogram of the chest shows a patent extracardiac Fontan conduit (*arrow*) and a single morphologic right ventricle (RV). Note the high vascular attenuation despite acquisition in a delayed venous phase (to ensure homogeneous Fontan opacification) facilitated by the use of 40 keV monoenergetic reconstruction.

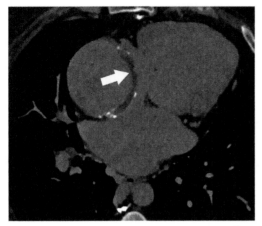

Fig. 23. Fontan thrombus post single ventricle palliation (right atrial appendage to pulmonary artery anastomosis) in a 53-year-old man. Oblique axial-reformatted image from a high-pitch helical, ECG-synchronized CT angiogram of the chest in the delayed venous phase shows a peripheral, partially calcified low attenuation filling defect (*arrow*) in the Fontan tunnel, compatible with chronic nonocclusive thrombus.

pericardial effusions, plastic bronchitis (airway casts), ascites, bowel and mesenteric edema, hepatomegaly, and cirrhosis with subsequent risk for hepatocellular carcinoma.[37,38] Although some of these abnormalities (eg, involving lymphatics and liver) are better characterized by MR imaging, CT including abdominal imaging where appropriate provides a ready alternative.[40]

SUMMARY

Cardiac CT now has an established and central role in the diagnosis, preoperative management, and postoperative monitoring of CHD patients from birth to adulthood. In unrepaired CHD, the primary goals of CT are to delineate the extracardiac vasculature, coronaries, and noncardiac structures, often achievable with rapid, free-breathing acquisitions. In repaired CHD, CT provides an excellent depiction of postoperative complications and a ready alternative to MR imaging for surveillance of ventricular size and function and vessel diameters when ECG-gating is used. Modern CT scanners incorporating dual-source detectors, multispectral imaging, and other innovations, along with robust postprocessing tools, have helped continue to expand the reach of CT in CHD while overcoming traditional downsides of radiation and iodinated contrast exposure. With continued technological advances, the utility of CT in CHD throughout the lifespan should only continue to grow.

CLINICS CARE POINTS

- Although echocardiography remains the first-line modality in congenital heart disease (CHD) imaging, cardiac computed tomography (CT) is superior for assessing the coronaries, extracardiac vasculature, lungs, and airways in the unrepaired patient.

- Dual-source CT technology allowing high-pitch acquisitions with rapid speed has helped overcome traditional sedation requirements in neonates and young children with CHD. Dual-energy CT with low kilovoltage monoenergetic reformats can help increase vascular attenuation.

- Achieving adequate contrast opacification can be challenging in CHD due to unique patient anatomy and physiology. In neonates, the injection rate should generally be tailored to achieve injection duration of 15 to 25 seconds and foot intravenous consider reducing superior vena cava (SVC) streak artifact. In the Fontan patient, delayed imaging is advised so as not to mistake upper/lower body venous mixing for thrombus.

- The segmental anatomic approach provides a framework for systematically reporting the vast number of potential congenital cardiovascular malformations. Although some entities such as a left SVC or benign anomalous coronary have little or no specific clinical consequence in isolation, they may alter the approach for certain procedures and thus should be noted.

- In repaired CHD, CT excels in evaluating the patency and integrity of shunts, conduits, and stents are other implanted material. When electrocardiographic-gating is used, CT facilitates the quantification of ventricular volumes, mass, and function, providing an alternative to cardiac MR imaging when contraindicated, suboptimal, or unfeasible.

DISCLOSURE

The author has nothing to disclose.

REFERENCES

1. Hoffman JI, Kaplan S. The incidence of congenital heart disease. J Am Coll Cardiol 2002;39(12):1890–900.
2. Liu A, Diller GP, Moons P, et al. Changing epidemiology of congenital heart disease: effect on outcomes and quality of care in adults. Nat Rev Cardiol 2023;20(2):126–37.

3. Mutluer FO, Çeliker A. General concepts in adult congenital heart disease. Balkan Med J 2018; 35(1):18–29.

4. Zucker EJ, Koning JL, Lee EY. Cyanotic congenital heart disease: essential primer for the practicing radiologist. Radiol Clin North Am 2017;55(4):693–716.

5. Watts JR Jr, Sonavane SK, Singh SP, et al. Pictorial review of multidetector CT imaging of the preoperative evaluation of congenital heart disease. Curr Probl Diagn Radiol 2013;42(2):40–56.

6. Lapierre C, Déry J, Guérin R, et al. Segmental approach to imaging of congenital heart disease. Radiographics 2010;30(2):397–411.

7. Gaca AM, Jaggers JJ, Dudley LT, et al. Repair of congenital heart disease: a primer–part 1. Radiology 2008;247(3):617–31.

8. Gaca AM, Jaggers JJ, Dudley LT, et al. Repair of congenital heart disease: a primer–part 2. Radiology 2008;248(1):44–60.

9. DiGeorge NW, El-Ali AM, White AM, et al. Pediatric cardiac CT and MRI: considerations for the general radiologist. AJR Am J Roentgenol 2020;215(6): 1464–73.

10. Pulerwitz TC, Khalique OK, Leb J, et al. Optimizing cardiac CT protocols for comprehensive acquisition prior to percutaneous MV and TV repair/replacement. JACC Cardiovasc Imaging 2020;13(3):836–50.

11. Hong SH, Goo HW, Maeda E, et al. Asian Society of Cardiovascular Imaging Congenital Heart Disease Study Group. User-friendly vendor-specific guideline for pediatric cardiothoracic computed tomography provided by the Asian Society of Cardiovascular Imaging Congenital Heart Disease Study Group: part 1. Imaging techniques. Korean J Radiol 2019; 20(2):190–204.

12. Rachoin JS, Wolfe Y, Patel S, et al. Contrast associated nephropathy after intravenous administration: what is the magnitude of the problem? Ren Fail 2021;43(1):1311–21.

13. Rapp JB, Biko DM, Siegel MJ. Dual-energy CT for pediatric thoracic imaging: A review. AJR Am J Roentgenol 2023. https://doi.org/10.2214/AJR.23. 29244.

14. Cao J, Bache S, Schwartz FR, et al. Pediatric applications of photon-counting detector CT. AJR Am J Roentgenol 2023;220(4):580–9.

15. Leng S, Bruesewitz M, Tao S, et al. Photon-counting detector CT: system design and clinical applications of an emerging technology. Radiographics 2019; 39(3):729–43.

16. Layden N, Brassil C, Jha N, et al. Cinematic versus volume rendered imaging for the depiction of complex congenital heart disease. J Med Imaging Radiat Oncol 2023. https://doi.org/10.1111/1754-9485.13518.

17. Dallas-Orr D, Penev Y, Schultz R, et al. Comparing computed tomography-derived augmented reality holograms to a standard picture archiving and communication systems viewer for presurgical planning: feasibility study. JMIR Perioper Med 2020;3(2):e18367.

18. Anwar S, Singh GK, Miller J, et al. 3D printing is a transformative technology in congenital heart disease. JACC Basic Transl Sci 2018;3(2):294–312.

19. Chen J, Wetzel LH, Pope KL, et al. FFRCT: current status. AJR Am J Roentgenol 2021;216(3):640–8.

20. Lantz J, Gupta V, Henriksson L, et al. Intracardiac flow at 4D CT: comparison with 4D flow MRI. Radiology 2018;289(1):51–8.

21. Scholtz JE, Ghoshhajra B. Advances in cardiac CT contrast injection and acquisition protocols. Cardiovasc Diagn Ther 2017;7(5):439–51.

22. Chan FP, Hanneman K. Computed tomography and magnetic resonance imaging in neonates with congenital cardiovascular disease. Semin Ultrasound CT MR 2015;36(2):146–60.

23. Karaosmanoglu AD, Khawaja RD, Onur MR, et al. CT and MRI of aortic coarctation: pre- and postsurgical findings. AJR Am J Roentgenol 2015;204(3):W224–33.

24. Goo HW, Siripornpitak S, Chen SJ, et al. Pediatric cardiothoracic CT guideline provided by the Asian Society of Cardiovascular Imaging Congenital Heart Disease Study Group: part 2. Contemporary clinical applications. Korean J Radiol 2021;22(8):1397–415.

25. Priya S, Thomas R, Nagpal P, et al. Congenital anomalies of the aortic arch. Cardiovasc Diagn Ther 2018;8(Suppl 1):S26–44.

26. Hanneman K, Newman B, Chan F. Congenital variants and anomalies of the aortic arch. Radiographics 2017;37(1):32–51.

27. Zucker EJ. Cross-sectional imaging of congenital pulmonary artery anomalies. Int J Cardiovasc Imaging 2019;35(8):1535–48.

28. Zucker EJ. Computed tomography in tetralogy of Fallot: pre- and postoperative imaging evaluation. Pediatr Radiol 2022;52(13):2485–97.

29. Kılıçkıran Avcı B, Karadağ B, Tüzün H, et al. Unilateral absence of the left pulmonary artery with patent ductus arteriosus and interrupted inferior vena cava. Turk Kardiyol Dern Ars 2014;42(5):399–402.

30. Dyer KT, Hlavacek AM, Meinel FG, et al. Imaging in congenital pulmonary vein anomalies: the role of computed tomography. Pediatr Radiol 2014;44(9): 1158–68 [quiz: 1155–7].

31. Pandey NN, Sinha M, Sharma A, et al. Anomalies of coronary artery origin: evaluation on multidetector CT angiography. Clin Imaging 2019;57:87–98.

32. Lincoln J, Garg V. Etiology of valvular heart disease-genetic and developmental origins. Circ J 2014;78(8): 1801–7.

33. Saef JM, Ghobrial J. Valvular heart disease in congenital heart disease: a narrative review. Cardiovasc Diagn Ther 2021;11(3):818–39.

34. Patel KP, Vandermolen S, Herrey AS, et al. Cardiac computed tomography: application in valvular

heart disease. Front Cardiovasc Med 2022;9: 849540.

35. Nikam R, Rapp J, Kandula A, et al. Congenital absence of pericardium. Ann Pediatr Cardiol 2020; 13(4):373–4.

36. Newman B. Congenital absence of the pericardium: pearls and pitfalls. Semin Ultrasound CT MR 2022; 43(1):47–50.

37. Raptis DA, Bhalla S. Current status of cardiac CT in adult congenital heart disease. Semin Roentgenol 2020;55(3):230–40.

38. Ojha V, Ganga KP, Kumar S. Computed tomography imaging of complications in postoperative cyanotic congenital heart diseases - a pictorial essay. Clin Imaging 2021;71:1–12.

39. Canan A, Ashwath R, Agarwal PP, et al. Multimodality imaging of transposition of the great Arteries. Radiographics 2021;41(2):338–60.

40. Ciliberti P, Ciancarella P, Bruno P, et al. Cardiac imaging in patients after Fontan palliation: which test and when? Front Pediatr 2022;10:87674.

Role of Radiology in Assessment of Postoperative Complications of Heart Transplantation

Mangun K. Randhawa, MD[a], Sadia Sultana, MD[a], Matthew T. Stib, MD[b], Prashant Nagpal, MD[c], Eriberto Michel, MD[d], Sandeep Hedgire, MD[a],*

KEYWORDS

- Orthotopic heart transplant • Cardiac transplant • Cardiac computed tomography
- Cardiac MR imaging

KEY POINTS

- Imaging is crucial in identifying periprocedural complications, allograft failure, rejection, biopsy complications, vasculopathy, and posttransplant infections and malignancies.
- Both rejection and coronary allograft vasculopathy (CAV) are cardiac-specific complications.
- Due to potential delays in developing clinical signs of critical posttransplant complications, such as allograft rejection and CAV, imaging plays an important role in their early detection, thereby affecting patient outcomes.
- MR imaging is particularly effective in identifying pericardial anomalies and signs of allograft rejection because it not only offers functional data but also myocardial tissue characterization.

INTRODUCTION

Heart transplantation is the treatment of choice for patients with end-stage heart failure. Recent advancements in surgical techniques and postoperative management, including immunosuppressant medication, have led to significant improvements in posttransplant survival rates. The median life expectancy after a heart transplant, conditional on surviving 1 year, has now been extended to 13 years.[1]

Orthotopic heart transplantation (OHT) is currently the primary method performed by transplant surgeons. The initial heart transplant used the simpler biatrial technique.[1] However, the bicaval method[2] is now preferred in most centers due to its anatomic advantages and fewer complications.

Despite the considerable success of heart transplantation, there are a variety of potential posttransplantation complications, including rejection, infections, graft failure, vasculopathy, and drug toxicity. Imaging technologies have revolutionized the approach to posttransplant complications, enabling early detection and management.[3–5]

This review article focuses on various imaging techniques and findings of posttransplant complications, emphasizing the importance of early detection for enhanced clinical decision-making.

NORMAL ANATOMY AND IMAGING TECHNIQUE

OHT results in unique anatomic changes. The biatrial technique involves preserving the native left and the right atrial cuff to which the donor's left

[a] Division of Cardiovascular Imaging, Department of Radiology, Massachusetts General Hospital, Boston, MA, USA; [b] Division of Cardiothoracic Imaging, Department of Radiology, Mayo Clinic Hospital, Phoenix, AZ, USA; [c] Division of Cardiovascular Imaging, Department of Radiology, University of Wisconsin-Madison, Madison, WI, USA; [d] Division of Cardiac Surgery, Department of Surgery, Massachusetts General Hospital, Boston, MA, USA

* Corresponding author. Massachusetts General Hospital, 175 Cambridge Street, Boston, MA 02114.
E-mail address: hedgire.sandeep@mgh.harvard.edu

Radiol Clin N Am 62 (2024) 453–471
https://doi.org/10.1016/j.rcl.2023.12.002
0033-8389/24/© 2023 Elsevier Inc. All rights reserved.

and right atria are sutured. This technique was initially preferred because it led to decreased allograft ischemic time.[6] However, the biatrial technique creates a larger common atrial chamber, identifiable by an enlarged atrial chamber on imaging, and can lead to atrial arrhythmias and tricuspid valve dysfunction.[7] In contrast, the bicaval technique (**Figs. 1** and **2**) is a modification of the biatrial method and involves preserving the recipient's right atrium. It aligns the recipient's superior and inferior vena cava with the donor heart's corresponding veins, thereby reducing complications such as tricuspid regurgitation and right atrial enlargement.[8] Radiological studies posttransplantation are vital for assessing anatomic integrity and identifying postoperative complications.

IMAGING MODALITIES

Various imaging techniques are available to accurately assess the potential range of postoperative complications following cardiac transplantation.

Table 1 showcases these modalities, each offering unique advantages and limitations in the detection and assessment of posttransplant complications.

Computed Tomography

The computed tomography (CT) acquisition protocol (**Table 2**) after cardiac transplantation is governed by the underlying clinical question.

Heart rate optimization is more difficult in patients following heart transplantation because cardiac allografts commonly experience resting tachycardia due to surgical denervation. The sinoatrial (SA node) node automaticity is no longer suppressed by the vagus nerve, and higher heart rates result in increased cardiac motion artifact. Additionally, the use of beta-blockers, calcium channel blockers, and ivabradine has less effect on heart transplant recipients, further complicating heart rate optimization.[9]

Advancements in CT technology, including the use of dual-source CT, have shortened acquisition time, significantly increasing the success of imaging heart transplant patients with high or variable heart rates. Some scanners can even acquire the entire heart in one heartbeat or in half a second time.[10] Vasodilating premedication also aids in evaluation of the coronary arteries.

CT can be performed with, with and without, or just without intravenous (IV) contrast. Noncontrast images, particularly in acute settings or for the first-time imaging of cardiac allograft, are useful to identify any hyperdense surgical material and to differentiate from hyperdense extraluminal hemorrhage. Intravenous iodinated contrast is used in the absence of severe kidney dysfunction or life-threatening contrast allergy (premedication regimens are available to reduce anaphylaxis risk). Contrast timing optimization is critical to ensure optimal visualization of the cardiac chambers.

Biphasic injections are standard in most of the tertiary centers, whereby the initial injection of contrast is immediately followed by a second injection, which is mixed with saline (usually 80:20 saline: contrast mix) in a proportion planned as per the clinical indication. If evaluation of the right heart chambers or pulmonary arterial anastomosis is required, the second injection can be a mix of 50:50 saline:contrast.[11] An alternative is to use an additional 30 cc of contrast to lengthen the bolus without using the second mixed bolus. The latter regime is used when dual rule out (coronary/cardiac pathology as well as pulmonary embolism) is required; however, the field of view will need to be extended cranially to the level of the clavicles to include the entire pulmonary arterial

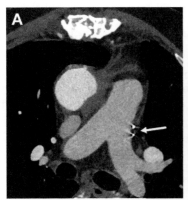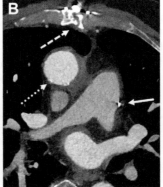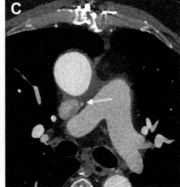

Fig. 1. Postcontrast axial CT Thorax of bicaval anastomotic technique showing median sternotomy (*dashed arrow*), (*B*) surgical material (demonstrated as focal high densities) used for aortic anastomosis (*dotted arrow*), (*A, B*) MPA anastomosis (*solid arrows*) and (*C*) SVC anastomosis (*double arrow*).

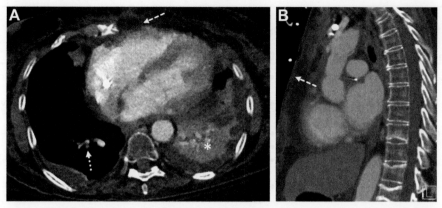

Fig. 2. (*A*) Axial and (*B*) sagittal postcontrast CT Thorax of a 50-year-old patient requiring partial sternal and rib resection (*dashed arrows*) to accommodate the cardiac allograft. Additionally, there is left lower lobe collapse (*asterisk*). Incidental subsegmental pulmonary embolism (*dotted arrow*) in the right lower lobe was also noted.

Table 1
Advantages and disadvantages of imaging modalities in diagnosing postheart transplant complications

Modality	Advantages	Disadvantages
Cardiac CT including CCTA	• Noninvasive • Both anatomic and functional assessment • CCTA offers high sensitivity and negative predictive value for detection of CAV • Relatively quick and widespread availability	• Exposure to radiation • Possible overestimation of the degree of vascular stenosis • Premedication may be needed before coronary imaging • Use of iodinated contrast material
Cardiac MR imaging (CMR)	• No ionizing radiation • Structural and functional assessment possible • Tissue characterization is possible using a variety of sequences such as T2 weighted imaging, T1 and T2 mapping, and delayed gadolinium enhancement	• Limited by patient factors • Relatively time-consuming and expensive • No coronary luminal assessment
Echocardiography	• Noninvasive • No radiation exposure • Relatively inexpensive and readily available • Both functional and structural assessment	• Inability to detect early coronary disease • Acoustic window dependent • Relatively limited in comprehensive assessment
ICA	• Gold standard for assessing coronary artery anatomy • Ability to concurrently diagnosis and treat lesions during the same procedure	• Invasive • Risk of procedural complications
PET-CT	• Myocardial perfusion imaging (MPI) • Evaluation of allograft related occult infection • Evaluation of malignancy	• Exposure to radiation • Limited availability

Table 2
Protocol for cardiac computed tomography acquisition

Parameter	Description
Premedication	• Nitroglycerine sublingual or patch if coronary arteries are to be evaluated • Use of rate controlling medication: often ineffective in heart transplant patients
Contrast material	• Intravenous Iodinated contrast - Biphasic injection • Injection 1: Contrast (rate 5.5–6.5 mL/s) • Injection 2: Saline and contrast mixed (80% + 20%) or 50% + 50% if right heart opacification is desired • Additional 30 mL contrast can be alternative to 50–50 mix of contrast and saline • Injection 3: Saline flash
Cardiac Gating	• Prospective ECG gating (diastolic or systolic imaging according to institutional protocols) • Retrospective gating: if ventricular function (both qualitative and quantitative) or valvular assessment is needed • High pitch Helical mode
Phases to be acquired	• Tailored for specific clinical question • Noncontrast, postcontrast arterial phase and delayed phase (usually 1 min delay)
Triggering	• Region of interest (ROI) placed over the ascending aorta • Either bolus triggering or timed bolus/test bolus can be used
Field of view	• Cardiac only CT: Carina to diaphragm • Cardiac and pulmonary arterial study: Extension to FOV to clavicles
Image acquisition	• Volumetric data spiral acquisition with overlap (retrospective gated) or step and shoot (prospective gated)
Postprocessing/image reconstruction	• Slice thickness 1 mm or less. • Axial, sagittal, and coronal reconstructions • Curved MPR for coronary arteries and aorta • 3D volume rendered images of the heart or blood vessels if needed

tree. Techniques such as bolus tracking and the newer dual-region-of-interest trackers ensure optimal contrast timing and visualization of the desired anatomy. A test bolus can also be used when cardiac output is a concern or in pediatric settings to minimize trigger delay.

The latest CT scanner generations, capable of scans within a single heartbeat,[10] highlight the need for exact timing of the contrast medium bolus. With the introduction of low tube voltage examinations and iterative reconstruction techniques, the radiation dose on the new generation scanners has further reduced.[12] Photon counting scanners are the latest CT imaging technology, resulting in even faster acquisition with higher spatial resolution and lower radiation doses.[13]

Electrocardiogram (ECG) gating is essential in minimizing cardiac motion artifacts and can be performed either prospectively or retrospectively. The advantage of prospectively triggered scans is a lower radiation dose but at the cost of more potential artifacts due to the "step and shoot" method.[14] This can be overcome if the scanner can acquire images in a single heartbeat or use retrospective gating where helical acquisition with overlap is possible.[15] Retrospective acquisition enables qualitative and quantitative function assessment.[16] Cardiac function can also be assessed with prospectively acquired images when padding is used.[17] High-pitch helical cardiac CT is an alternative to reduce radiation dose; however, a heart rate of less than 60 beats per minute is a requirement in this technique.[18]

In cases where acute hemorrhage is suspected, special attention should be given to carefully considering the number of phases needed (eg, noncontrast, arterial, and delayed phases). The presence of a contrast blush on the arterial phase with changes in the morphology of the blush or an increase in volume on the delayed phase is

Table 3
Protocol for cardiac MR imaging acquisition

Parameter	Description
Localizers	Axial, coronal and sagittal
Planning of chamber views and cine images for wall motion and quantitative functional assessment of LV and RV	Planes: 2ch, 3ch, 4ch cine and short axis cine stack Technique: SSFP cine or GRE
Parametric mapping	T1 mapping and T2 mapping Normal range is scanner specific, therefore, will require setting up the scanner specific range of normal values
T2-weighted imaging (using single or dual echo)	To assess myocardial edema, short axis acquisition in multiple slices
[a]MR angiogram of aorta and pulmonary artery and pulmonary veins	MRA aorta can be performed with or without contrast. Accurate bolus timing is required for optimal contrast opacification of the vessel of interest
Late gadolinium imaging	10 min after administration of intravenous gadolinium
Extra-long TI in long axis planes	Can be added for suspected intracardiac thrombus
Postcontrast T1 mapping	Useful for assessment of ECV
[a]Myocardial tagging	Can be used for assessing pericardial adhesions in constrictive pericarditis
[a]Real-time imaging in inspiration and expiration	Ventricular interdependence in constrictive pericarditis

[a] Optional: can be performed if clinically indicated.

indicative of active hemorrhage in the immediate postoperative period. Additionally, delayed acquisition can be helpful in distinguishing mixing artifacts from left atrial appendage thrombus.[19]

Cardiac Magnetic Resonance Imaging

Although the first modalities of choice to evaluate cardiac function and coronary artery disease are echocardiography and coronary CT angiography (CCTA), respectively, in recent years, cardiac magnetic resonance (CMR) imaging has become an increasingly important tool in evaluating allograft rejection.[20] In addition to providing a dynamic functional assessment of the right and left ventricles and the valves, the promising aspect of CMR is the ability of tissue characterization through T2-weighted sequences, T1 mapping, T2 mapping, and postcontrast late gadolinium imaging.[21,22] The relevant protocols are mentioned in **Table 3**.

Typical CMR sequences include steady-state free precession (SSFP) or gradient echo (GRE) cine imaging for dynamic visualization as well as quantitative right and left ventricular volumes and functions. Segmented cine SSFP images are acquired using a breath-hold technique in short axis (cine stack of multiple slices from base to apex) and long axis views (2-chamber, 3-chamber,

4-chamber, left ventricular outflow tract [LVOT]). Additionally, phase contrast flow can be used for valvular assessment or shunt analysis. Myocardial tagging and real-time cine imaging can aid in evaluating constrictive pericarditis in conjunction with pericardial enhancement on late gadolinium imaging.

For allograft rejection, T2-weighted sequences, T1 and T2 mapping, as well as late gadolinium-enhancement sequences are valuable. Dual echo T2 sequence can be used as a qualitative assessment of myocardial edema. Because there may be subjective bias in qualitative T2-weighted images, quantitative assessment with T2 mapping sequences can be applied where global edema from acute inflammation can be calculated. Marie and colleagues found a high level of correlation between increased values of T_2 (≥ 56 ms) and detection of biopsy-proven moderate acute rejections ($\geq$ International Society for Heart and Lung Transplantation [ISHLT] grade 2) with statistically significant sensitivity, 89% and specificity, 70%.[23,24]

However, T2 elevation can be due to several different etiologies, such as myocarditis, acute ischemia or infarction, acute inflammation such as sarcoidosis, or autoimmune conditions and drug reactions. However, in appropriate clinical settings where rejection is the main consideration due to a constellation of other clinical parameters, T2 elevation may be extremely helpful in deciding to titrate immunosuppression therapy.

There is a strong correlation between CMR findings and positive endomyocardial biopsy (EMB) when the combination of right ventricular end-diastolic volume index and myocardial edema values (T2 relaxation time) was used with excellent sensitivity, 93%; specificity, 78%; positive predictive value, 52%; and negative predictive valve, 98%.[25,26]

The importance of using T_1 mapping in diagnosing cardiac allograft rejection noninvasively is increasingly understood. Imran and colleagues found that the sensitivity, specificity, and negative predictive value were 93%, 79%, and 99%, respectively.[27,28] T_1 mapping detects interstitial edema and fibrosis, which are important markers of acute and chronic rejection.[27] Extracellular volume (ECV) is calculated using precontrast and postcontrast T1 mapping of myocardium and blood pool with concurrent hematocrit of the patient considered. Vermes and colleagues found that the sensitivity, specificity, and diagnosis accuracy for basal ECV: (cut off 32%) were 86%, 85%, and 85%, respectively.[29]

In addition to diagnostic value, there have been studies showing prognostic implications of CMR. Quantification of ECV and T2 mapping in heart transplant patients were independently associated with cardiac and noncardiac outcomes in a study by Chaikriangkrai and colleagues.[30,31]

The addition of late gadolinium-enhancement images for tissue characterization provides a superior confidence level in diagnosing allograft rejection.[32] Myocardial enhancement may involve both right and left ventricles.[33] Diffuse subepicardial enhancement has also been seen in the context of allograft failure.[34] Moreover, a subendocardial pattern of enhancement might help to exclude the isolated or concomitant presence of myocardial infarction from obstructive coronary artery disease.

Echocardiography

Echocardiography plays a pivotal role in the postoperative assessment of heart transplant recipients. It is used intraoperatively and immediately posttransplant to detect early graft dysfunction.[35] Notably, echocardiography can detect changes in both systolic and diastolic function, with diastolic parameters being more sensitive to acute cellular rejection (ACR). Techniques such as tissue Doppler imaging and 2-dimensional speckle tracking echocardiography further enhance the detection of myocardial deformation and rejection.[36]

Invasive Coronary Angiography

Invasive coronary angiography (ICA) remains the primary method for monitoring coronary arteries for cardiac allograft vasculopathy (CAV) after heart transplantation.[37] Due to the denervation of the donor's heart during procurement, these patients may not experience ischemic pain, especially shortly after transplantation. Coupled with the aggressive progression of CAV, this necessitates regular angiographic assessments. Despite its importance, angiography has limitations, especially in detecting early stage disease and microvascular lesions. In contrast, intravascular ultrasound (IVUS) is emerging as a superior tool for CAV screening.[38] IVUS offers visualization of the vessel wall, proving more sensitive than angiography in detecting early CAV.[39]

Positron Emission Tomography

PET is frequently used in heart transplantation to detect complications such as CAV.[40] PET, using tracers such as N-13 ammonia, O-15 water, or Rb-82, can measure both resting and peak myocardial blood flow and myocardial flow reserve (MFR), allowing for the detection of abnormalities in both the epicardial vessels and the microvasculature.[41] Global MFR, as assessed by PET, is a potent predictor of cardiac events.[42] Studies have shown that PET's flow quantification aligns well with invasive coronary flow measures, offering high sensitivity and specificity for CAV detection.[43]

Radiography

Although not as detailed or specific as other advanced imaging techniques, chest radiographs can noninvasively provide quick and valuable insights into potential posttransplant complications such as identifying signs of pulmonary edema, pleural effusions, or infection.[44] Additionally, they can be used to monitor the position of surgical hardware, such as sternal wires or pacing leads, and to detect any postoperative pneumothorax.

POST HEART TRANSPLANT COMPLICATIONS

Multiple complications can develop following heart transplantation. These complications, which are enlisted in **Table 4**, can be broadly categorized based on their cause into periprocedural (procedure-related), allograft-related, and immunosuppression-related complications.

Periprocedural Complications

Procedure-related complications in cardiac surgery can develop due to the transplant itself or

Table 4
Classification of post heart transplant complications based on etiology

Periprocedural (Procedure-related)	Allograft-related	Immunosuppression-related
• Bleeding	• Primary graft failure	• Drug toxicity
• Thrombosis	• Allograft rejection	• Opportunistic infections
• Infection	• CAV	• PTLD
• Pulmonary edema	• Valvular complications	• Malignancy
• Pericardial constriction	• Vascular complications	

the supportive procedures performed before or after surgery. OHT recipients are more prone to surgical wound complications compared with other patients. This heightened susceptibility can be attributed to various factors, including poor baseline health, immunosuppression, and the presence of life-support devices that have the potential to act as sources of infection.[45]

Perioperative bleeding and thrombosis

Bleeding is a known complication associated with periprocedural interventions and cardiac surgery that can occur at any time during the procedure or during the early postoperative period.

Following sternotomy, retrosternal hematomas and fluid collections can be expected.[46] Imaging findings (**Figs. 3** and **4**) include high attenuation (30–80 HU) on CT,[47] mediastinal widening in the case of mediastinal hemorrhage, and hemopericardium. During evaluation, it is imperative to carefully assess for active extravasation within the hematoma, which may present as a high-attenuation blush within the hematoma on contrast-enhanced CT. Differentiating this from a pseudoaneurysm is crucial, which typically seems as a contained, round, or oval collection with contrast enhancement, often

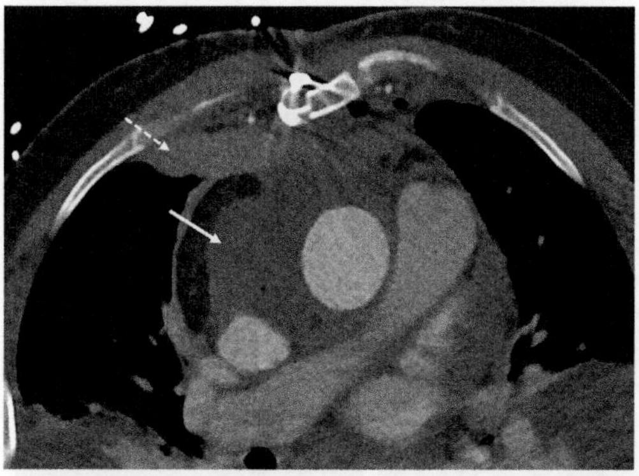

Fig. 3. Contrast-enhanced axial chest CT image showing a low attenuation periaortic fluid collection (*solid arrow*) as well as a retrosternal hyperdense collection consistent with a hematoma (dashed *arrow*) in a patient following an autologous OHT.

connected to a vessel. However, it is important to note that most fluid collections, including hematomas, tend to resolve within 6 to 8 weeks.

Strategies to prevent and manage hemorrhage encompass preoperative optimization, intraoperative monitoring, targeted hemostatic interventions, and postoperative care.[48,49] It should be noted that the use of prophylactic anticoagulants and antiplatelet medications to reduce thrombotic complications may increase the risk of perioperative bleeding.[50,51] Although there is increased thrombogenicity during the perioperative period,[52,53] balancing the use of these medications with the risk of complications is important.

Infections

Infectious complications are a common occurrence after cardiac surgery, affecting up to 20% of cases.[54] These represent the most frequent type of complication associated with cardiac transplants and can manifest at any stage during the postoperative period.[55]

The initial phase following transplantation is crucial and carries a high risk due to the extensive immunosuppression and the vulnerability of the transplant recipient.[56]

Throughout the posttransplant period, a predictable pattern of common pathogens responsible for these infections can be observed. Gram-negative bacteria, particularly *Escherichia coli* and *Pseudomonas aeruginosa*, are responsible for more than 50% of infections following heart transplantation, whereas gram-positive bacteria, notably *Staphylococcus* species, are isolated in around one-third of the cases.[21] The incidence of nosocomial and donor-derived infections is highest within the initial month after transplantation, followed by opportunistic infections that may stem from the reactivation of latent infections during the first 6 months.[55,57] In the early phase (first 30 days), the most frequent complications include wound infections and followed by pneumonia and urinary tract infections in the midphase (30–180 days). Typically, after the first year following transplantation, opportunistic infections become less common, and infections

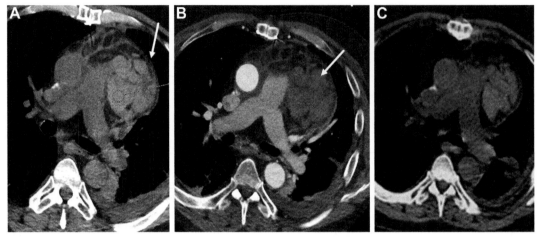

Fig. 4. (*A*, *B*) Axial CT Thorax 3 months posttransplantation demonstrates a middle mediastinal hematoma (*arrows*) adjacent to the main pulmonary artery. The patient was admitted for chest pain, with no recent interventions reported. (*A*) Noncontrast image showing hyperdense fluid (80 HU) consistent with hematoma. (*B*) No features of active contrast extravasation on arterial phase. (*C*) PET-CT without corresponding FDG avidity, excluding an infective process.

caused by pathogens in the community become more frequent among these patients.[58]

In heart transplant recipients, the cause of pneumonia varies over time. In the initial month following cardiac transplant, bacterial infections from hospital-acquired pathogens such as *Pseudomonas aeruginosa* and *Staphylococcus aureus* are common. From 1 to 6 months, opportunistic pathogens (such as *Pneumocystis jirovecii* and cytomegalovirus) emerge due to immunosuppression. After 6 months, community-acquired pathogens such as *Streptococcus pneumoniae* become prevalent.[58]

Mediastinitis is a rare but serious complication after heart transplantation, with an incidence reported to range from 2.5% to 7.5%.[59] Radiologically, mediastinitis can manifest as ill-defined mediastinal fat stranding, pneumomediastinum, or and/or rim-enhancing abscess (**Fig. 5**).[60] The presence of sternal dehiscence (see **Fig. 5**), particularly when accompanied by certain features, such as a sternal gap greater than 3 mm, substernal fluid or air, and abscess formation, are poor prognostic signs.[61] Radiography can be the first imaging modality to suggest mediastinitis when there are new changes in the alignment of the sternal wires. However, wire migration may not be present, and CT should be performed when there is high clinical suspicion, preferably with IV contrast.[62]

Allograft-related Complications

Cardiac allograft vasculopathy
CAV is a significant complication affecting the survival of heart transplant recipients, even though

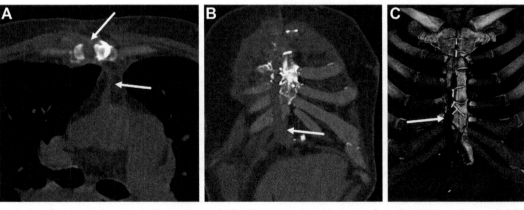

Fig. 5. (*A*, *B*) Axial and coronal CT images, and (*C*) volume-rendered images of mediastinitis and sternal dehiscence (*arrows*) in the early posttransplant period.

the incidence has declined since the early days of heart transplantation. The prevalence of CAV is reported to be 7.8% in the first year posttransplantation, increasing to 30% within 5 years and peaking at 50% within 10 years, according to the ISHLT registry.[29,63]

Unlike the conventional atherosclerotic process, CAV is thought to be immune-mediated, characterized by a rapid yet clinically silent progression. Research suggests that donor coronary artery endothelium expressing HLA-DR + stimulates recipient T cells, leading to a local immunologic response. Subsequent cytokine release in the coronary arteries of allografted hearts may influence smooth muscle cell proliferation and matrix accumulation.[64]

In contrast to traditional coronary atherosclerotic disease, which is predominantly focal and affects the proximal arteries, CAV exhibits both proximal eccentric disease and distal concentric narrowing of the coronary vessels. This results in a phenomenon known as "distal pruning."[65] The disease involving the proximal vessels is atherosclerotic in nature and inherited from the donor, whereas the more distal disease is immune-mediated and acquired by the recipient.[66,67]

Typically, ischemic graft failure results from extensive, diffuse intimal hyperplastic lesions that develop in allograft arteries and eventually impair luminal flow (Fig. 6). In terms of diagnosis, ICA has been considered the gold standard. However, coronary computed tomography angiography (CTA) has emerged as a promising noninvasive alternative, offering comparable accuracy, cost-effectiveness, and detailed anatomic information.[55] Notably, coronary artery calcium has been proposed as a potential marker for atherosclerotic heart disease in transplant recipients.[68] The lack of coronary artery calcification has been associated with a low prevalence of CAV.[69] Moreover, the combination of CT-myocardial perfusion imaging (MPI) and CTA has shown excellent diagnostic performance for early detection, offering a powerful noninvasive screening technique.[70]

Treatment strategies for CAV are primarily preventative. However, for nonobstructive disease, medical management with immunosuppressive, lipid-lowering agents, and antiplatelet drugs remains the mainstay of treatment.[71] Obstructive disease necessitates revascularization procedures, of which PCI is found to be the main technique.[72] Five-year mortality was found to be 17% on a meta-analysis by El-Andari and colleagues.[73] For advanced CAV not amenable to revascularization, medical management, and retransplantation are 2 viable options.[74] A retrospective cohort study involving more than 4500 participants from the ISHLT Registry found that overall long-term survival

is similar between persistent CAV treatment and retransplantation. However, retransplantation might improve survival in some cases, particularly in individuals with systolic dysfunction.[75]

Cardiac allograft rejection

Cardiac allograft rejection plays a pivotal role in determining the long-term prognosis of heart transplant recipients. It encompasses hyperacute, acute cellular, and acute antibody-mediated pathophysiologic processes. Notably, allograft rejection is responsible for approximately 12% of deaths occurring in the intermediate postoperative period.[76] The first year following heart transplantation carries the highest risk of allograft rejection, with peak incidences observed between weeks 2 and 12.[51,55,58]

The most prevalent form of rejection, affecting 20% to 40% of patients during the first year post-transplant, is acute cellular rejection (ACR).[58,77,78] In contrast, hyperacute allograft rejection occurs within the first few days after transplantation due to preformed recipient antibodies targeting antigens expressed on the donor vascular endothelium, mainly human leukocyte antigens.[78]

Acute antibody-mediated rejection, occurring in 10% to 20% of patients within the first year, is less frequent compared with ACR.[58,78,79] Because most patients remain asymptomatic in the early stages of rejection, frequent monitoring is essential during the early posttransplantation period.[79]

Unlike kidney and liver transplantation, heart transplant rejection has traditionally lacked clinically validated biomarkers for its identification. However, the advent of Food and Drug Administration-approved noninvasive surveillance tools such as AlloMap (CareDx, Brisbane, CA, USA) has shown promise in detecting signs of acute rejection (AR) in this patient population.[80] Despite this, EMB remains the current gold standard for the diagnosis and surveillance of rejection.[79,81] However, EMB carries certain risks, with complication rates ranging from 1% to 14%.[78,79,82]

Echocardiographic characteristics, such as increased wall thickness (caused by myocardial edema), left ventricular size, and ejection fraction, are not sufficiently sensitive for detecting rejection and cannot be solely relied on for screening.[82]

In recent research by Butler and colleagues, cardiac MR imaging demonstrated excellent sensitivity and negative predictive value for EMB-positive rejection (93% and 98%, respectively) when using parameters such as T2 prolongation and right ventricular end-diastolic volume index, thereby establishing its potential as a reliable noninvasive tool for detecting cardiac transplant rejection.[25] Cardiac MR imaging, the leading

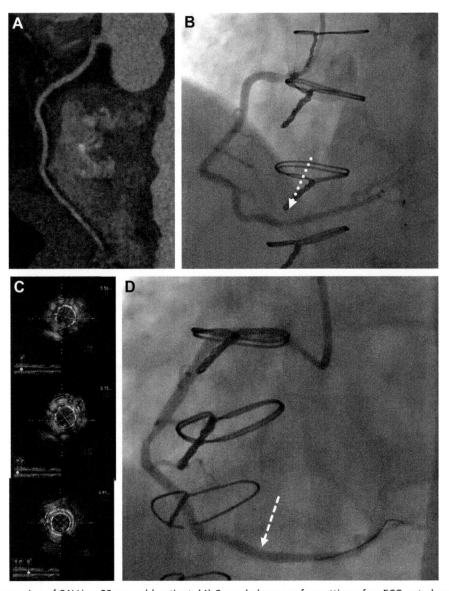

Fig. 6. Progression of CAV in a 28-year-old patient. (*A*) Curved planner reformatting of an ECG-gated coronary CT angiogram performed 1 year posttransplant reveals a normal right coronary artery. (*B*) An invasive angiogram performed a year later showed significant stenosis in the mid-right coronary artery (*dotted arrow*) due to progressive CAV. (*C*) Concurrent IVUS demonstrated increased intimal thickening and luminal constriction. (*D*) Resolution of RCA stenosis (*dashed arrow*) post-angioplasty.

noninvasive imaging modality to detect rejection, not only offers functional data akin to traditional echocardiography but also excels in myocardial tissue characterization, aiding in the detection of rejection signs such as T2 signal hyperintensity, increased left ventricular myocardial mass, and delayed myocardial contrast enhancement.[83]

An integrated CMR technique using T2 mapping and ECV (**Fig. 7**) quantification in heart transplant patients has shown high diagnostic accuracy (100%) for detecting AR and avoided the need for EMB in 63% of patients.[84] This approach may offer a noninvasive and effective means of monitoring allograft status and aiding in the timely detection of rejection episodes.

Primary graft failure

Primary graft failure, which accounts for 40.5% of fatalities within the first 30 days following transplantation, remains the most common cause of death in heart transplant recipients.[55] This condition is characterized by ventricular failure leading to hemodynamic compromise and cardiogenic shock, often necessitating the use of intravascular

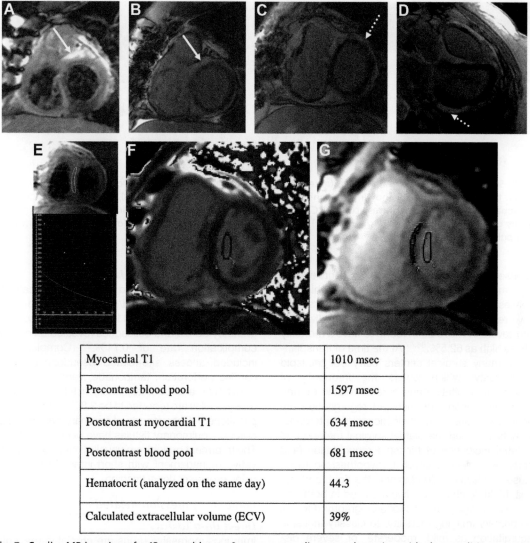

Myocardial T1	1010 msec
Precontrast blood pool	1597 msec
Postcontrast myocardial T1	634 msec
Postcontrast blood pool	681 msec
Hematocrit (analyzed on the same day)	44.3
Calculated extracellular volume (ECV)	39%

Fig. 7. Cardiac MR imaging of a 42-year-old man, 9 years postcardiac transplantation with abnormalities concerning for allograft rejection. (*A*) A basal short-axis image of double inversion recovery T2-sequence showing subepicardial hyperintensity, consistent with edema (*solid arrow*). (*B*) Corresponding circumferential subepicardial enhancement on LGE images at the same level (*solid arrow*). (*C*) Basal short-axis view and (*D*) 3-chamber view showing extensive circumferential subepicardial late gadolinium enhancement (dotted *arrows*) (*E*) T2 map at the midsegment in short-axis view displays T2 prolongation. (*F, G*) Precontrast and postcontrast T1 mapping, respectively, with regions of interest (ROI)s drawn in the myocardium and blood pool to calculate ECV, which was 39%.

inotropic drugs and circulatory assist devices.[77,85] Unfortunately, only half of the patients requiring extracorporeal membrane oxygenation during the initial week survive to discharge.[58] The pathophysiology of graft failure involves a complex interplay of technical, recipient, and donor factors, and as such, its precise mechanisms are not fully understood.[83] Radiographs and CT scans commonly reveal nonspecific signs of graft failure, such as pulmonary edema and pleural effusion (**Fig. 8**). Hemodynamic compromise is evident through low cardiac output, low cardiac index, and elevated filling pressures. Echocardiographic findings often show reduced right and left ventricular systolic function, with or without chamber dilation, along with frequent tricuspid regurgitation.

Valvular complications
The most frequent valvular problem following OHT, with a reported incidence of 19% to 84%,[86,87] is tricuspid regurgitation. Although many episodes of tricuspid regurgitation are minor and clinically

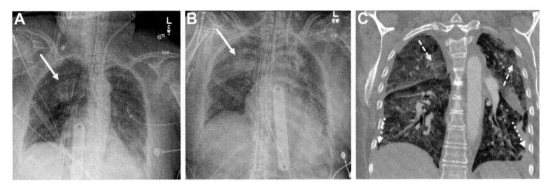

Fig. 8. Sequential plain chest radiographs (anterior-posterior projection) of a 60-year-old woman, 25 days post-cardiac transplantation. (*A, B*) Showing worsening perihilar opacification (solid *arrows*), indicative of progressive pulmonary edema. (*C*) Postcontrast coronal CT Thorax demonstrating diffuse interlobular septal thickening, patchy ground glass opacities (*dashed arrows*) and trace bilateral pleural effusions (*dotted arrows*) consistent with pulmonary edema.

inconsequential, about one-third of patients experience moderate-to-severe regurgitation, which increases morbidity and frequently necessitates valve replacement or repair. Untreated individuals with severe TR have been found to have a mortality rate as high as 62.5%.[86,87] At the time of transplantation, many surgical centers carry out tricuspid annuloplasty, which lowers the frequency of tricuspid regurgitation and cardiac-related mortality.[88] The reasons for tricuspid regurgitation are many. Compared with their bicaval counterparts, patients who had the biatrial surgical method had a higher incidence of tricuspid regurgitation (and mitral insufficiency), which is hypothesized to be caused by tissue redundancy in the right (and left) atria. Multiple characteristics are used in both cardiac MR imaging and echocardiography (**Fig. 9**), the primary imaging modality, to classify tricuspid regurgitation as mild, moderate, or severe disease.[89] Repetitive EMBs are another cause frequently stated in studies reporting a correlation between the number of EMBs performed and the incidence of substantial tricuspid regurgitation.[78]

Other cardiac and vascular complications

Posttransplant cardiac and vascular complications can be related to EMB and/or invasive coronary angiographies. A study of 2117 EMB on cardiac allografts by Saraia and colleagues revealed an overall complication rate of 0.71%.[68] Complications included access site-related pseudoaneurysms, cardiac perforation, tamponade, various forms of arrhythmia, and coronary artery fistulas. Coronary artery fistulas are reported to be 2.8% of those complications.[68] Case reports of coronary-cameral and coronary pulmonary fistulas have been reported.[69] The treatment options are usually limited to conservative management with short-interval follow-ups using cross-sectional imaging.

Immunosuppression Related

Direct drug toxicity

Immunosuppressive drugs are crucial in preventing organ rejection following transplantation but they carry potential risks and side effects in terms of both disease onset (eg, diabetes or hypertension) and possible iatrogenic disorders (eg, cancer

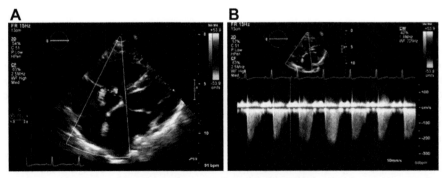

Fig. 9. Echo images of a 63-year-old patient after a cardiac transplant demonstrating moderate tricuspid regurgitation during systole (*A*) color Doppler and (*B*) spectral Doppler.

or infections).[90] The most commonly used drugs include calcineurin inhibitors, mammalian target of rapamycin (mTOR) inhibitors, corticosteroids, and antimetabolites.

Calcineurin inhibitors are most commonly used and can lead to nephrotoxicity, pulmonary toxicity (**Fig. 10**), neurotoxicity, hypertension, and metabolic disturbances.[91] Additionally, other immunosuppressive drugs such as corticosteroids and antimetabolites have their own specific toxicities. Close monitoring and personalized management are crucial to minimize drug toxicity while maintaining effective immunosuppression.

Chronic kidney disease (CKD) affects up to 50% of patients at year 5, with 6% requiring dialysis by year 10 after a heart transplant.[55,92,93] Risk factors include age, female gender, pretransplant GFR, tobacco use, pretransplant hypertension/diabetes, ischemic cardiomyopathy, retransplantation, and acute kidney insufficiency.[23,25,55,93–95] Calcineurin inhibitor use, while nephrotoxic, has conflicting evidence regarding its contribution to CKD.[23,27,30,92] CKD can cause an up to 4-fold increase in mortality, with recipients on dialysis having even higher rates.[93,95] Although renal dysfunction minimally affects mortality within the first 5 years, its impact grows beyond that period.[55]

Opportunistic infections

Opportunistic infections (OIs) following cardiac transplants and other forms of organ transplantation are a significant concern due to the immunosuppressive therapy that recipients undergo. These infections can have an insidious onset and atypical clinical manifestations, making early diagnosis and timely treatment crucial for successful outcomes.[96] OIs are most common in the early posttransplantation period or with increased immunosuppression, largely because of impaired T-cell function.[97] The risk for any type of infection changes throughout the transplant course and is greatly influenced by the degree and duration of immunosuppression.[98]

The use of thin slices in CT is important in detecting pulmonary infections (**Fig. 11**). The imaging appearances on CT are not significantly different compared with the other nontransplant patients, for example, patchy airspace consolidations, nodules (centrilobular or tree in bud) lobar consolidation, multifocal ground glass changes, masses with or without associated pleural effusions, and mediastinal lymphadenopathy. However, some pathognomonic features on CT, such as the "halo sign" in a posttransplant patient with immunosuppression, suggest a fungal cause such as pulmonary aspergillosis.

The use of metabolic imaging with 18F-fluorodeoxyglucose (FDG) positron emission tomography/computed tomography (PET/CT) has been increasingly recognized in optimizing the diagnosis of invasive infection, monitoring the response to therapy, and guiding the duration of antimicrobial therapy or the need to escalate to surgical intervention.[72]

Posttransplant lymphoproliferative disorder

Posttransplant lymphoproliferative disorder (PTLD) is a spectrum of lymphoid conditions associated with the use of potent immunosuppressive drugs.[99,100] PTLD has an incidence rate of up to 9% within 5 years in adult heart transplant recipients, with 35% of cases occurring during the first year.[101] The disorder is associated with the Epstein-Barr Virus (EBV) in 50% of cases,[102,103] and pretransplant testing for EBV has been found to reduce the frequency of PTLD in the pediatric population.[104] PTLD is reported to be more common in lung transplants, followed by liver and cardiac, and is lowest with kidney transplants.[105] Clinical manifestations can include masses and lymph node enlargement (**Fig. 12**), and in some cases, splenomegaly. Treatment often involves a

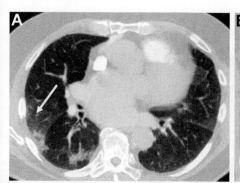
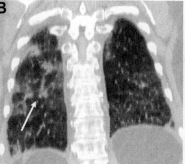
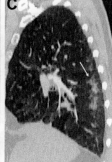

Fig. 10. CT images of a 69-year-old patient who underwent a heart transplant 12 years ago and was on Sirolimus. (*A*) Axial, (*B*) coronal, and (*C*) sagittal images showing bilateral multifocal, predominantly peripheral and basal patchy consolidations and ground glass opacities (*arrows*) as well as reticulation, features concerning for drug toxicity due to Sirolimus.

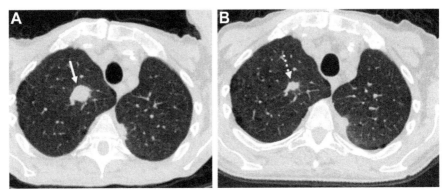

Fig. 11. *Rhizopus* infection in a 59-year-old patient postheart transplant. (*A*) An axial noncontrast CT scan (lung window) reveals an irregular solid nodule in the right upper lobe (*solid arrow*). (*B*) Follow-up CT Thorax after a course of antifungal treatment demonstrates a noticeable reduction in the nodule's size (*dotted arrow*).

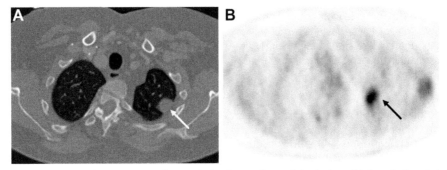

Fig. 12. (*A*) Axial CT scan without contrast (lung window) reveals a solid subpleural left apical nodule (*white arrow*). (*B*) Corresponding axial PET-CT images show intense FDG uptake (*black arrow*). Subsequent biopsy of this lesion confirmed the presence of EBV and lymphoma based on histopathological analysis.

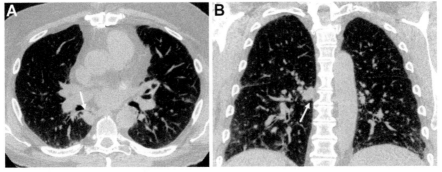

Fig. 13. (*A*) Axial and (*B*) coronal CT scans (lung window) of a 72-year-old individual following cardiac transplant showing a subpleural nodule in the medial right lower lobe (*arrows*). Endobronchial biopsy revealed *Cryptococcus neoformans* infection.

reduction in immunosuppression, which can conflict with graft survival.[101]

Malignancy

Malignancies pose a significant threat to long-term survival in heart transplant patients. Individuals who receive cardiac transplants have a 4 times higher risk of developing malignancies than people of the same age, sex, and ethnicity.[106] This increased risk is largely attributed to immunosuppressive therapy, which is essential to prevent organ rejection but can inadvertently increase the risk of carcinogenesis.[107] The most observed malignancies reported in heart transplant patients are gastrointestinal, skin, and hematological, followed by respiratory (**Fig. 13**), head and neck, and breast cancer.[106] Regular preventive screening is crucial, which includes clinical, biochemical, and imaging assessment. In cases of malignancies in this patient population, medical treatments (chemotherapies, immunotherapies, and so forth) and surgical treatments can be effective but carry higher risks for complications than in nontransplant patients.[108]

SUMMARY

The role of diagnostic imaging in the assessment of post-heart transplant complications is essential. The advancement of modern imaging technologies holds promising potential in enhancing the sensitivity and specificity for early and accurate detection of graft-related complications, particularly with the increasing number and survival of orthotopic heart transplant patients. Radiologists, cardiologists, and cardiac surgeons must possess a comprehensive understanding of imaging modalities, as well as the spectrum of normal and abnormal appearances in detecting perioperative and postoperative complications related to surgery, drugs, and allograft. The ultimate aim is to provide the heart transplant patient population with the optimal care to minimize morbidities and improve survival rates.

CLINICS CARE POINTS

- Cardiac CT is a reliable tool for identifying most posttransplant complications.
- Cardiac MR imaging excels in assessing pericardial conditions and potential allograft rejection.
- Recognition of rejection and CAV is vital because they are unique to cardiac transplantation.

REFERENCES

1. Lower RR, Shumway NE. Studies on orthotopic homotransplantation of the canine heart. Surg Forum 1960;11:18–9.
2. el Gamel A, Yonan NA, Grant S, et al. Orthotopic cardiac transplantation: a comparison of standard and bicaval Wythenshawe techniques. J Thorac Cardiovasc Surg 1995;109(4):721–9 [discussion: 9–30].
3. Anthony C, Imran M, Pouliopoulos J, et al. Cardiovascular Magnetic Resonance for Rejection Surveillance After Cardiac Transplantation. Circulation 2022;145(25):1811–24.
4. Ajluni SC, Mously H, Chami T, et al. Non-invasive Imaging in the Evaluation of Cardiac Allograft Vasculopathy in Heart Transplantation: A Systematic Review. Curr Probl Cardiol 2022;47(8):101103.
5. Sciaccaluga C, Ghionzoli N, Mandoli GE, et al. The role of non-invasive imaging modalities in cardiac allograft vasculopathy: an updated focus on current evidences. Heart Fail Rev 2022;27(4):1235–46.
6. Jacob S, Sellke F. Is bicaval orthotopic heart transplantation superior to the biatrial technique? Interact Cardiovasc Thorac Surg 2009;9(2):333–42.
7. Angermann CE, Spes CH, Tammen A, et al. Anatomic characteristics and valvular function of the transplanted heart: transthoracic versus transesophageal echocardiographic findings. J Heart Transplant 1990;9(4):331–8.
8. Schnoor M, Schäfer T, Lühmann D, et al. Bicaval versus standard technique in orthotopic heart transplantation: A systematic review and meta-analysis. J Thorac Cardiovasc Surg 2007;134(5):1322–31.e7.
9. Shah NR, Blankstein R, Villines T, et al. Coronary CTA for Surveillance of Cardiac Allograft Vasculopathy. Current Cardiovascular Imaging Reports 2018;11(11):26.
10. Achenbach S, Anders K, Kalender WA. Dual-source cardiac computed tomography: image quality and dose considerations. Eur Radiol 2008;18:1188–98.
11. Rajiah PS, Reddy P, Baliyan V, et al. Utility of CT and MRI in Tricuspid Valve Interventions. Radiographics 2023;43(7):e220153.
12. Scholtz J-E, Ghoshhajra B. Advances in cardiac CT contrast injection and acquisition protocols. Cardiovasc Diagn Ther 2017;7(5):439–51.
13. Ahmed Z, Campeau D, Gong H, et al. High-pitch, high temporal resolution, multi-energy cardiac imaging on a dual-source photon-counting-detector CT. Medical physics 2023;50(3):1428–35.
14. Horiguchi J, Kiguchi M, Fujioka C, et al. Radiation dose, image quality, stenosis measurement, and CT densitometry using ECG-triggered coronary

64-MDCT angiography: a phantom study. Am J Roentgenol 2008;190(2):315–20.

15. Becker CR, Knez A, Ohnesorge B, et al. Imaging of noncalcified coronary plaques using helical CT with retrospective ECG gating. Am J Roentgenol 2000; 175(2):423–4.

16. Mochizuki T, Hosoi S, Higashino H, et al. Assessment of coronary artery and cardiac function using multidetector CT. Seminars Ultrasound, CT MRI 2004;25(2):99–112.

17. Feuchtner G, Goetti R, Plass A, et al. Dual-step prospective ECG-triggered 128-slice dual-source CT for evaluation of coronary arteries and cardiac function without heart rate control: a technical note. Eur Radiol 2010;20(9):2092–9.

18. Masuda T, Funama Y, Nakaura T, et al. Radiation dose reduction method combining the ECG-Edit function and high helical pitch in retrospectively-gated CT angiography. Radiography 2022;28(3): 766–71.

19. Pavitt C, Lazoura O, Lindsay A, et al. 148 The Use of Cardiac CT for the Detection of Left Atrial Appendage Thrombus: A Quality Improvement Project. Heart 2014;100(Suppl 3):A86–7.

20. Dolan RS, Rahsepar AA, Blaisdell J, et al. Multiparametric cardiac magnetic resonance imaging can detect acute cardiac allograft rejection after heart transplantation. JACC (J Am Coll Cardiol): Cardiovascular Imaging 2019;12(8 Part 2):1632–41.

21. Almenar L, Igual B, Martínez-Dolz L, et al. Utility of cardiac magnetic resonance imaging for the diagnosis of heart transplant rejection. Transplant Proc 2003;35(5):1962–4.

22. Butler CR, Thompson R, Haykowsky M, et al. Cardiovascular magnetic resonance in the diagnosis of acute heart transplant rejection: a review. J Cardiovasc Magn Reson 2009;11(1):7.

23. Lachance K, White M, de Denus S. Risk Factors for Chronic Renal Insufficiency Following Cardiac Transplantation. Ann Transplant 2015;20:576–87.

24. Marie PY, Angioï M, Carteaux JP, et al. Detection and prediction of acute heart transplant rejection with the myocardial T2 determination provided by a black-blood magnetic resonance imaging sequence. J Am Coll Cardiol 2001;37(3):825–31.

25. Lázaro IS, Bonet LA, Martínez-Dolz L, et al, editors. Effect of hypertension, diabetes, and smoking on development of renal dysfunction after heart transplantation. Transplantation proceedings. Elsevier; 2008.

26. Butler CR, Savu A, Bakal JA, et al. Correlation of cardiovascular magnetic resonance imaging findings and endomyocardial biopsy results in patients undergoing screening for heart transplant rejection. J Heart Lung Transplant 2015;34(5):643–50.

27. Groetzner J, Kaczmarek I, Schulz U, et al. Mycophenolate and sirolimus as calcineurin inhibitor-free immunosuppression improves renal function better than calcineurin inhibitor-reduction in late cardiac transplant recipients with chronic renal failure. Transplantation 2009;87(5):726–33.

28. Imran M, Wang L, McCrohon J, et al. Native T1 Mapping in the Diagnosis of Cardiac Allograft Rejection: A Prospective Histologically Validated Study. JACC Cardiovasc Imaging 2019;12:1618–28.

29. Kobashigawa J, Zuckermann A, Macdonald P, et al. Report from a consensus conference on primary graft dysfunction after cardiac transplantation. J Heart Lung Transplant 2014;33(4):327–40.

30. Manito N, Rabago G, Palomo J, et al, editors. Improvement in chronic renal failure after mycophenolate mofetil introduction and cyclosporine dose reduction: four-year results from a cohort of heart transplant recipients. Transplantation proceedings. Elsevier; 2011.

31. Chaikriangkrai K, Abbasi MA, Sarnari R, et al. Prognostic Value of Myocardial Extracellular Volume Fraction and T2-mapping in Heart Transplant Patients. JACC Cardiovasc Imaging 2020;13(7): 1521–30.

32. Krieghoff C, Barten MJ, Hildebrand L, et al. Assessment of sub-clinical acute cellular rejection after heart transplantation: comparison of cardiac magnetic resonance imaging and endomyocardial biopsy. Eur Radiol 2014;24(10):2360–71.

33. Şimşek E, Nalbantgil S, Ceylan N, et al. Diagnostic performance of late gadolinium enhancement in the assessment of acute cellular rejection after heart transplantation. Anatol J Cardiol 2016;16(2): 113–8.

34. Almufleh A, Garuba H, Mielniczuk LM, et al. Diffuse Subepicardial Late Gadolinium Enhancement After Heart Transplant: A Potentially Ominous Finding. Can J Cardiol 2018;34(12):1687.e3-7.

35. Thorn EM, de Filippi CR. Echocardiography in the Cardiac Transplant Recipient. Heart Fail Clin 2007;3(1):51–67.

36. Pieper GM, Shah A, Harmann L, et al. Speckle-tracking 2-dimensional strain echocardiography: a new noninvasive imaging tool to evaluate acute rejection in cardiac transplantation. J Heart Lung Transplant 2010;29(9):1039–46.

37. Shahandeh N, Kashiyama K, Honda Y, et al. Invasive Coronary Imaging Assessment for Cardiac Allograft Vasculopathy: State-of-the-Art Review. Journal of the Society for Cardiovascular Angiography & Interventions 2022;1(4):100344.

38. Nelson LM, Rossing K, Ihlemann N, et al. Intravascular ultrasound-guided selection for early noninvasive cardiac allograft vasculopathy screening in heart transplant recipients. Clin Transplant 2020; 34(12):e14124.

39. Torres HJ, Merello L, Ramos SA, et al. Prevalence of Cardiac Allograft Vasculopathy Assessed With

Coronary Angiography Versus Coronary Vascular Ultrasound and Virtual Histology. Transplant Proc 2011;43(6):2318–21.

40. Chih S, Wiefels CC, Beanlands RS, editors. PET assessment of cardiac allograft vasculopathy. Seminars in Nuclear Medicine. Elsevier; 2021.

41. Grupper A, Gewirtz H, Kushwaha S. Reinnervation post-heart transplantation. Eur Heart J 2018; 39(20):1799–806.

42. Feher A, Miller EJ. PET myocardial blood flow for post-transplant surveillance and cardiac allograft vasculopathy in heart transplant recipients. Curr Cardiol Rep 2022;24(12):1865–71.

43. Bravo PE, Bergmark BA, Vita T, et al. Diagnostic and prognostic value of myocardial blood flow quantification as non-invasive indicator of cardiac allograft vasculopathy. Eur Heart J 2017;39(4): 316–23.

44. Long B, Brady WJ, Gragossian A, et al. A primer for managing cardiac transplant patients in the emergency department setting. Am J Emerg Med 2021;41:130–8.

45. Brink JG, Hassoulas J. The first human heart transplant and further advances in cardiac transplantation at Groote Schuur Hospital and the University of Cape Town - with reference to : the operation. A human cardiac transplant : an interim report of a successful operation performed at Groote Schuur Hospital, Cape Town. Cardiovasc J Afr 2009; 20(1):31–5.

46. Raphael J, Mazer CD, Subramani S, et al. Society of Cardiovascular Anesthesiologists Clinical Practice Improvement Advisory for Management of Perioperative Bleeding and Hemostasis in Cardiac Surgery Patients. Anesth Analg 2019;129(5): 1209–21.

47. Jeong H-G, Bang JS, Kim BJ, et al. Hematoma Hounsfield units and expansion of intracerebral hemorrhage: A potential marker of hemostatic clot contraction. Int J Stroke 2021;16(2):163–71.

48. Engelman DT, Ben Ali W, Williams JB, et al. Guidelines for Perioperative Care in Cardiac Surgery: Enhanced Recovery After Surgery Society Recommendations. JAMA Surgery 2019;154(8): 755–66.

49. Tibi P, McClure RS, Huang J, et al. STS/SCA/AmSECT/SABM Update to the Clinical Practice Guidelines on Patient Blood Management. Ann Thorac Surg 2021;112(3):981–1004.

50. Baumann Kreuziger L, Karkouti K, Tweddell J, et al. Antithrombotic therapy management of adult and pediatric cardiac surgery patients. J Thromb Haemost 2018;16(11):2133–46.

51. Ho S, Reddy GP. Cardiovascular imaging. Korean J Radiol 2011;1229(6929):2005–8330.

52. Elboudwarej O, Patel JK, Liou F, et al. Risk of deep vein thrombosis and pulmonary embolism after heart transplantation: clinical outcomes comparing upper extremity deep vein thrombosis and lower extremity deep vein thrombosis. Clin Transplant 2015;29(7):629–35.

53. Alvarez-Alvarez RJ, Barge-Caballero E, Chavez-Leal SA, et al. Venous thromboembolism in heart transplant recipients: incidence, recurrence and predisposing factors. J Heart Lung Transplant 2015;34(2):167–74.

54. Cove ME, Spelman DW, MacLaren G. Infectious complications of cardiac surgery: a clinical review. J Cardiothorac Vasc Anesth 2012;26(6):1094–100.

55. Lund LH, Khush KK, Cherikh WS, et al. The Registry of the International Society for Heart and Lung Transplantation: Thirty-fourth Adult Heart Transplantation Report-2017; Focus Theme: Allograft ischemic time. J Heart Lung Transplant 2017; 36(10):1037–46.

56. Sutaria N, Sylvia L, DeNofrio D. Immunosuppression and Heart Transplantation. Handb Exp Pharmacol 2022;272:117–37.

57. Fishman JA. Infection in solid-organ transplant recipients. N Engl J Med 2007;357(25):2601–14.

58. Alba A, Bain E, Ng N, et al. Complications after heart transplantation: hope for the best, but prepare for the worst. Int J Transplant Res Med 2016;2(2):2–22.

59. Sénéchal M, LePrince P, Tezenas du Montcel S, et al. Bacterial mediastinitis after heart transplantation: clinical presentation, risk factors and treatment. J Heart Lung Transplant 2004;23(2):165–70.

60. Tabotta F, Ferretti GR, Prosch H, et al. Imaging features and differential diagnoses of non-neoplastic diffuse mediastinal diseases. Insights Imaging 2020;11(1):111.

61. Li AE, Fishman EK. Evaluation of complications after sternotomy using single- and multidetector CT with three-dimensional volume rendering. AJR Am J Roentgenol 2003;181(4):1065–70.

62. Akman C, Kantarci F, Cetinkaya S. Imaging in mediastinitis: a systematic review based on aetiology. Clin Radiol 2004;59(7):573–85.

63. Yusen RD, Edwards LB, Dipchand AI, et al. The Registry of the International Society for Heart and Lung Transplantation: Thirty-third Adult Lung and Heart–Lung Transplant Report—2016; Focus Theme: Primary Diagnostic Indications for Transplant. J Heart Lung Transplant 2016;35(10): 1170–84.

64. Salomon RN, Hughes CC, Schoen FJ, et al. Human coronary transplantation-associated arteriosclerosis. Evidence for a chronic immune reaction to activated graft endothelial cells. Am J Pathol 1991;138(4):791–8.

65. Tuzcu EM, De Franco AC, Goormastic M, et al. Dichotomous pattern of coronary atherosclerosis 1 to 9 years after transplantation: insights from

systematic intravascular ultrasound imaging. J Am Coll Cardiol 1996;27(4):839–46.

66. Estep JD, Shah DJ, Nagueh SF, et al. The role of multimodality cardiac imaging in the transplanted heart. JACC (J Am Coll Cardiol): Cardiovascular Imaging 2009;2(9):1126–40.

67. Skorić B, Čikeš M, Ljubas Maček J, et al. Cardiac allograft vasculopathy: diagnosis, therapy, and prognosis. Croat Med J 2014;55(6):562–76.

68. Günther A, Andersen R, Gude E, et al. The predictive value of coronary artery calcium detected by computed tomography in a prospective study on cardiac allograft vasculopathy in heart transplant patients. Transpl Int 2018;31(1):82–91.

69. Sharma V, Agarwal S, Grover T, et al. Coronary allograft vasculopathy in post-heart transplant patients: pathogenesis and role of cardiac computed tomography in diagnosis-a comprehensive review. Ann Med Surg (Lond) 2023;85(7):3531–7.

70. Ahn Y, Koo HJ, Hyun J, et al. CT Coronary Angiography and Dynamic CT Myocardial Perfusion for Detection of Cardiac Allograft Vasculopathy. JACC Cardiovasc Imaging 2023;16(7):934–47.

71. Spitaleri G, Farrero Torres M, Sabatino M, et al. The pharmaceutical management of cardiac allograft vasculopathy after heart transplantation. Expet Opin Pharmacother 2020;21(11):1367–76.

72. Longhitano A, Alipour R, Khot A, et al. The role of 18F-Fluorodeoxyglucose Positron Emission Tomography/Computed Tomography (FDG PET/CT) in assessment of complex invasive fungal disease and opportunistic co-infections in patients with acute leukemia prior to allogeneic hematopoietic cell transplant. Transpl Infect Dis 2021;23(3):e13547.

73. El-Andari R, Bozso SJ, Fialka NM, et al. Coronary Artery Revascularization in Heart Transplant Patients: A Systematic Review and Meta-Analysis. Cardiology 2022;147(3):348–63.

74. Pober JS, Chih S, Kobashigawa J, et al. Cardiac allograft vasculopathy: current review and future research directions. Cardiovasc Res 2021; 117(13):2624–38.

75. Barghash MH, Pinney SP. Heart Retransplantation: Candidacy, Outcomes, and Management. Curr Transplant Rep 2020;7(1):12–7.

76. Usman AA, Taimen K, Wasielewski M, et al. Cardiac magnetic resonance T2 mapping in the monitoring and follow-up of acute cardiac transplant rejection: a pilot study. Circulation: Cardiovascular Imaging 2012;5(6):782–90.

77. Mangini S, Alves BR, Silvestre OM, et al. Heart transplantation. Einstein (Sao Paulo) 2015;13: 310–8.

78. Costanzo MR, Dipchand A, Starling R, et al. The International Society of heart and lung transplantation Guidelines for the care of heart transplant recipients. Elsevier; 2010. p. 914–56.

79. Strecker T, Rösch J, Weyand M, et al. Endomyocardial biopsy for monitoring heart transplant patients: 11-years-experience at a german heart center. Int J Clin Exp Pathol 2013;6(1):55.

80. Crespo-Leiro MG, Stypmann J, Schulz U, et al. Clinical usefulness of gene-expression profile to rule out acute rejection after heart transplantation: CARGO II. Eur Heart J 2016;37(33):2591–601.

81. Chi N-H, Chou N-K, Tsao C-I, et al, editors. Endomyocardial biopsy in heart transplantation: schedule or event? Transplantation proceedings. USA: Elsevier; 2012.

82. Lu W, Zheng J, Pan X-D, et al. Diagnostic performance of cardiac magnetic resonance for the detection of acute cardiac allograft rejection: a systematic review and meta-analysis. J Thorac Dis 2015;7(3):252.

83. Smith JD, Stowell JT, Martínez-Jiménez S, et al. Evaluation after orthotopic heart transplant: what the radiologist should know. Radiographics 2019; 39(2):321–43.

84. Vermes E, Pantaléon C, Auvet A, et al. Cardiovascular magnetic resonance in heart transplant patients: diagnostic value of quantitative tissue markers: T2 mapping and extracellular volume fraction, for acute rejection diagnosis. J Cardiovasc Magn Reson 2018;20(1):59.

85. Dronavalli VB, Rogers CA, Banner NR. Primary cardiac allograft dysfunction—validation of a clinical definition. Transplantation 2015;99(9):1919.

86. Berger Y, Har Zahav Y, Kassif Y, et al. Tricuspid valve regurgitation after orthotopic heart transplantation: prevalence and etiology. Journal of Transplantation 2012;2012.

87. Kwon MH, Shemin RJ. Tricuspid valve regurgitation after heart transplantation. Ann Cardiothorac Surg 2017;6(3):270.

88. Jeevanandam V, Russell H, Mather P, et al. Donor tricuspid annuloplasty during orthotopic heart transplantation: long-term results of a prospective controlled study. Ann Thorac Surg 2006;82(6): 2089–95.

89. Zoghbi WA, Adams D, Bonow RO, et al. Recommendations for noninvasive evaluation of native valvular regurgitation: a report from the American Society of Echocardiography developed in collaboration with the Society for Cardiovascular Magnetic Resonance. J Am Soc Echocardiogr 2017;30(4):303–71.

90. Kasiske BL, Zeier MG, Chapman JR, et al. KDIGO clinical practice guideline for the care of kidney transplant recipients: a summary. Kidney Int 2010; 77(4):299–311.

91. Nogueiras-Álvarez R, Mora-Cuesta VM, Cifrián-Martínez JM, et al. Calcineurin inhibitors' impact on cardiovascular and renal function, a descriptive study in lung transplant recipients from the North of Spain. Sci Rep 2022;12(1):21207.

92. Janus N, Launay-Vacher V, Sebbag L, et al. Renal insufficiency, mortality, and drug management in heart transplant. Results of the CARIN study. Transpl Int 2014;27(9):931–8.

93. Kida Y. Chronic renal failure after transplantation of a nonrenal organ. N Engl J Med 2003;349(26): 2563–5. author reply.

94. González-Vílchez F, Arizon J, Segovia J, et al, editors. Chronic renal dysfunction in maintenance heart transplant patients: the ICEBERG study. Transplantation Proceedings. USA: Elsevier; 2014.

95. Thomas HL, Banner NR, Murphy CL, et al. Incidence, determinants, and outcome of chronic kidney disease after adult heart transplantation in the United Kingdom. Transplantation 2012;93(11):1151–7.

96. Guo Y, Zhu Z, Cai W, et al. Intracerebral opportunistic infections caused by immunosuppressants after orthotopic liver transplantation: Report of two cases and literature review. Front Immunol 2022; 13:1003254.

97. Ferdjallah A, Young JH, MacMillan ML. A Review of Infections After Hematopoietic Cell Transplantation Requiring PICU Care: Transplant Timeline Is Key. Front Pediatr 2021;9:634449.

98. Cheung H, Azar MM, Gan G, et al. 1099. Opportunistic Infections Among Long Term Survivors of Kidney Transplantation: Defining Risk Factors. Open Forum Infect Dis 2020;7(Suppl 1):S579–80.

99. Nourse JP, Jones K, Gandhi MK. Epstein-Barr Virus-related post-transplant lymphoproliferative disorders: pathogenetic insights for targeted therapy. Am J Transplant 2011;11(5):888–95.

100. Dierickx D, Habermann TM. Post-Transplantation Lymphoproliferative Disorders in Adults. N Engl J Med 2018;378(6):549–62.

101. Asleh R, Alnsasra H, Habermann TM, et al. Post-transplant Lymphoproliferative Disorder Following Cardiac Transplantation. Front Cardiovasc Med 2022;9:787975.

102. Kotton CN, Huprikar S, Kumar D. Transplant Infectious Diseases: A Review of the Scientific Registry of Transplant Recipients Published Data. Am J Transplant 2017;17(6):1439–46.

103. Luskin MR, Heil DS, Tan KS, et al. The Impact of EBV Status on Characteristics and Outcomes of Posttransplantation Lymphoproliferative Disorder. Am J Transplant 2015;15(10):2665–73.

104. Chang YC, Young RR, Mavis AM, et al. Epstein-Barr Virus DNAemia and post-transplant lymphoproliferative disorder in pediatric solid organ transplant recipients. PLoS One 2022;17(10):e0269766.

105. McKenna M, Epperla N, Ghobadi A, et al. Real-world evidence of the safety and survival with CD19 CAR-T cell therapy for relapsed/refractory solid organ transplant-related PTLD. Br J Haematol 2023;202(2):248–55.

106. Lateef N, Farooq MZ, Latif A, et al. Prevalence of Post-Heart Transplant Malignancies: A Systematic Review and Meta-Analysis. Curr Probl Cardiol 2022;47(12):101363.

107. Gutierrez-Dalmau A, Campistol JM. Immunosuppressive therapy and malignancy in organ transplant recipients: a systematic review. Drugs 2007; 67(8):1167–98.

108. Crespo-Leiro MG, Villa-Arranz A, Manito-Lorite N, et al. Lung cancer after heart transplantation: results from a large multicenter registry. Am J Transplant 2011;11(5):1035–40.

The Role of Artificial Intelligence in Cardiac Imaging

Check for updates

Carlotta Onnis, MD[a,b], Marly van Assen, PhD[a], Emanuele Muscogiuri, MD[a,c], Giuseppe Muscogiuri, MD, PhD[d], Gabrielle Gershon, BSc[a], Luca Saba, MD[b], Carlo N. De Cecco, MD, PhD[a,e],*

KEYWORDS

- Artificial intelligence • Cardiac imaging • Machine learning • Deep learning
- Cardiac computed tomography • Cardiac magnetic resonance • Clinical workflow

KEY POINTS

- Main areas of artificial intelligence (AI) applicability in cardiac imaging are detection, quantification, and characterization of cardiac disease.
- AI has been successfully used to perform time-consuming tasks, such as segmentation and post-processing, optimization of data acquisition and reconstruction, and grading of disease severity.
- AI can aid physicians in better understanding the patient's cardiac health.
- Integration of AI applications into clinical workflow will have a great impact on costs, wider usability, and optimization of workflow efficiency.

INTRODUCTION

Cardiovascular disease (CVD) remains the number one cause of death worldwide, and the number of annual deaths is expected to increase in the near future[1]; thus it is not surprising that a great deal of effort is being put forth to advance cardiac imaging. Simultaneously, artificial intelligence (AI) has made great advances in the medical imaging field.

The 2 main approaches that have been used in medical imaging, including cardiac applications, are machine learning (ML) and deep learning (DL). ML uses computer algorithms to identify patterns in large data sets with a multitude of variables. ML is usually built from test inputs, makes data-driven predictions, and has been used for diagnostic or prognostic outcomes prediction. ML relies on the principle that a set of weak base classifier can be combined in a single strong classifier when their weighting is adjusted. Thus, a series of base classifier predictions and a weighting distribution are produced. The predictions are subsequently combined by weighted majority voting with a resulting overall classifier as a continuous estimate of predicted risk. ML requires 3 steps: training, where it learns characteristics of

[a] Translational Laboratory for Cardiothoracic Imaging and Artificial Intelligence, Department of Radiology and Imaging Sciences, Emory University, 100 Woodruff Circle, Atlanta, GA 30322, USA; [b] Department of Radiology, Azienda Ospedaliero Universitaria (A.O.U.), di Cagliari–Polo di Monserrato, SS 554 km 4,500 Monserrato, Cagliari 09042, Italy; [c] Division of Thoracic Imaging, Department of Radiology, University Hospitals Leuven, Herestraat 49, Leuven 3000, Belgium; [d] Department of Diagnostic and Interventional Radiology, Papa Giovanni XXIII Hospital, Piazza OMS, 1, Bergamo BG 24127, Italy; [e] Division of Cardiothoracic Imaging, Department of Radiology and Imaging Sciences, Emory University, Emory University Hospital, 1365 Clifton Road Northeast, Suite AT503, Atlanta, GA 30322, USA

* Corresponding author. Division of Cardiothoracic Imaging, Department of Radiology and Imaging Sciences, Emory University Hospital, 1365 Clifton Road Northeast, Suite AT503, Atlanta, GA 30322.
E-mail address: carlo.dececco@emory.edu
Twitter: @CarlottaOnnis (C.O.); @marly_van_assen (M.A.); @GiuseppeMuscog (G.M.); @gabbygershon (G.G.); @lucasabaITA (L.S.); @DeCeccoCN (C.N.D.C.)

Radiol Clin N Am 62 (2024) 473–488
https://doi.org/10.1016/j.rcl.2024.01.002

data; validation, where it validates the learned characteristics in a separate data set; and testing, where the accuracy of the ML model is evaluated.

DL methods, a subgroup of ML, are more advanced AI methods that, unlike classic ML that requires hand-engineered feature extraction, directly interrogates the data, learns the features by which to classify it, and performs tasks such as segmentation, classification, detection, or outcome prediction. DL works through multilayered neural networks to transform input images into outputs; it uses weighted connections between nodes that are iteratively adjusted through exposure to training data by back-propagating a corrective error signal through the network.[2,3] DL, being at its core represented by convolutional neural networks (CNNs), lends itself to be particularly suitable for large data sets with many features, such as imaging data sets, and it has been widely applied to radiology. Within cardiac imaging (Table 1), CNNs have been used to perform detection tasks, such as coronary plaque. CNN uses a bounding box that searches for the target in the input images, then another CNN model discriminates if the subimages found are true or false targets, and then coordinates of true detected targets are given as output. CNN has also been applied to segmentation, for example, segmentation of cardiac chambers, coronary arteries, or atherosclerotic plaques, by using encoder–decoder–based neural networks, and classification, where CNN gives category labels as outputs.

GENERAL ARTIFICIAL INTELLIGENCE APPLICATIONS
Image Acquisition and Reconstruction

Computed tomography (CT) and MR image acquisition and reconstruction can benefit from AI techniques. For example, AI can improve the image acquisition and reconstruction time in MR or improve the CT image quality at low-dose radiation.

CT exposes patients to radiation, and research has focused on the application of AI to reduce the dose. Low-dose CT ensures less radiation exposure, but it is characterized by intrinsic severe artifacts that undermine its reliability. CT vendors have introduced iterative reconstruction techniques to reduce dose and noise, but there are concerns over loss of anatomic details, and long reconstruction times. AI has been applied to overcome these problems that limit accuracy and feasibility. AI-based high-quality reconstruction methods have been developed, such as those based on CNN. Some of these AI-based image denoising methods based on CNN-quality enhancement have attained

commercial availability.[4] Other approaches to denoise low-dose CT involve wavelet decomposition and processing by a neural network[5] and generative adversarial network, which uses DL to reduce image noise on both low-dose CT and nonenhanced cardiac CT, in order to obtain quality similar to conventional-dose CT.[6] Compared with iterative reconstruction, the strength of AI-based reconstruction relies on its ability to retrieve missing details and enhance the quality of output images, by learning from complex prior information. Greffier and colleagues[7] assessed the impact on quality and dose reduction of a DL-image reconstruction (DLIR) algorithm compared with a vendor's iterative reconstruction algorithm (adaptive statistical iterative reconstruction-V [ASiR-V] at 50% strength; GE Healthcare; Waukesha, WI, USA). They concluded that the DLIR reduced noise, improved spatial resolution, and optimized radiation dose, without perceived image alteration, commonly reported with iterative methods. Similarly, Bernard and colleagues[8] evaluated radiation dose and image quality of coronary CT angiography (CCTA) using a DLIR model compared with a hybrid iterative reconstruction algorithm: they showed that DLIR reduced radiation dose by about 40% and improved quality by about 50% (Fig. 1). Last, AI can perform image quality assessment evaluating the input image and producing a map, a metric of image quality, as output. CNNs are used to learn a similarity score between a reference and a reconstructed noisy image; the learned similarity is then considered a quality reference for the noisy image.[9]

With regards to cardiac magnetic resonance (CMR), optimal plane positioning is a crucial step to obtain high-diagnostic-quality images, and it traditionally required experienced technologists and time. Thus, AI-aided recognition of imaging planes has been developed to guide image scan, optimizing workflow and providing high-quality, highly reproducible images, with increased time efficiency and minimal user input.[10] Different studies have suggested AI models with acceptable accuracy,[11,12] and more recent studies have also shown reduced number of breath-holds.[13] Moreover, CMR acquisition time is long and often poorly tolerated by the patient; hence, effort has been put on developing AI technologies that could improve this aspect while maintaining a high spatiotemporal resolution. State-of-the-art software, such as compressed sensing (CS), is a widely used example of it, which, however, requires high computational power and is not always applicable to accelerated cine CMR images owing to motional changes in cardiac volume between frames.[14] To enable progress beyond CS-based

Table 1
Clinical applications of artificial intelligence in cardiac imaging

Clinical Application	Description	Advantage
Image acquisition		
Radiation dose reduction	DL-based reconstruction method	Improved image quality
CMR plane positioning	AI-aided plane recognition	High-quality, highly reproducible images
CMR acquisition time reduction	DL-aided acceleration of cine sequences	Reduced number of breath-holds
Image optimization		
Denoising	DL-based reduction of image noise and artifacts	Optimized image quality
Enhancement	Optimization of nonenhanced images	No need of contrast media
Outcome prediction		
MACE risk assessment	Integration of clinical and imaging data to ML	Better assessment than clinical and imaging data alone
Coronary artery disease		
Coronary calcium	Semiautomated and automated calcium scoring algorithms	Quantification of CAC from ECG- and non-ECG-gated CT
Plaque characterization	DL-based CAD-RADS assessment and high-risk features evaluation	Reduced postprocessing time and improved outcome prediction
CT-FFR	ML FFR calculation	Reduced processing time and costs
Epicardial fat	AI-based segmentation and quantification	Reduced postprocessing time and improved CV risk assessment
Evaluation of infarcted myocardium	AI-aided detection, segmentation, and analysis on noncontrast CMR images	No need of contrast media, reduced postprocessing time, and improved outcome prediction
Myocardial function		
Volume analysis	Automated segmentation	Reduced postprocessing time
Myocardial strain	Strain quantification from cine-to-tagged images	Wider availability and reduced processing time
Valve disease		
Classification	Grading of disease from phase-contrast CMR images	Reduced postprocessing time and improved outcome prediction
Cardiomyopathies		
Classification	Detection of diagnostic features and LGE evaluation	Improved prognostic prediction
Congenital heart disease		
Image acquisition	AI-aided acquisition and reconstruction	Reduced time of acquisition and postprocessing

reconstruction approach, DL methods have been proposed and have shown great performance in terms of quality and time, in a research setting. For example, CINENet[15] is a DL network that enabled highly accelerated cine sequences in a single breath-hold using spatiotemporal convolutions, and ESPIRiT,[16] another DL reconstruction

framework, also showed higher image quality, contributing to improved segmentation.

Image Optimization

Image quality is central to diagnostic capabilities, and AI algorithms can assess it. This is particularly

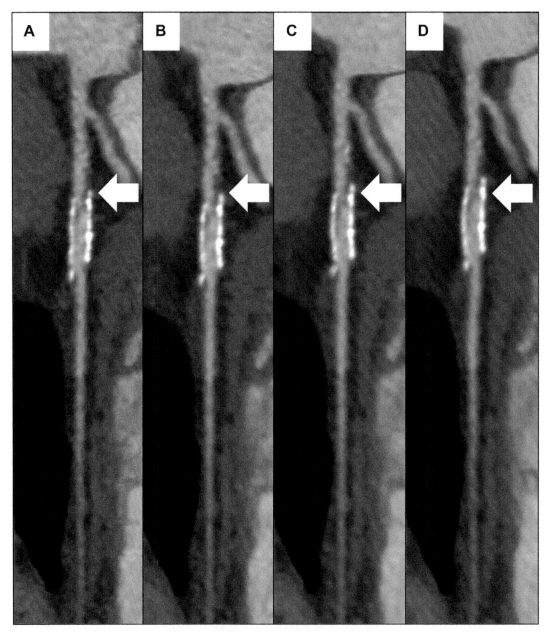

Fig. 1. A 57-year-old male patient who underwent CCTA following a positive stress ECG. CCTA shows severe in-stent restenosis (*arrow*) after previous stenting of the proximal left descending artery. Left descending artery is reconstructed using ASiR-V 50% (*A*), low-grade DLIR (*B*), medium-grade DLIR (*C*), and high-grade DLIR (*D*). DLIR reconstruction (GE Healthcare, Waukesha, WI, USA) is a DL algorithm reconstruction that allows the reduction of image noise. The DLIR application results in a significant reduction of the images noise without affecting the im-age signal and contrast. (*B–D*) A progressive reduction of the image noise can be appreciated.

true when it comes to noise, motion, or aliasing ar-tifacts, which can negatively impact both CT and MR imaging quality. AI has been applied in this setting to optimize image quality. For example, CMR is deeply affected by motion artifacts, which can be caused by intended or accidental (respira-tion and cardiac motion) patient movement, and it can benefit from retrospective AI-aided artifact correction. A generative adversarial network has been used to pursue this goal, demonstrating feasibility resulting in near-realistic motion-free im-ages.[17] A generative adversarial network com-bines 2 CNNs that work against each other to progressively refine their algorithms in order to give more accurate results. After the network has been trained with paired motion-free and motion-corrupted images, it can be a useful tool to remove motion artifacts from images.[18]

The ability of AI to reduce artifacts has been applied to CT as well. In particular, CNNs have proven to be useful in reducing metal artifacts in various settings, from cardiac CTs with artifacts and moving pacemakers[19] to ear CTs with artifacts from cochlear implants.[20] Metal artifact reduction methods based on DL are mostly supervised methods trained on synthetic-artifact CT images, which limit their applicability to unlabeled CTs. Both semisupervised[21] and fully unsupervised[22] methods have been developed to disentangle metal artifacts while addressing this problem, and they showed good generalizability for real-artifacts CT images.

Last, AI plays a promising role in contrast enhancement optimization. Recent studies focused on its ability to optimize image enhancement without the administration of contrast media. As shown by Zhang and colleagues,[23] virtual native enhancement, in the assessment of myocardial scar, demonstrated superior image quality compared with late gadolinium enhancement (LGE), excellent agreement between the 2 methods, and also with the histopathologic comparison. Thus, AI has proven useful to avoid gadolinium contrast administration with a dual advantage: reduced scan time and costs and reduced risks of contrast media adverse effects for patients.

ARTIFICIAL INTELLIGENCE APPLICATIONS IN CARDIAC COMPUTED TOMOGRAPHY
Coronary Artery Disease

Coronary calcium
Coronary artery calcium (CAC) score has been recognized as a predictor of future cardiovascular (CV) events and mortality.[24] Its measurement on cardiac CT can be obtained manually, with time-consuming segmentation, and semiautomatically or fully automatically, with DL-based algorithms. Several semiautomated and automated calcium scoring algorithms have been proposed,[25] and they have been applied to either electrocardiogram (ECG)-gated CT[26] or non-ECG-gated CT[27] scans with excellent accuracy comparable to expert readings and significant improvement in the workflow. The possibility to measure CAC score from noncontrast, non-ECG-gated CT scans has broadened the number of patients whose score, and consequent CV risk, can be evaluated without the need of dedicated cardiac CAC scan. In their study, van Velzen and colleagues[28] used a DL method for automatic calcium scoring across a wide variety of CT scan types, and they found that the method was robust with high performance. In addition, van Assen and colleagues[29] used a DL-based, fully automated calcium quantification on ECG and non-ECG-gated chest CT; they obtained good correlation compared with reference standards (manual evaluation and Agatston score) and shorter evaluation time. Other DL algorithms have been successfully applied to CCTA scans to measure CAC score avoiding additional scans and consequent additional radiation exposure.[30,31]

Plaque characterization
CCTA plays an important role in the noninvasive evaluation of coronary artery disease (CAD). Thanks to its high negative-predictive value, it allows us to effectively exclude the presence of obstructive CAD. Moreover, CCTA allows quantification of stenosis and grading according to the Coronary Artery Disease Reporting And Data System (CAD-RADS) and also allows assessment of high-risk plaque features,[32] included in the CAD-RADS 2.0.[33] AI has been applied to optimize the extraction of these features, thereby reducing postprocessing time by performing these tasks in an automated but accurate manner (**Fig. 2**). CNN-based models have been developed to classify CCTAs in the correct CAD-RADS category, using expert readers' grading as a reference standard. These CNN-based models have shown promising results, with performance similar to those achieved by the radiologist.[34–37] DL has also been applied to CCTA to increase its diagnostic performance and specificity in detecting functionally significant stenosis. DL models have been applied to identify patients with functionally significant stenoses who underwent CCTA and invasive coronary angiography (ICA) with fractional flow reserve (FFR) measurement, used as a reference standard. The DL model analyzed the presence of ischemic changes in the left ventricle myocardium and classified patients as having a nonsignificant or significant stenosis, resulting in improved discrimination compared with CCTA-based degree of stenosis only.[38,39] Recently, Lin and colleagues[40] showed that DL-based luminal stenosis severity has excellent agreement not only with expert readers but also with intravascular ultrasound, as well as DL-based CAD-RADS category agrees closely with expert CCTA read and ICA.

Beyond quantification of stenosis, CCTA also allows atherosclerotic plaque evaluation and vessel remodeling assessment. Several automated methods have been developed to perform these

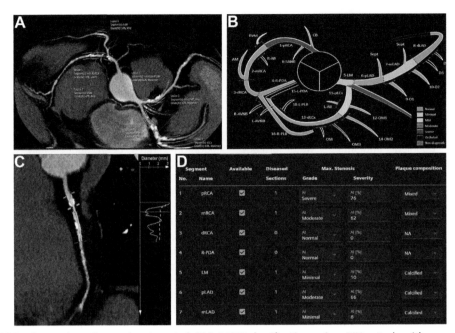

Fig. 2. CCTA plaque detection and automated CAD-RADS classification using AIHeart algorithm, an AI-based research prototype from Siemens Healthineers, Erlangen, Germany. (A) Identification of coronary plaque. (B) Classification of severity through a color-coded map. (C) Analysis of a single lesion, with a graph of the vessel diameter throughout. (D) Results of AIHeart analysis for all coronary segments, with plaque composition, stenosis grade and severity, and available manual correction. pRCA, proximal right coronary artery; mRCA, mid RCA; dRCA, distal RCA; R/L-PDA, posterior descending artery from the right/left; LM, left main; pLAD, proximal left anterior descending; mLAD, mid LAD, dLAD, distal LAD; D1-D3, diagonal branches 1 to 3; OM1-3, obtuse marginal branches 1 to 3; pLCx, proximal left circumflex; dLCx, distal LCx; AM, acute marginal branch; R-/L-PLB, posterior-lateral branch from the right/left; Sept, septal branches; R-/L-AB, right/left atrial branches; SANB, sinoatrial nodal branch; R-/L-AVNB, atrio-ventricular nodal branch from the right/left.

tasks, which would otherwise require time-consuming manual evaluation and challenging its clinical applicability to workflow.[41] AI-augmented software programs are able to automatically perform quantitative plaque analysis, with evaluation of plaque burden, calcified/noncalcified plaque, and high-risk features. Much of AI-assisted software has been validated against invasive or histologic data.[42] Total coronary plaque burden is a prognostic marker that correlates with disease severity, and noncalcified plaque burden is an indicator of more vulnerable/active plaque.[43] AI-based quantification methods allow for a rapid and standardized analysis of plaque burden, thereby reducing measurement variability that would affect the evaluation of plaque progression, another important prognostic factor.[44] Various software to perform AI-based plaque quantification has been developed and has obtained Food and Drug Administration approval.[45] For example, Cleerly (Cleerly Healthcare, New York, NY, USA) is a recent AI-assisted, fully automated software. It uses a series of validated CNN models to assess image quality, label, and segment and analyze the coronary

tree and contours, outputting degree of stenosis, plaque volume, remodeling index, and plaque characteristics, such as low-density noncalcified plaque. Cleerly (Cleerly Healthcare, New York, NY, USA) recently showed high-diagnostic performance for stenosis severity and high correlation to quantitative coronary angiography, in accordance with the prior multicenter CLARIFY trial.[37,46] Another software is VascuCAP (Elucid Bioimaging, Wenham, MA, USA). It is a computer-assisted, semiautomated approach that performs structural and plaque component quantification, with evaluation of lipid-rich necrotic core, matrix, calcified plaque, as well as stenosis degree, plaque volume, and remodeling index (**Fig. 3**). Both of these examples allow the radiologist to perform quality control and manual adjustment if necessary.

Moreover, AI-based models were demonstrated to be useful in prognostic prediction: quantification of total, noncalcified, and low-attenuation plaque burden. These AI-based tools have been shown to significantly improve prediction of lesion-specific ischemia by FFR over stenosis grading alone.[47] AI-based plaque characterization has

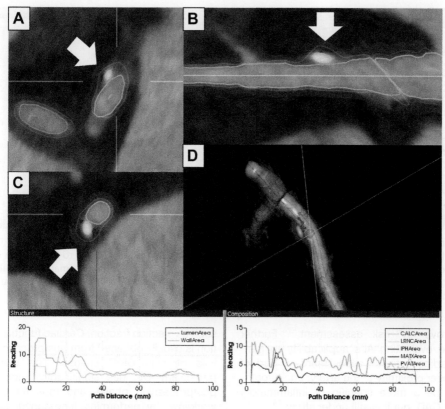

Fig. 3. A 61-year-old female patient with multiple CV risk factors who underwent CCTA. Analysis was performed via a DL-based software, Elucid Vascucap (Elucid Bioimaging, Wenham, MA, USA). (*A–C*) Cross-sectional images show color-coded plaque analysis of the left anterior descending artery (LAD): arrows pointing at a calcified plaque (*turquoise*) with spot of intraplaque hemorrhage (*brown*), and perivascular adipose tissue surrounding the vessel (*yellow*). (*D*) Color-coded 3D reconstruction of the vessel, with planes indicating the level at which images *A–C* were taken. Graphs showing structure and composition of the vessel.

also shown improved prognostic stratification, demonstrating better major adverse cardiovascular events (MACE) prognostication than clinical risk factors alone, increasing accuracy from 0.629 to 0.872.[48]

Computed tomography–fractional flow reserve
Even though CCTA mainly provides anatomic information, thanks to CT-FFR, it can provide functional assessment as well. However, it requires complex computer fluid dynamics computations, which are time-consuming and costly. ML has recently been applied to a CT-FFR calculation (FFR$_{ML}$) as opposed to a computational fluid dynamics (FFR$_{CFD}$) -based approach in order to shorten execution times (**Fig. 4**). As shown by Tesche and colleagues,[49] FFR$_{ML}$ required significantly shorter processing time when compared with FFR$_{CFD}$, while performing equally in detecting ischemia. Moreover, FFR$_{ML}$ closely reproduces FFR$_{CFD}$ calculations, assesses the hemodynamic severity of coronary stenosis, correlating with

invasive FFR results, and improves diagnostic accuracy and positive-predictive value of CCTA on a per-vessel and per-patient level.[50] However, CT reconstruction algorithms influence FFR$_{ML}$ analysis results; thus, further studies are needed.[51] Recent studies have shown that FFR$_{ML}$ can be useful in outcome prediction: the combined use of FFR$_{ML}$ and CCTA-derived plaque features improves predictive value for MACE over stenosis grading alone.[52,53]

Epicardial fat
Epicardial adipose tissue (EAT) is the metabolically active fat depot that surrounds coronary arteries. It is known that it is related to CV events owing to its local proinflammatory, proatherogenic effect on vasculature.[54] AI can assist in segmentation and quantification of EAT. Semiautomated and fully automated models have been developed to measure epicardial fat from nonenhanced, calcium scoring CT.[55,56] This AI-based approach has proven to be a time-saving and reliable tool that

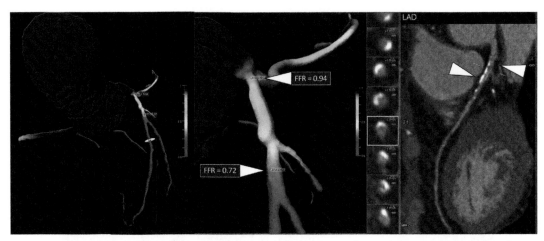

Fig. 4. Coronary CT-FFR analysis with ML-based research prototype from Siemens Healthineers, Erlangen, Germany. The analysis shows severe stenosis in the proximal LAD, with a drop of CT-FFR to 0.72, which is considered functionally significant (abnormal if less than 0.75). *Arrowheads* indicate the proximal and distal markers used for CT-FFR assessment. Normal value of CT-FFR proximally to the lesion (0.94) and abnormal value distally (0.72) can be observed.

may improve CV risk assessment.[57] Further studies are evaluating AI's applicability to pericoronary adipose tissue assessment—a part of EAT, in closer proximity to the artery, and hypothesized to be a more specific proinflammatory marker for CAD, but it is still under study.[58]

ARTIFICIAL INTELLIGENCE APPLICATIONS IN CARDIAC MR IMAGING
Volumes Analysis

One of the key advantages of CMR is to quantitatively assess cardiac function by measuring reproducible, less operator-dependent parameters, such as ejection fraction. Cardiac function evaluation is usually obtained from postprocessing analysis of cine CMR images. The use of AI, particularly DL, has significantly improved the postprocessing phase, and thus the radiology workflow, by performing time-consuming activities, such as manual segmentation (**Figs. 5** and **6**). Tao and colleagues[59] used CNN to perform fully automated quantification of left ventricle function from short-axis cine CMR images, and they obtained high accuracy when tested against a multivendor, multicenter data set. In addition, their trained CNN was able to process a complete cine CMR data set (approximately 300 images) in

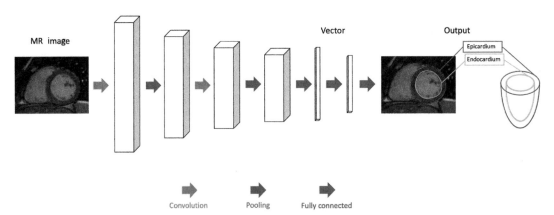

Fig. 5. A CNN for automated CMR ventricular segmentation. The CMR image is used as input by the CNN, which learns hierarchical features through a stack of convolution and pooling procedures, generating spatial features maps. These maps are flattened into a vector through fully connected layers, yielding the output, that is, the segmentation of the left ventricle (LV). As depicted in the output section, the algorithm learns the spatial features corresponding to endocardium and epicardium, thus obtaining a geometric model of the LV and performing automated segmentation.

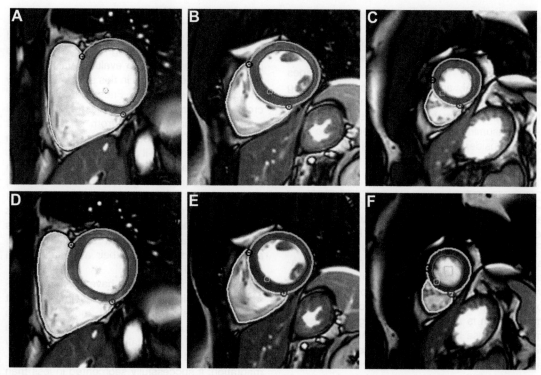

Fig. 6. Reconstruction of biventricular volumes obtained using a DL algorithm (Circle Cardiovascular Imaging,[42] Calgary, Canada) that automatically identified the best diastole, systole, the epicardial border of left ventricle, and the endocardial border of both left and right ventricle. Automated segmentation of left ventricle (epicardial border: *green*; endocardial border: *red*) and right ventricle (endocardial border: *yellow*) volumes and mass in diastole using DL reconstruction on basal (*A*), midventricle (*B*), and apical (*C*), in comparison with the myocardial borders manually drawn by human reader (*D–F*). The DL algorithm provides an accurate quantification of the ventricular volumes and mass in just a few seconds compared with several minutes from manual tracing.

approximately 1 second, free of any user intervention. Similarly, Ruijsink and colleagues[60] developed a fully automated DL-based framework for quality-controlled cardiac function analysis, without the need for direct clinician action; more recently, Evertz and colleagues[61] showed that a fully automated biventricular volumetric assessment was able to efficiently predict risk of CV death in patients undergoing transcatheter aortic valve replacement when compared with manual approach, with a significant time saving, which would improve and optimize clinical management.

Volume and function assessment is not limited to the left ventricle. AI algorithms have been applied also to whole-heart segmentation tasks. Automated CNN models performed whole-heart segmentation on short axis, long-axis four-chamber view, and both sets of images together, with similar accuracy to manual analysis, indicating feasibility and time-saving advantage of this approach.[62,63] However, accuracy is shown to be slightly lower for right chambers and basal slices, mainly because of higher morphologic complexity and variability of this anatomic regions, which cause more difficulties in segmentation, even for expert clinicians.[64,65]

Moreover, recent studies have drawn attention to AI-based methods to assess myocardial strain, a prognostic and diagnostic marker of CVDs, which represents radial, circumferential, and longitudinal deformation of myocardium from relaxed to contractile state.[66] CMR-based strain is usually obtained from tagged images, which are not routinely included in the workflow because of their need of time-consuming analysis and specific software; however, AI has been a useful tool to speed the process and make myocardial strain more widely available.[67] Some studies have developed AI models that automate strain analysis from tagged images, but these models still require manual input for initialization of reference points.[68,69] More recently, Dhaene and colleagues[70] addressed this problem by developing a DL algorithm that segments the myocardium from tagged images obtained from cine images through a cine-to-tagged transformation, and they showed a performance comparable to existing networks for cine images.

Thus, AI has proven to be a reliable tool that improves operator-dependency, speeds postprocessing phase, and optimizes CMR images assessment. AI, and DL in particular, is being widely implemented to improve radiology workflows by performing volume analysis, an otherwise time-consuming task that would require the clinician a considerable amount of time.

Ischemic Heart Disease

Of the multiple clinical applications of AI, its use to assess and evaluate ischemic heart disease, the leading cause of death globally, is noteworthy. Particularly, AI is being used to detect, segment, and analyze infarcted myocardium, and its application in myocardial viability studies has shown advantages over the traditional diagnostic evaluation of LGE and T1 mapping.[71] Detection of viable myocardium is a key step for prognosis assessment, because it represents the muscle that can recover after revascularization. Recent studies[72,73] applied texture analysis to cardiac cine MR images in order to differentiate between infarcted nonviable, viable, remote, or normal myocardium. Texture analysis has been successfully applied to noncontrast CMR images as well, giving an alternative to LGE,[74] particularly important for those patients with severe renal impairment.

With regards to segmentation, AI has been used to perform semiautomated and fully automated segmentation of myocardial infarction (MI), mainly with the use of DL-based algorithms using CNN-based networks,[75,76] enabling quantification of disease severity without time-consuming manual image annotation. Zabihollahy and colleagues[77,78] showed that CNN provided fully automated segmentation of myocardial scar from 3-dimensional (3D) LGE images, outperforming alternative approaches, including the manual one. In addition, Kotu and colleagues[79,80] suggested an automatic scar segmentation method based on texture analysis and Bayes classification, and they found comparable results to manual segmentation.

Once the scar is detected and segmented, its analysis provides useful prognostic information. Scar burden with LGE has been shown to predict all-cause mortality,[81] sudden cardiac death, and ventricular arrhythmias, especially in patients with ventricular dysfunction.[82,83] AI has been applied to fibrosis analysis with the aim of improving processing time, variability, and generalizability. Moreover, ML-based LGE analysis, compared with human-based, has proven to predict MACE, especially when dense scar is detected.[84]

Valve Disease

CMR, thanks to phase-contrast sequences and the possibility of obtaining specific anatomic planes, has been used to evaluate valves' anatomy. AI has been applied in this setting to classify and grade valve diseases. Fries and colleagues[85] created a DL model that satisfactorily classified aortic valve malformations from phase-contrast CMR images. They used weak supervision to train a DL model and used it to classify bicuspid aortic valve in unlabeled MR imaging sequences from the UK Biobank. Using health outcome data, they found that the model identified individuals at increased risk of MACE. In addition, ML models have been used to identify different phenotypes of bicuspid valve-associated aortopathy (root, ascending, and arch) and their association with specific clinical findings.[86]

Moreover, advances in AI have improved automated processing of phase-contrast images. Bratt and colleagues[87] tested an ML model for aortic flow analysis using this type of sequence. The model tracked aortic valve borders to quantify aortic flow and was compared with manual segmentation; it successfully segmented in less than 0.01 minutes per case compared with 3.96 minutes per case of the manual approach. Aortic flow is particularly important to assess forward and regurgitant flow, enabling CMR diagnosis and grading of aortic regurgitation. Regarding mitral valve assessment, CMR uses 2 acquisition techniques to quantify mitral regurgitation: 2-dimensional phase-contrast across the aortic valve and short-axis cine of the left ventricle to obtain aortic forward flow and left ventricle stroke volume, respectively. The subtraction of the two indirectly gives a measurement of mitral regurgitant flow. AI, as previously mentioned, has been applied to both acquisition techniques in order to automatically segment and quantify flow and volume.

Cardiomyopathies

CMR plays an increasingly important role in the diagnosis, management planning, and prognosis of cardiomyopathies. AI has been applied to this setting for the detection of specific diagnostic features, and LGE evaluation, which has a prognostic relevance in diseases such as hypertrophic cardiomyopathy (HCM), and disease classification. Ammar and colleagues[88] used a DL network and a classifier ensemble to segment and classify images from CMR of healthy patients, HCM, dilated cardiomyopathy (DCM), abnormal right ventricle, and MI, and they reported excellent accuracy. Radiomic texture analysis combined with AI algorithms has played a role in cardiomyopathy classification as well. Its diagnostic ability has been shown to be high, as seen in the study by Neisius and colleagues,[89] which aimed to perform radiomic analysis of native T1 images in order to differentiate between hypertensive and HCMs. Moreover, Fahmy and colleagues[90] developed an AI-based screening model that uses radiomics and DL features to identify patients with HCM without scar before the administration of contrast; the combined DL-Radiomics model outperformed the DL or radiomics models alone, indicating the potential of the combination of these 2 approaches. Fahmy and colleagues[91] also developed a DL model that combined LGE and cine images to improve accuracy of scar quantification among patients with HCM.

Moreover, AI has been applied to prognostic evaluation and risk stratification. Chen and colleagues[92] used an ML model to effectively predict risk of CV events in patients with DCM at 1-year follow-up. Zhou and colleagues[93] applied DL to detect the risk of having a genetic mutation in patients with HCM, and the DL model, especially if combined with Toronto genotype score, improved mutation-risk prediction and showed high diagnostic performance. Finally, DL has been successfully used in the setting of other cardiomyopathies: detection and classification of cardiac amyloidosis,[94,95] aiding diagnosis of left ventricular noncompaction,[96] and arrhythmogenic right ventricular cardiomyopathy.[97]

Congenital Heart Disease

CMR is widely used in the evaluation of congenital heart disease (CHD), and many studies have applied AI in this setting for acquisition speed-up and image reconstruction, with the aim to make CMR more suitable for the pediatric population and image processing easier despite the complex anatomy of these patients. For example, Karimi-Bidhendi and colleagues[98] used a fully automated DL method to segment right and left ventricles in patients with CHD, and the model showed strong agreement with manual segmentation. One other study[99] aimed to reduce scan time by acquiring images at lower resolution and subsequently processed the images by an ML network that recovered the high-resolution features from the rapidly acquired whole-heart images. The authors found good recovery of features and high diagnostic accuracy and confidence.

OUTCOME PREDICTION

The significant number of imaging markers of CV risk, such as CAC score, plaque features, adipose tissue, and radiomics, are being incorporated to traditional clinical risk factors, in order to create predictive models that can increase the performance of current risk score and prognostic models. AI plays an important role in this process, enabling the consideration of clinical and imaging data together while including a larger number of clinical parameters. Several fusion models have been developed to combine multiple resources, and they have been successfully applied to CVD risk and severity assessment, acute CVD detection, and CVD phenotyping.[100] CNNs can be used to extract clinical data from electronic medical records, radiology notes, imaging studies, and clinical notes, whereas ML algorithms, by integrating clinical and imaging data, have been shown to improve prediction of disease and evaluate prognosis[101] (**Fig. 7**). ML has been used to predict 5-year all-cause mortality in patients undergoing CCTA; the ML risk score combining clinical and CCTA data exhibited a significantly higher

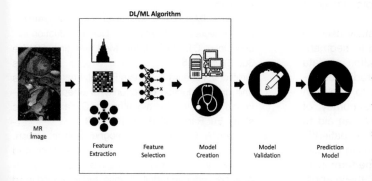

Fig. 7. A DL/ML algorithm based on CMR images texture analysis. The images are used as the input after being processed (eg, segmented and elaborated for analysis), and they are fed to the proposed algorithm, which automatically performs feature extraction, obtaining features of different orders. The features are subsequently selected and reduced, creating a radiomic signature model, possibly integrating such data also with electronic medical records (EMR). The model is further validated, thus creating finally a prediction model, the latter possibly being used to perform different tasks (eg, myocardial scar detection, pathology classification). ML and DL can be involved in different steps of the texture analysis process or automatize most of the workflow. The automated combination of advanced imaging features and EMR can provide more accurate and rapid prediction models to be applied in clinical practice.

area under the curve for outcome prediction when compared with the two alone.[102] The ML approach was also used to predict 3-year risk of MACE by combining myocardial perfusion single-photon emission CT data with clinical data, and it showed high predictive accuracy.[103] Fusion models are not limited to clinical and imaging data alone, but can include other types of data, such as genetic data, which can be used to predict 10-year risk of ischemic heart disease together with medical records.[104] Overall, a significant effort has been put into the development of various multimodality AI models that can improve patient care and CVD assessment.

SUMMARY

Continuous technical advancement is driving the implementation of AI into radiology, and recent literature has witnessed an increase in the number of publications regarding AI applicability in every field of imaging, including cardiac imaging. Literature shows that many AI-based algorithms are being applied to cardiac CT and MR and are partly already integrated into clinical application. The main areas of AI applicability are detection, quantification, and characterization of cardiac disease.

Although great progress has already been made, most of the AI models developed still present limitations, such as narrow focus and limited generalizability, that need to be addressed before AI can be clinically applied with confidence.[105] It is predicted that AI will aid radiologists by performing time-consuming tasks, saving resources that can be used for more difficult/rare cases where AI is expected to fail, therefore improving workflow. A limitation of AI is the lack of intuition, cognition, and reasoning—human skills that the radiologists will always apply to judge AI performance and to check for possible errors in difficult cases.

In summary, AI has been successfully used to perform time-consuming tasks, such as segmentation and postprocessing, optimization of data acquisition and reconstruction, and grading of disease severity. AI has been proven to show an improvement, in terms of time and accuracy, of human work, and therefore, serves as an aid to physicians in better understanding of the patient's cardiac health. Several AI applications in cardiac imaging demonstrate human-level performance, and it is likely that, in the near future, these applications will be further improved to be integrated into clinical workflow; this will have a great impact on costs, wider usability, and optimization of workflow efficiency.

CLINICS CARE POINTS

- Artificial intelligence can be applied to cardiac imaging postprocessing, significantly decreasing time and improving accuracy.
- Artificial intelligence can improve cardiac disease quantification and repeatability, directly impacting patients' cardiac health.
- Artificial intelligence solutions will improve clinical workflow and efficiency in cardiac imaging.

DISCLOSURE

Dr C.N. De Cecco receives funding from Siemens Healthineers, Germany and is a consultant of Bayer and Xeos. Dr M. van Assen receives funding from Siemens Healthineers.

REFERENCES

1. Benjamin EJ, Muntner P, Alonso A, et al. Heart Disease and Stroke Statistics—2019 Update: A Report From the American Heart Association. Circulation 2019;139(10):e56–528.
2. Chartrand G, Cheng PM, Vorontsov E, et al. Deep Learning: A Primer for Radiologists. Radiographics 2017;37(7):2113–31.
3. Cheng PM, Montagnon E, Yamashita R, et al. Deep Learning: An Update for Radiologists. Radiographics 2021;41(5):1427–45.
4. FDA Cleared AI Algorithms. American College of Radiology Data Science Institute. Available at: https://aicentral.acrdsi.org/. [Accessed 20 June 2023].
5. Kang E, Min J, Ye JC. A deep convolutional neural network using directional wavelets for low-dose X-ray CT reconstruction. Med Phys 2017;44(10):e360–75.
6. Wolterink JM, Leiner T, Viergever MA, et al. Generative Adversarial Networks for Noise Reduction in Low-Dose CT. IEEE Trans Med Imaging 2017;36(12):2536–45.
7. Greffier J, Hamard A, Pereira F, et al. Image quality and dose reduction opportunity of deep learning image reconstruction algorithm for CT: a phantom study. Eur Radiol 2020;30(7):3951–9.
8. Bernard A, Comby P-O, Lemogne B, et al. Deep learning reconstruction versus iterative reconstruction for cardiac CT angiography in a stroke imaging protocol: reduced radiation dose and improved image quality. Quant Imag Med Surg 2021;11(1):392–401.
9. Patwari M, Gutjahr R, Raupach R, et al. Measuring CT Reconstruction Quality with Deep Convolutional

Neural Networks. Lect Notes Comput Sc 2019; 11905:113–24.

10. Slomka PJ, Dey D, Sitek A, et al. Cardiac imaging: working towards fully-automated machine analysis & interpretation. Expert Rev Med Devices 2017; 14(3):197–212.

11. Blansit K, Retson T, Masutani E, et al. Deep Learning-based Prescription of Cardiac MRI Planes. Radiology Artificial intelligence 2019;1(6): e180069.

12. Frick M, Paetsch I, Harder Cd, et al. Fully automatic geometry planning for cardiac MR imaging and reproducibility of functional cardiac parameters. J Magn Reson Imag : JMRI 2011;34(2):457–67.

13. Edalati M, Zheng Y, Watkins MP, et al. Implementation and prospective clinical validation of AI-based planning and shimming techniques in cardiac MRI. Med Phys 2022;49(1):129–43.

14. Yoon H, Kim KS, Kim D, et al. Motion adaptive patch-based low-rank approach for compressed sensing cardiac cine MRI. IEEE Trans Med Imaging 2014;33(11):2069–85.

15. Küstner T, Fuin N, Hammernik K, et al. CINENet: deep learning-based 3D cardiac CINE MRI reconstruction with multi-coil complex-valued 4D spatio-temporal convolutions. Sci Rep 2020;10(1):13710.

16. Sandino CM, Lai P, Vasanawala SS, et al. Accelerating cardiac cine MRI using a deep learning-based ESPIRiT reconstruction. Magn Reson Med 2021;85(1):152–67.

17. Küstner T, Armanious K, Yang J, et al. Retrospective correction of motion-affected MR images using deep learning frameworks. Magn Reson Med 2019;82(4):1527–40.

18. Armanious K, Jiang C, Fischer M, et al. MedGAN: Medical image translation using GANs. Comput Med Imaging Graph 2020;79:101684.

19. Lossau Née Elss T, Nickisch H, Wissel T, et al. Learning metal artifact reduction in cardiac CT images with moving pacemakers. Med Image Anal 2020;61:101655.

20. Wang J, Zhao Y, Noble JH, Dawant BM. Conditional Generative Adversarial Networks for Metal Artifact Reduction in CT Images of the Ear. Med Image Comput Comput Assist Interv 2018;11070:3–11.

21. Shi Z, Wang N, Kong F, et al. A semi-supervised learning method of latent features based on convolutional neural networks for CT metal artifact reduction. Med Phys 2022;49(6):3845–59.

22. Liao H, Lin W-A, Zhou SK, et al. Artifact Disentanglement Network for Unsupervised Metal Artifact Reduction. IEEE Trans Med Imaging 2020;39(3):634–43.

23. Zhang Q, Burrage MK, Shanmuganathan M, et al. Artificial Intelligence for Contrast-Free MRI: Scar Assessment in Myocardial Infarction Using Deep Learning–Based Virtual Native Enhancement. Circulation 2022;146(20):1492–503.

24. Yeboah J, McClelland RL, Polonsky TS, et al. Comparison of novel risk markers for improvement in cardiovascular risk assessment in intermediate-risk individuals. JAMA 2012;308(8):788–95.

25. Wolterink JM, Leiner T, de Vos BD, et al. An evaluation of automatic coronary artery calcium scoring methods with cardiac CT using the orCaScore framework. Med Phys 2016;43(5):2361.

26. Martin SS, van Assen M, Rapaka S, et al. Evaluation of a Deep Learning-Based Automated CT Coronary Artery Calcium Scoring Algorithm. JACC Cardiovasc Imaging 2020;13(2 Pt 1):524–6.

27. Lessmann N, Van Ginneken B, Zreik M, et al. Automatic Calcium Scoring in Low-Dose Chest CT Using Deep Neural Networks With Dilated Convolutions. IEEE Trans Med Imaging 2018;37(2):615–25.

28. Van Velzen SGM, Lessmann N, Velthuis BK, et al. Deep Learning for Automatic Calcium Scoring in CT: Validation Using Multiple Cardiac CT and Chest CT Protocols. Radiology 2020;295(1): 66–79.

29. Van Assen M, Martin SS, Varga-Szemes A, et al. Automatic coronary calcium scoring in chest CT using a deep neural network in direct comparison with non-contrast cardiac CT: A validation study. Eur J Radiol 2021;134:109428.

30. Mu D, Bai J, Chen W, et al. Calcium Scoring at Coronary CT Angiography Using Deep Learning. Radiology 2022;302(2):309–16.

31. Wolterink JM, Leiner T, de Vos BD, et al. Automatic coronary artery calcium scoring in cardiac CT angiography using paired convolutional neural networks. Med Image Anal 2016;34:123–36.

32. Feuchtner G, Kerber J, Burghard P, et al. The high-risk criteria low-attenuation plaque <60 HU and the napkin-ring sign are the most powerful predictors of MACE: a long-term follow-up study. Eur Heart J Cardiovasc Imaging 2017;18(7):772–9.

33. Cury RC, Leipsic J, Abbara S, et al. CAD-RADS™ 2.0 - 2022 Coronary Artery Disease-Reporting and Data System: An Expert Consensus Document of the Society of Cardiovascular Computed Tomography (SCCT), the American College of Cardiology (ACC), the American College of Radiology (ACR), and the North America Society of Cardiovascular Imaging (NASCI). J Cardiovasc Comput Tomogr 2022;16(6):536–57.

34. Muscogiuri G, Chiesa M, Trotta M, et al. Performance of a deep learning algorithm for the evaluation of CAD-RADS classification with CCTA. Atherosclerosis 2020;294:25–32.

35. Paul JF, Rohnean A, Giroussens H, et al. Evaluation of a deep learning model on coronary CT angiography for automatic stenosis detection. Diagn Interv Imaging 2022;103(6):316–23.

36. Huang Z, Xiao J, Wang X, et al. Clinical Evaluation of the Automatic Coronary Artery Disease Reporting

and Data System (CAD-RADS) in Coronary Computed Tomography Angiography Using Convolutional Neural Networks. Acad Radiol 2023;30(4): 698–706.

37. Choi AD, Marques H, Kumar V, et al. CT Evaluation by Artificial Intelligence for Atherosclerosis, Stenosis and Vascular Morphology (CLARIFY): A Multicenter, international study. J Cardiovasc Comput Tomogr 2021;15(6):470–6.

38. Zreik M, Lessmann N, van Hamersvelt RW, et al. Deep learning analysis of the myocardium in coronary CT angiography for identification of patients with functionally significant coronary artery stenosis. Med Image Anal 2018;44:72–85.

39. van Hamersvelt RW, Zreik M, Voskuil M, et al. Deep learning analysis of left ventricular myocardium in CT angiographic intermediate-degree coronary stenosis improves the diagnostic accuracy for identification of functionally significant stenosis. Eur Radiol 2019;29(5):2350–9.

40. Lin A, Manral N, McElhinney P, et al. Deep learning-enabled coronary CT angiography for plaque and stenosis quantification and cardiac risk prediction: an international multicentre study. The Lancet Digital Health 2022;4(4):e256–65.

41. van Assen M, von Knebel Doeberitz P, Quyyumi AA, et al. Artificial intelligence for advanced analysis of coronary plaque. Eur Heart J Suppl 2023; 25(Supplement_C):C112–7.

42. Williams MC, Earls JP, Hecht H. Quantitative assessment of atherosclerotic plaque, recent progress and current limitations. J Cardiovasc Comput Tomogr 2022;16(2):124–37.

43. Williams MC, Kwiecinski J, Doris M, et al. Low-Attenuation Noncalcified Plaque on Coronary Computed Tomography Angiography Predicts Myocardial Infarction. Circulation 2020;141(18): 1452–62.

44. Lee SE, Chang HJ, Sung JM, et al. Effects of Statins on Coronary Atherosclerotic Plaques: The PARADIGM Study. JACC Cardiovasc Imaging 2018;11(10):1475–84.

45. Available at:Artificial intelligence and machine learning (AI/ML)-Enabled medical Devices https://www.fda.gov/medical-devices/software-medical-device-samd/artificial-intelligence-and-machine-learning-aiml-enabled-medical-devices. [Accessed 21 June 2023].

46. Griffin WF, Choi AD, Riess JS, et al. AI Evaluation of Stenosis on Coronary CTA, Comparison With Quantitative Coronary Angiography and Fractional Flow Reserve: A CREDENCE Trial Substudy. JACC Cardiovasc Imaging 2023;16(2):193–205.

47. Diaz-Zamudio M, Dey D, Schuhbaeck A, et al. Automated Quantitative Plaque Burden from Coronary CT Angiography Noninvasively Predicts Hemodynamic Significance by using Fractional Flow Reserve in Intermediate Coronary Lesions. Radiology 2015;276(2):408–15.

48. Van Assen M, Varga-Szemes A, Schoepf UJ, et al. Automated plaque analysis for the prognostication of major adverse cardiac events. Eur J Radiol 2019;116:76–83.

49. Tesche C, De Cecco CN, Baumann S, et al. Coronary CT Angiography-derived Fractional Flow Reserve: Machine Learning Algorithm versus Computational Fluid Dynamics Modeling. Radiology 2018;288(1):64–72.

50. Coenen A, Kim Y-H, Kruk M, et al. Diagnostic Accuracy of a Machine-Learning Approach to Coronary Computed Tomographic Angiography–Based Fractional Flow Reserve. Circ Cardiovasc Imaging 2018;11(6):e007217.

51. Mastrodicasa D, Albrecht MH, Schoepf UJ, et al. Artificial intelligence machine learning-based coronary CT fractional flow reserve (CT-FFRML): Impact of iterative and filtered back projection reconstruction techniques. J Cardiovasc Comput Tomogr 2019;13(6):331–5.

52. von Knebel Doeberitz PL, De Cecco CN, Schoepf UJ, et al. Impact of Coronary Computerized Tomography Angiography-Derived Plaque Quantification and Machine-Learning Computerized Tomography Fractional Flow Reserve on Adverse Cardiac Outcome. Am J Cardiol 2019;124(9):1340–8.

53. von Knebel Doeberitz PL, De Cecco CN, Schoepf UJ, et al. Coronary CT angiography-derived plaque quantification with artificial intelligence CT fractional flow reserve for the identification of lesion-specific ischemia. Eur Radiol 2019;29(5): 2378–87.

54. Mahabadi AA, Berg MH, Lehmann N, et al. Association of epicardial fat with cardiovascular risk factors and incident myocardial infarction in the general population: the Heinz Nixdorf Recall Study. J Am Coll Cardiol 2013;61(13):1388–95.

55. Dey D, Wong ND, Tamarappoo B, et al. Computer-aided non-contrast CT-based quantification of pericardial and thoracic fat and their associations with coronary calcium and Metabolic Syndrome. Atherosclerosis 2010;209(1):136–41.

56. Commandeur F, Goeller M, Betancur J, et al. Deep Learning for Quantification of Epicardial and Thoracic Adipose Tissue From Non-Contrast CT. IEEE Trans Med Imaging 2018;37(8):1835–46.

57. Zhang L, Sun J, Jiang B, et al. Development of artificial intelligence in epicardial and pericoronary adipose tissue imaging: a systematic review. Eur J Hybrid Imaging 2021;5(1):14.

58. Ma R, Fari R, van der Harst P, et al. Evaluation of pericoronary adipose tissue attenuation on CT. Br J Radiol 2023;96(1145):20220885.

59. Tao Q, Yan W, Wang Y, et al. Deep Learning-based Method for Fully Automatic Quantification of Left

Ventricle Function from Cine MR Images: A Multi-vendor, Multicenter Study. Radiology 2019;290(1): 81–8.

60. Ruijsink B, Puyol-Antón E, Oksuz I, et al. Fully Automated, Quality-Controlled Cardiac Analysis From CMR: Validation and Large-Scale Application to Characterize Cardiac Function. JACC Cardiovasc Imaging 2020;13(3):684–95.

61. Evertz R, Lange T, Backhaus SJ, et al. Artificial Intelligence Enabled Fully Automated CMR Function Quantification for Optimized Risk Stratification in Patients Undergoing Transcatheter Aortic Valve Replacement. J Interv Cardiol 2022;2022:1–9.

62. Arai H, Kawakubo M, Sanui K, et al. Assessment of Bi-Ventricular and Bi-Atrial Areas Using Four-Chamber Cine Cardiovascular Magnetic Resonance Imaging: Fully Automated Segmentation with a U-Net Convolutional Neural Network. Int J Environ Res Public Health 2022;19(3). https://doi.org/10.3390/ijerph19031401.

63. Bai W, Sinclair M, Tarroni G, et al. Automated cardiovascular magnetic resonance image analysis with fully convolutional networks. J Cardiovasc Magn Reson 2018;20(1):65.

64. Bernard O, Lalande A, Zotti C, et al. Deep Learning Techniques for Automatic MRI Cardiac Multi-Structures Segmentation and Diagnosis: Is the Problem Solved? IEEE Trans Med Imaging 2018; 37(11):2514–25.

65. Penso M, Moccia S, Scafuri S, et al. Automated left and right ventricular chamber segmentation in cardiac magnetic resonance images using dense fully convolutional neural network. Comput Methods Programs Biomed 2021;204:106059.

66. Amzulescu MS, De Craene M, Langet H, et al. Myocardial strain imaging: review of general principles, validation, and sources of discrepancies. Eur Heart J Cardiovasc Imaging 2019;20(6): 605–19.

67. Ibrahim E-SH. Myocardial tagging by Cardiovascular Magnetic Resonance: evolution of techniques–pulse sequences, analysis algorithms, and applications. J Cardiovasc Magn Reson 2011;13(1):36.

68. Ferdian E, Suinesiaputra A, Fung K, et al. Fully Automated Myocardial Strain Estimation from Cardiovascular MRI-tagged Images Using a Deep Learning Framework in the UK Biobank. Radiology Cardiothoracic imaging 2020;2(1):e190032.

69. Loecher M, Hannum AJ, Perotti LE, Ennis DB. Arbitrary Point Tracking with Machine Learning to Measure Cardiac Strains in Tagged MRI. Funct Imaging Model Heart 2021;12738:213–22.

70. Dhaene AP, Loecher M, Wilson AJ, et al. Myocardial Segmentation of Tagged Magnetic Resonance Images with Transfer Learning Using Generative Cine-To-Tagged Dataset Transformation. Bioengineering 2023;10(2):166.

71. Katikireddy CK, Samim A. Myocardial viability assessment and utility in contemporary management of ischemic cardiomyopathy. Clin Cardiol 2022;45(2):152–61.

72. Larroza A, López-Lereu MP, Monmeneu JV, et al. Texture analysis of cardiac cine magnetic resonance imaging to detect nonviable segments in patients with chronic myocardial infarction. Med Phys 2018;45(4):1471–80.

73. Avard E, Shiri I, Hajianfar G, et al. Non-contrast Cine Cardiac Magnetic Resonance image radiomics features and machine learning algorithms for myocardial infarction detection. Comput Biol Med 2022;141:105145.

74. Zhang N, Yang G, Gao Z, et al. Deep Learning for Diagnosis of Chronic Myocardial Infarction on Nonenhanced Cardiac Cine MRI. Radiology 2019-06-01 2019;291(3):606–17.

75. Chen Z, Lalande A, Salomon M, et al. Automatic deep learning-based myocardial infarction segmentation from delayed enhancement MRI. Comput Med Imaging Graph 2022;95:102014.

76. Heidenreich JF, Gassenmaier T, Ankenbrand MJ, et al. Self-configuring nnU-net pipeline enables fully automatic infarct segmentation in late enhancement MRI after myocardial infarction. Eur J Radiol 2021;141:109817.

77. Zabihollahy F, Rajan S, Ukwatta E. Machine Learning-Based Segmentation of Left Ventricular Myocardial Fibrosis from Magnetic Resonance Imaging. Curr Cardiol Rep 2020;22(8). https://doi.org/10.1007/s11886-020-01321-1.

78. Zabihollahy F, Rajchl M, White JA, et al. Fully automated segmentation of left ventricular scar from 3D late gadolinium enhancement magnetic resonance imaging using a cascaded multi-planar U-Net (CMPU-Net). Med Phys 2020;47(4):1645–55.

79. Kotu LP, Engan K, Skretting K, et al. Segmentation of Scarred Myocardium in Cardiac Magnetic Resonance Images. ISRN Biomedical Imaging 2013; 2013:1–12.

80. Kotu LP, Engan K, Eftestol T, et al. Segmentation of scarred and non-scarred myocardium in LG enhanced CMR images using intensity-based textural analysis. Annu Int Conf IEEE Eng Med Biol Soc 2011;2011:5698–701.

81. Kwon DH, Asamoto L, Popovic ZB, et al. Infarct characterization and quantification by delayed enhancement cardiac magnetic resonance imaging is a powerful independent and incremental predictor of mortality in patients with advanced ischemic cardiomyopathy. Circ Cardiovasc Imaging 2014;7(5):796–804.

82. Zegard A, Okafor O, de Bono J, et al. Myocardial Fibrosis as a Predictor of Sudden Death in Patients With Coronary Artery Disease. J Am Coll Cardiol 2021;77(1):29–41.

83. Disertori M, Rigoni M, Pace N, et al. Myocardial Fibrosis Assessment by LGE Is a Powerful Predictor of Ventricular Tachyarrhythmias in Ischemic and Nonischemic LV Dysfunction. JACC Cardiovasc Imaging 2016;9(9):1046–55.

84. Ghanbari F, Joyce T, Lorenzoni V, et al. AI Cardiac MRI Scar Analysis Aids Prediction of Major Arrhythmic Events in the Multicenter DERIVATE Registry. Radiology 2023;307(3):e222239.

85. Fries JA, Varma P, Chen VS, et al. Weakly supervised classification of aortic valve malformations using unlabeled cardiac MRI sequences. Nat Commun 2019;10(1). https://doi.org/10.1038/s41467-019-11012-3.

86. Wojnarski CM, Roselli EE, Idrees JJ, et al. Machine-learning phenotypic classification of bicuspid aortopathy. J Thorac Cardiovasc Surg 2018;155(2):461–9.e4.

87. Bratt A, Kim J, Pollie M, et al. Machine learning derived segmentation of phase velocity encoded cardiovascular magnetic resonance for fully automated aortic flow quantification. J Cardiovasc Magn Reson 2019;21(1). https://doi.org/10.1186/s12968-018-0509-0.

88. Ammar A, Bouattane O, Youssfi M. Automatic cardiac cine MRI segmentation and heart disease classification. Comput Med Imaging Graph 2021;88:101864.

89. Neisius U, El-Rewaidy H, Nakamori S, et al. Radiomic Analysis of Myocardial Native T. JACC Cardiovasc Imaging 2019;12(10):1946–54.

90. Fahmy AS, Rowin EJ, Arafati A, et al. Radiomics and deep learning for myocardial scar screening in hypertrophic cardiomyopathy. J Cardiovasc Magn Reson 2022;24(1). https://doi.org/10.1186/s12968-022-00869-x.

91. Fahmy AS, Rowin EJ, Chan RH, et al. Improved Quantification of Myocardium Scar in Late Gadolinium Enhancement Images: Deep Learning Based Image Fusion Approach. J Magn Reson Imag 2021;54(1):303–12.

92. Chen R, Lu A, Wang J, et al. Using machine learning to predict one-year cardiovascular events in patients with severe dilated cardiomyopathy. Eur J Radiol 2019;117:178–83.

93. Zhou H, Li L, Liu Z, et al. Deep learning algorithm to improve hypertrophic cardiomyopathy mutation prediction using cardiac cine images. Eur Radiol 2021;31(6):3931–40.

94. Martini N, Aimo A, Barison A, et al. Deep learning to diagnose cardiac amyloidosis from cardiovascular magnetic resonance. J Cardiovasc Magn Reson 2020;22(1). https://doi.org/10.1186/s12968-020-00690-4.

95. Germain P, Vardazaryan A, Labani A, et al. Deep Learning to Classify AL versus ATTR Cardiac Amyloidosis MR Images. Biomedicines 2023;11(1). https://doi.org/10.3390/biomedicines11010193.

96. Rodríguez-de-Vera JM, Bernabé G, García JM, et al. Left ventricular non-compaction cardiomyopathy automatic diagnosis using a deep learning approach. Comput Methods Programs Biomed 2022;214:106548.

97. Bourfiss M, Sander J, De Vos BD, et al. Towards automatic classification of cardiovascular magnetic resonance Task Force Criteria for diagnosis of arrhythmogenic right ventricular cardiomyopathy. Clin Res Cardiol 2023;112(3):363–78.

98. Karimi-Bidhendi S, Arafati A, Cheng AL, et al. Fully-automated deep-learning segmentation of pediatric cardiovascular magnetic resonance of patients with complex congenital heart diseases. J Cardiovasc Magn Reson 2020;22(1). https://doi.org/10.1186/s12968-020-00678-0.

99. Steeden JA, Quail M, Gotschy A, et al. Rapid whole-heart CMR with single volume super-resolution. J Cardiovasc Magn Reson 2020;22(1):56.

100. Amal S, Safarnejad L, Omiye JA, et al. Use of Multi-Modal Data and Machine Learning to Improve Cardiovascular Disease Care. Front Cardiovasc Med 2022;9:840262.

101. Rajkomar A, Oren E, Chen K, et al. Scalable and accurate deep learning with electronic health records. NPj Digital Medicine 2018;1(1). https://doi.org/10.1038/s41746-018-0029-1.

102. Motwani M, Dey D, Berman DS, et al. Machine learning for prediction of all-cause mortality in patients with suspected coronary artery disease: a 5-year multicentre prospective registry analysis. Eur Heart J 2017;38(7):500–7.

103. Betancur J, Otaki Y, Motwani M, et al. Prognostic Value of Combined Clinical and Myocardial Perfusion Imaging Data Using Machine Learning. JACC Cardiovasc Imaging 2018;11(7):1000–9.

104. Zhao J, Feng Q, Wu P, et al. Learning from Longitudinal Data in Electronic Health Record and Genetic Data to Improve Cardiovascular Event Prediction. Sci Rep 2019;9(1):717.

105. Ng D, Du H, Yao MM-S, et al. Today's radiologists meet tomorrow's AI: the promises, pitfalls, and unbridled potential. Quant Imag Med Surg 2021;11(6):2775–9.

Role of Computed Tomography in Cardiac Electrophysiology

Sadia Sultana, MD[a], Cian P. McCarthy, MB, BCh, BAO, SM[b],
Mangun Randhawa, MD[a], Jinjin Cao, MD[c], Anushri Parakh, MBBS, MD[a],
Vinit Baliyan, MBBS, MD[a],*

KEYWORDS

- Cardiac electrophysiology, • Cardiac computed tomography, • Atrial fibrillation

KEY POINTS

- For preablation planning, cardiac CT delineates pulmonary venous anatomy, excludes left atrial appendage thrombi, and identifies relevant anatomic variants.
- One should be mindful of device-related measurements specific to the device planned to be used.
- In assessing specific complications such as cardiac implantable electronic device lead perforation and lead-associated thrombus, cardiac CT is a valuable imaging modality.
- Cardiac CT can be used for assessing myocardial scar, especially in cases where MR imaging is unavailable or contraindicated.

INTRODUCTION

Cardiac electrophysiology (EP) is a subspecialty of cardiology focusing on diagnosing and treating arrhythmias or abnormal heart rhythms. The prevalence of arrhythmias such as atrial fibrillation (AF) has been increasing[1]; and it is estimated that 1 in 5 individuals will experience AF over their lifetime even.[2] Simultaneously, there has been an increase in the volume of EP procedures that treat arrhythmias, such as pulmonary vein isolation (PVI) and cardiac implantable electronic device (CIED) implantation.[3]

Cardiac computed tomography (CT) is a noninvasive imaging modality that can provide a detailed assessment of the heart's anatomy and function. Significant advancements have been made during the past decades in CT technology, resulting in improved spatial resolution, increased temporal resolution, and decreased radiation dosage.[4] Accordingly, during the past decade,

there has been a substantial and consistent increase in cardiac CT utilization for the evaluation of various cardiac conditions.[5,6]

In recent years, there has been an increasing interest in the use of cardiac CT for EP. This noninvasive imaging modality holds significant value in this patient population for several compelling reasons. First, CT provides comprehensive anatomic information. This is pivotal in planning EP interventions, such as PVI or left atrial appendage closure. Second, CT is an essential tool for detecting cardiac thrombi, which can occur as a complication of AF.[7] Third, there has been a steady increase in the use of CT to evaluate the coronary arteries for the presence of coronary artery disease, which can affect antiarrhythmic agent selection.[8] Fourth, there is increasing evidence that CT may help assess myocardial fibrosis, which can be a potential substrate for arrhythmias. Finally, CT assumes a crucial role in the early detection of various complications following EP procedures.

[a] Division of Cardiovascular Imaging, Department of Radiology, Massachusetts General Hospital, Boston, MA, USA; [b] Division of Cardiology, Department of Medicine, Massachusetts General Hospital, Boston, MA, USA; [c] Division of Abdominal Imaging, Department of Radiology, Massachusetts General Hospital, Boston, MA, USA
* Corresponding author. Massachusetts General Hospital, 175 Cambridge Street, Boston, MA 02114.
E-mail address: vbaliyan@mgh.harvard.edu

Radiol Clin N Am 62 (2024) 489–508
https://doi.org/10.1016/j.rcl.2023.12.016

In this article, we will review the strengths of cardiac CT over other imaging modalities and the contemporary role of cardiac CT for EP.

STRENGTHS OF CARDIAC COMPUTED TOMOGRAPHY

Cardiac CT has several advantages over other imaging modalities used in EP. These advantages include the following:

- *High-spatial resolution anatomic images*: Cardiac CT provides high-resolution anatomic images of the heart. This is not only helpful in planning EP procedures but also useful in assessing postprocedure results and complications.
- *Noninvasive*: Cardiac CT is a noninvasive imaging modality, which makes it a generally safe and convenient option for patients.
- *Wide availability:* As a widely available and easy-to-access modality in most hospitals and imaging centers, CT has become popular among patients and physicians.
- *Short scan times:* Cardiac CT is a quick test where image acquisition is faster than a single breath-hold.

CONTEMPORARY ROLES OF CARDIAC CT FOR EP
Left Atrial Appendage Thrombus Evaluation

Background: Due to the risk of left atrial appendage thrombi formation as a complication of AF, an evaluation of the left atrial appendage is frequently needed before electrical or chemical cardioversion and invasive EP procedures such as PVI and percutaneous left atrial appendage closure. Transesophageal echocardiogram (TEE) is considered the gold standard imaging modality for evaluating left atrial appendage thrombi. Nevertheless, it poses risks such as esophageal injury and requires sedation, which may result in complications.[9]

Role of cardiac CT for evaluating left atrial appendage thrombi: Cardiac CT has emerged as an alternative imaging modality to TEE in assessing left atrial appendage thrombi. In a meta-analysis of 27 studies including 6960 patients, the summary sensitivity, specificity, positive posterior probability, and negative posterior probability of early cardiac CT compared with TEE for diagnosing left atrial thrombus was 0.95, 0.89, 19.11%, and 0.16%, respectively.[10] When combined with delayed imaging, the sensitivity increased to 0.98, specificity to 1.00, positive posterior probability to 95.76%, and negative posterior probability decreased to 0.12%.[10]

CT protocol for left atrial appendage thrombus evaluation: Cardiac CT for the evaluation of left atrial appendage thrombus may be performed using an electrocardiogram (ECG)-gated prospective axial sequential scan. The sensitivity and specificity of identifying left atrial appendage thrombus using ECG-gated CT is 100% and 88%, respectively.[11] Non-ECG-gated CT however has much lower sensitivity of 63.6% and specificity of 81.8%.[12] A biphasic or triphasic contrast protocol may be used with the bolus tracking placed in the ascending aorta (AscAo) to trigger the scan (**Fig. 1**). It is necessary to obtain a 1-minute delayed phase image of the entire left atrial appendage to differentiate slow flow in the appendage from the thrombus. Some literatures showed comparison of Hounsfield unit (HU) densities in the left atrial appendage (LAA) to the AscAo in the same axial plane and LAA/AscAo ratios greater than 0.75 demonstrate 100% negative predictive value.[13]

Relevant anatomy and reporting: A thrombus seems as a hypoattenuating filling defect in the left atrial appendage, which persists on delayed phase imaging (**Figs. 2 and 3**). The size and number of thrombi should be reported.

Pulmonary Vein Isolation for Atrial Fibrillation

Background: AF is the most common sustained arrhythmia in adults, and it is estimated that 1 in 5 individuals will experience AF over their lifetime.[2] It is associated with a 1.5-fold increased risk of mortality and a 2.3-fold increased risk of stroke.[14] For most individuals, AF is precipitated by ectopic beats originating from the pulmonary vein ostia.[15] Once diagnosed, the management of this arrhythmia typically focuses on symptom management through heart rate and rhythm control and the prevention of thromboembolism. Recent evidence supports earlier rhythm control for patients with AF,[16] and during the past decade, there has been a substantial increase in the use of PVI ablation to treat symptomatic AF.[3] PVI is a percutaneous procedure during which an electrophysiologist electrically isolates the ostial walls of the pulmonary veins from the atria using radiofrequency ablation or cryoablation, thereby preventing the trigger of AF. PVI has higher efficacy than antiarrhythmic medications at preventing AF reoccurrence.[17] Nevertheless, PVI ablation requires careful preprocedure planning and is associated with complications such as pulmonary vein stenosis (**Fig. 4**),[18] and, more rarely, atrioesophageal fistula formation.[19]

Role of cardiac CT in preablation planning: Delineation of the pulmonary venous anatomy before ablation is important as anatomy variation is

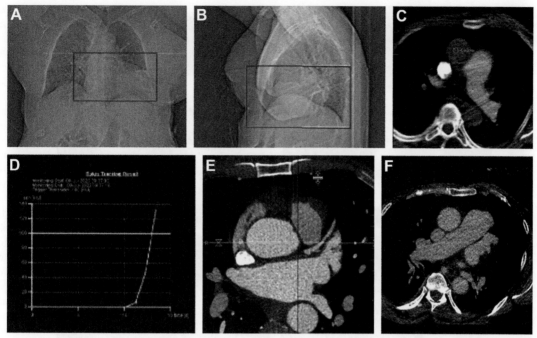

Fig. 1. (*A, B*) Antero-posterior and lateral scout. (*C, D*) Region of interest in the AscAo for bolus-triggered CT post-intravenous contrast injection. Axial CT (*E*) arterial phase, and (*F*) 1-minute delayed phase images.

common and may result in incomplete PVI, associated with higher AF recurrence rates.[20] Knowledge of the pulmonary vein ostia locations, their orientations, and branching patterns is essential to reduce the risk of pulmonary vein stenosis and avoid missing a branch that requires ablation. Pulmonary venous anatomy can be identified using angiography at the time of the PVI but this can be cumbersome and, accordingly, preprocedural cardiac CT has gained popularity. Beyond delineation of pulmonary venous anatomy, cardiac CT can exclude left atrial appendage thrombus, which is a contraindication to proceeding with ablation until thrombus resolution has occurred. Cardiac CT is also useful for identifying relevant anatomic variants, such as the top-pulmonary vein and the presence of an S-shaped sinoatrial nodal artery. The study can inform the proximity of the pulmonary veins to the esophagus.

Cardiac CT protocol for PVI planning: Protocols for PVI planning may vary from institution to institution. At our institution, a prospectively ECG-triggered axial-sequential scan is performed with images acquired during an expiration breath hold at end-systole/early diastole. A triphasic contrast bolus technique is used; the saline flush minimizes artifacts from contrast in the superior vena cava and right atrium. Institutions must use a consistent approach for image acquisition and pulmonary vein measurement because pulmonary vein ostia

size varies across the cardiac cycle. Ostia are, on average, 33% smaller during atrial systole than late atrial diastole.[21] Measurements should be performed using multiplanar reformatted images orthogonal to the pulmonary vein ostia. A delayed phase scan of the heart should be performed 1 minute after the arterial phase.

Relevant anatomy and reporting: Approximately 70% of the population have 4 pulmonary veins[22–24]; the right superior pulmonary vein (RSPV) usually drains the right upper and middle lung lobes, the right inferior pulmonary vein (RIPV) usually drains the right lower lung lobe, the left superior pulmonary vein (LSPV) typically drains the left upper lung lobe and the left inferior pulmonary vein (LIPV) drains the left lower lung lobe (**Figs. 5** and **6**). However, variations are common and may include an accessory pulmonary vein (**Fig. 7**) or a pulmonary trunk (**Figs. 8** and **9**). An accessory pulmonary vein, which is more common on the right side,[25] is characterized by an additional atrio-pulmonary venous junction beyond the superior and inferior pulmonary veins. Accessory veins on the right may include a right middle pulmonary vein (draining part or all of the right middle lobe), a superior segment right lower lobe vein, or a top vein, which enters the left atrium roof superomedial to the RSPV.[26] Accessory veins on the left are less common and, when present, usually drain some or all of the lingula.[26] In addition to accessory veins, early branching or

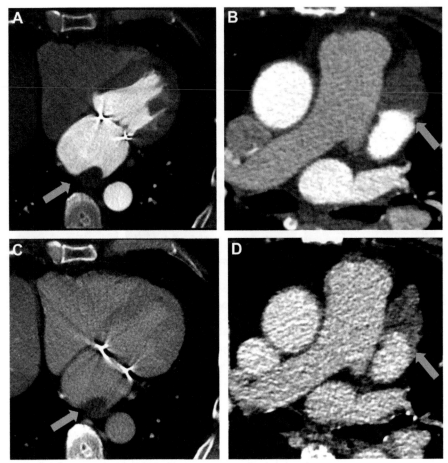

Fig. 2. Postcontrast axial cardiac CT images showing persistent well-defined hypoattenuating filling defects consistent with thrombus (*arrows*) on arterial (*A, B*) and delayed (*C, D*) images. The thrombus is attached to the posterior wall of the left atrium in one patient (*A, C*) and is within the left atrial appendage in another patient (*B, D*).

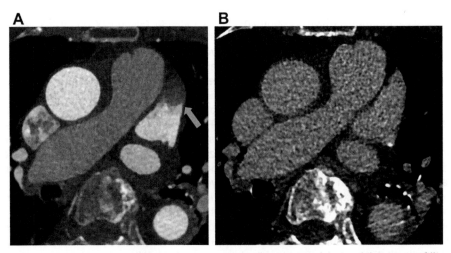

Fig. 3. An 86-year-old woman's precardioversion axial images of cardiac CT showing (*A*) apparent filling defect in the left atrial appendage (*arrow*) but (*B*) complete opacification of the left atrial appendage on the delayed phase implying slow filling of contrast.

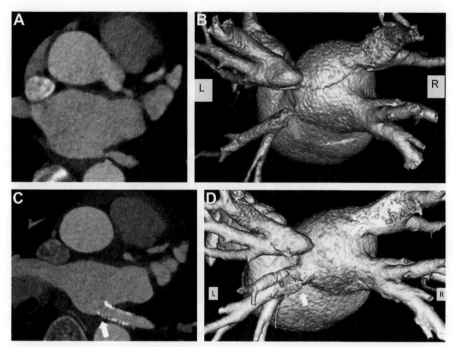

Fig. 4. Postcontrast CT images of a 41-year-old patient with PVI complicated by stenosis of the LIPV (*blue arrows*) on (*A*) axial 2D, and (*B*) 3D volume-rendered images. This was treated by transcatheter placement of a stent (*white arrows*), (*C*) axial 2D image, and (*D*) 3D volume rendered image.

"ostial veins" may be identified as branches draining within 5 mm of the atrio-pulmonary venous juncture. Identification of both accessory pulmonary veins and ostial veins is clinically significant because they pose a higher risk of pulmonary vein stenosis with ablation. Pulmonary vein trunks, when present, usually occur on the left side, with pulmonary veins draining the left lung, converging into one trunk, and entering the left atrium. Pulmonary vein anomalies such as partial or total anomalous pulmonary venous should also be reported. In addition, systemic venous variants vascular

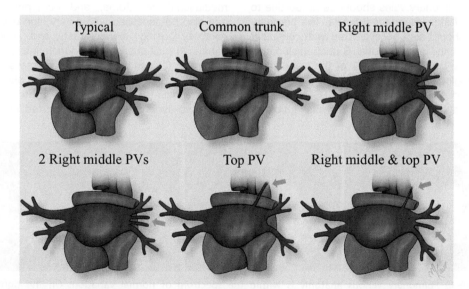

Fig. 5. Representation of anatomic variants of pulmonary veins. Specific variants are highlighted by blue arrows. PV, pulmonary vein.

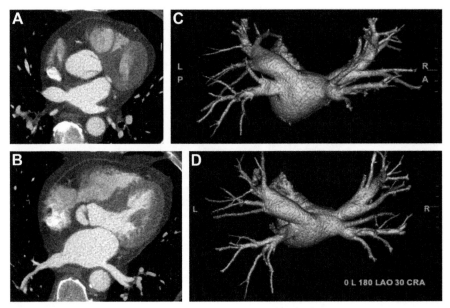

Fig. 6. (A–D) Contrast-enhanced cardiac CT (axial images on top row; 3D volume rendered images on bottom 2 rows) demonstrating pulmonary venous anatomy within the spectrum of normal.

anomalies, such as azygous continuation of the inferior vena cava, interrupted inferior vena cava, and persistent left superior vena cava, which are relevant for vascular access during the procedure should be noted.

The left atrial appendage should be evaluated for thrombi, with delayed imaging assisting in differentiating thrombi from sluggish flow. In addition, the interatrial septum should be scrutinized for a patent foramen ovale and atrial septal defects. The relationship between the esophagus and the pulmonary veins should be noted due to the risk of atrio-esophageal fistula. The coronary arteries should also be evaluated with particular attention to the presence of an S-shaped sinoatrial nodal artery, present in 10% of the population, which originates from the left circumflex coronary artery and courses between the LSPV and the left atrial appendage because it is susceptible to injury during ablation.[27] Finally, CT is also helpful in identifying congenital anomalies such as cor-triatriatum sinister.

Post-PVI cardiac CT: Complications of PVI occur in approximately 5% of patients and may include vascular complications, pericardial effusion or tamponade (up to 0.3%), or stroke/transient ischemic attack (TIA; up to 0.9%; **Figs. 10 and 11**).[28,29] Fortunately, complication rates have been declining.[28] In acute settings, periprocedural complications such as acute aortic syndrome, mediastinal hematoma, and hemopericardium can also be assessed with a very high degree of reliability using noncontrast and contrast-enhanced multiphase imaging techniques.

Cardiac CT can be beneficial for assessing pulmonary vein or left atrial dissection, pulmonary vein stenosis (reported incidence up to 4.4%),[29] and atrio-esophageal fistula (reported incidence

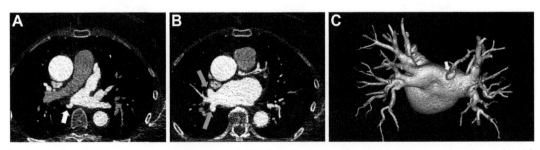

Fig. 7. (A–C) Pulmonary venous anatomy is within the spectrum of normal variation. On the right side: SPV + MPV + IPV with small right accessory pulmonary vein (*blue arrows*) and right top pulmonary vein (*white arrows*).

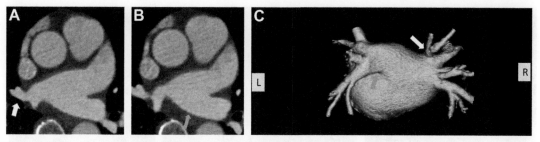

Fig. 8. (*A–C*) Pulmonary venous anatomy is within the spectrum of normal variation. On the right side: "top" pulmonary vein variant (*white arrows*). On the left side: Trunk (*blue arrows*).

up to 0.05%).[30] Pulmonary vein stenosis is characterized by a narrowing/stenosis of one or more of the pulmonary veins (see **Fig. 4**). It may be classified as mild (20%–50%), moderate (50%–69%), or severe (≥70%). Comparison of the post-PVI cardiac CT to the pre-PVI CT is particularly helpful for making the diagnosis. The presence and extent of symptoms can vary depending on the severity of stenosis. When symptoms occur, patients may experience shortness of breath or, if venous infarctions occur, pleuritic chest pain and/or hemoptysis.[31] Pulmonary vein balloon angioplasty and stenting are therapeutic options for symptomatic patients[32] (see **Fig. 4**).

Atrio-esophageal fistula is a rare but dreaded complication of PVI characterized by an abnormal connection between the left atrium and the esophagus (**Fig. 12**). This complication is associated with a high mortality rate due to air emboli, sepsis, and hematemesis. CT may reveal mediastinitis predominantly in the atrial-esophageal region with mediastinal fat and fluid collections or gas locules. Infarcts or sequelae of septic or air emboli may also be seen. Management usually includes a combination of antibiotics and urgent surgery.[30]

Percutaneous Left Atrial Appendage Closure

Background: A feared complication of AF is the formation of left atrial thrombi, which may embolize, causing cerebrovascular events. The vast majority (~90%) form in the left atrial appendage.[33] Percutaneous closure of the left atrial appendage has emerged as a prophylactic intervention for the prevention of thromboembolic events, alongside other methods such as surgical excision and ligation of the left atrial appendage (**Figs. 13 and 14**).[34,35] The 2019 American Heart Association/American College of Cardiology/Heart Rhythm Society focused update of the 2014 Guideline for the Management of Patients with Atrial Fibrillation advises that percutaneous left atrial appendage closure may be considered in patients with AF at an increased risk of stroke who have contraindications to long-term anticoagulation.[36]

Role of cardiac CT in planning left atrial appendage closure: Preprocedural imaging is essential for the evaluation of the shape and size of the left atrial appendage, its proximity to adjacent structures, and the presence of left atrial appendage thrombus, which is a contraindication to closure. A TEE is often used for this purpose but cardiac CT has emerged as an alternative

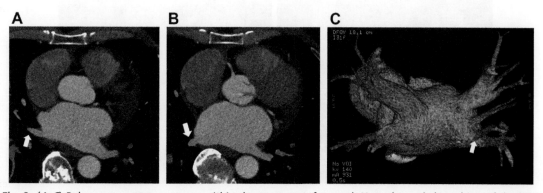

Fig. 9. (*A–C*) Pulmonary venous anatomy within the spectrum of normal. Note the early branching of the RIPV (*arrows*).

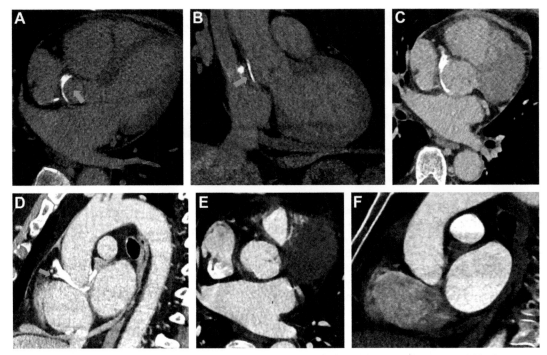

Fig. 10. Cardiac CT of a 67-year-old man who had an abandoned ablation procedure due to difficulty maneuvering the sheath into the atrium (septal puncture). Noncontrast (*A, B*) and postcontrast (*C, D*) demonstrates persistent contrast (used during the ablation procedure) around the aortic root (*arrows*). Twenty-four hours delayed images (*E, F*) showing resolution of the findings consistent with atrial wall perforation and extravasation during procedure. (*Image courtesy of* Dr Jonathan Weir-McCall, Royal Papworth Hospital, Cambridge, UK.)

noninvasive option with high spatial and temporal resolution.

CT protocol for planning left atrial appendage closure: Cardiac CT for left atrial appendage closure planning may be performed using retrospective ECG gating or systolic phase prospective ECG gating (preferred due to arrhythmias). A biphasic or triphasic contrast protocol may be used with AscAo bolus tracking for triggering. Similar to PVI planning, images are acquired during an expiratory breath hold, and a 1-minute delayed phase image of the heart should be obtained to evaluate for thrombus.

Relevant anatomy and reporting: Left atrial appendages can vary in shape, size, and number of lobes. Several distinct types of appendages have

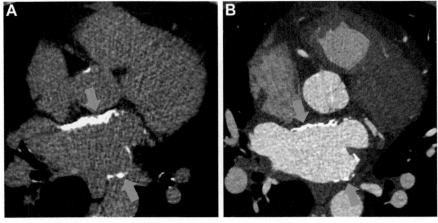

Fig. 11. A 63-year-old man who underwent PVI for persistent AF 10 years ago. ECG-gated cardiac CT demonstrates coarse calcification of the left atrial wall (*arrows*). (*A*) Noncontrast CT, (*B*) postcontrast CT.

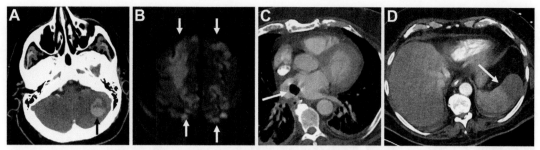

Fig. 12. A 75-year-old man with past medical history of AF on anticoagulation underwent left atrial ablation procedure. He was subsequently admitted with presyncope, developed fevers, and found to have streptococcal bacteremia. He later developed worsening mental status. Axial images of noncontrast CT head (*A*) shows acute left cerebellar hemorrhage (*black arrow*) and MR image of brain (*B*) shows extensive ischemic stroke (*white arrows*). Postcontrast CT chest (*C*) demonstrated air in the left atrial cavity (*white arrow*) suggesting atrial-esophageal fistula and (*D*) a splenic infarct (*white arrow*) in the upper abdomen. The constellation of findings is likely related to recent PV ablation complicated by atrial-esophageal fistula with subsequent bacteremia and embolic infarcts in the brain and spleen.

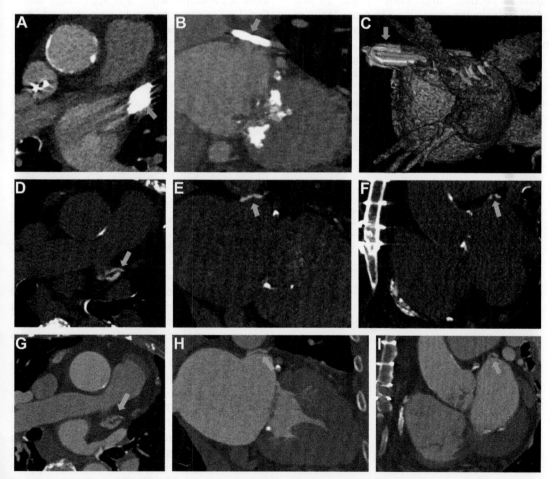

Fig. 13. Axial (*A*), sagittal (*B*), and volume rendered 3D (*C*) images in a 75-year-old woman with a left atrial appendage (*blue arrows*) closure with clips. Noncontrast images (*D–F*) and postcontrast images (*G–I*) of a 75-year-old woman after surgical excision of left atrial appendage with hyperdense surgical material (*green arrows*).

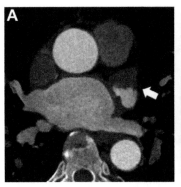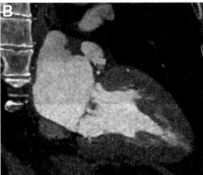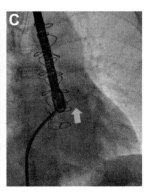

Fig. 14. Axial and sagittal postcontrast cardiac CT images of a 69-year-old man who underwent surgical replacement of aortic valve and left atrial appendage LAA ligation. (*A*) There is partial thrombosis at the appendage tip (*white arrow*) and (*B*) persistent opacification of the appendage via communication (*blue arrow*) with the left atrial chamber. Fluoroscopic image (*C*) showing the communication that was later closed using an Amplatz device (*green arrow*).

been described according to their appearance: "windsock," "chicken-wing," "cactus," "cauliflower," "bilobed," and "cone" (**Figs. 15** and **16**).[37] Notably, the most common type, "chicken wing," is associated with the lowest incidence of stroke.[38]

Accurately measuring the left atrial appendage is critical for ensuring correct device sizing (**Figs. 17** and **18**). Oversizing could result in appendage rupture, whereas undersizing could result in peridevice leaks (in up to 20% cases)[39] or embolization.

Measurement requirements differ across devices, including ostium size, landing zone diameter, left atrial appendage length, and appendage depth. Ostial measurements should be performed using 2-dimensional oblique transverse measurement when the appendage is largest (end-systole).[40] Landing zone location also differs across devices, and therefore, the correct location should be identified for the specific device before measurement. Beyond the ostium and landing zone size, the left atrial appendage length or depth must be measured depending on the device.

In addition to the appendage shape and size measurements, the distance from the appendage to the coumadin ridge, pulmonary venous anatomy, anatomy of adjacent structures including coronary arteries, and presence or absence of a left atrial appendage thrombus should be reported.

Postclosure cardiac CT: As an alternative to TEE, cardiac CT can be useful for assessing for device-related thrombus or peridevice leaks postclosure. A well-positioned closure device (**Fig. 19**) will be snugly positioned in the left atrial appendage, and endothelialization occurs over weeks or months. However, peridevice leaks (**Figs. 20** and **21**) are common, reported up to 31% combining all available devices.[41] When peridevice leak is severe (>5 mm), they are referred to as incomplete closure. In addition to leaks, CT helps diagnose device-related thrombus. This refers to the development of a thrombus on the atrial surface of the device. On CT, it may be visualized as a hypoattenuating lesion on the atrial surface of the device on arterial phase imaging, which persists on delayed-phase images. It is associated with an increased risk of thromboembolic events and necessitates initiation of anticoagulation.[42]

Fig. 15. Diagrammatic representation of the morphologic variations of left atrial appendage.

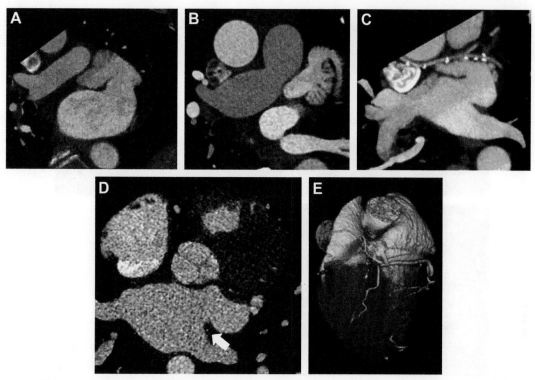

Fig. 16. Oblique planar reformatted postcontrast CT images demonstrating examples of special considerations: (*A*) anatomic variant, the "chicken wing" type with a sharp bend, (*B*) cauliflower type with a tapering tip, which can be contraindicated for device placement. (*C*) A coronary bypass graft coursing anterior to and abutting the left atrial appendage, which may be injured during lariat suture placement. (*D, E*) "S" shaped sinoatrial (SA nodal) artery (*white arrows*) originates from the right coronary artery, coursing along the left atrial wall and close to the LIPV.

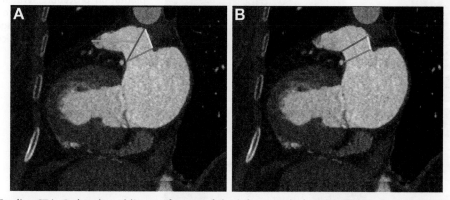

Fig. 17. Cardiac CT in 2-chamber oblique reformat of the left ventricle for LAA closure device planning. The orange line represents the ostium of the LAA. (*A*) Watchman device planning: Landing zone (*yellow line*), the landing zone diameter (*blue line*), and length of the LAA (*green line*). (*B*) Amplatzer cardiac plug and Amulet device planning: Depth of the LAA (*green line*); landing zone (*blue line*), which is perpendicular to the walls of the LAA. For Amplatzer cardiac plug and amulet devices, a distance of 10 mm and 1215 mm, respectively, measured distal to the ostium of the LAA (*yellow line*).

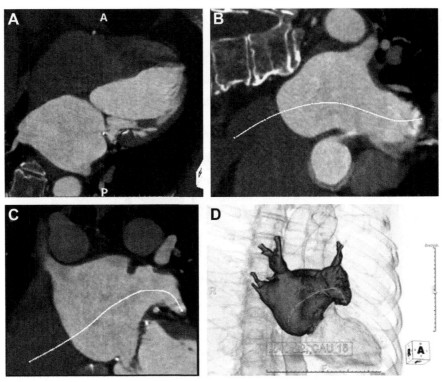

Fig. 18. Two-dimensional axial and oblique reformatted and volume rendered CT images showing a simulation of left atrial appendage closure procedure providing an evaluation of the interatrial septum for puncture planning (*A*), (*B*), and (*C*) and procedural fluoroscopic angles (*D*).

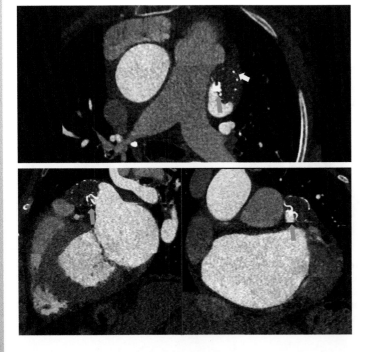

Fig. 19. Axial and sagittal and coronal oblique postcontrast CT images in a 73-year-old woman after a successful deployment of Watchman device implantation procedure: Watchman device in place (*blue arrows*), completely excluded left atrial appendage (*white arrows*) without any intradevice or peridevice contrast leak.

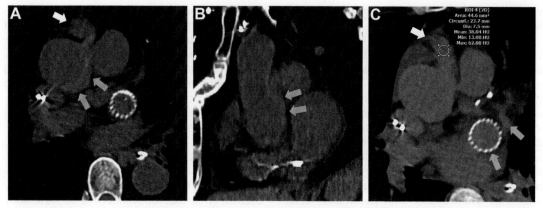

Fig. 20. A 60-year-old man developed chest pain after deployment of a Watchman device. Noncontrast multiplanar reformatted CT images (*A, B*) demonstrate a hyperdense crescent sign consistent with intramural hematoma (*blue arrow*) at the level of the aortic root and AscAo with a small volume of periaortic hematoma (*white arrow*) more pronounced anteriorly (with mean HU of 38). (*C*) Postintravenous contrast 1-minute delayed images show intradevice and peridevice leaks (*green arrows*).

Complications of Cardiac Implantable Electronic Devices

Background: Approximately 10% of individuals who receive a CIED experience a complication.[43] These can include minor complications such as hematomas or wound infections or major complications such as pneumothorax requiring intervention, lead perforation (incidence up to 3%), deep vein thrombosis (incidence up to 2% cases), stroke, or myocardial infarction.[43,44]

Role of cardiac CT in evaluation for CIED complications: Due to its high spatial and temporal resolution and compatibility with CIED devices, cardiac CT can be beneficial for assessing specific CIED complications such as lead-associated deep vein thrombosis and CIED lead perforation. To be able to exclude lead-associated thrombosis, the Z-axis coverage has to be extended superiorly to include subclavian veins, brachiocephalic veins, and the superior vena cava so that the entire course of the lead can be followed from the entry point to the distal tip in the cardiac chambers.

Cardiac CT protocol for CIED complications: ECG-gated retrospective helical protocol is preferable for assessing lead perforation because it permits visualization of the lead throughout the cardiac cycle. A triphasic contrast bolus technique can be used with a 50:50 contrast mix for second phase to optimize right heart chamber visualization. A contrast bolus tail of a 50:50 mix provides adequate opacification of the right heart and avoids streak artifacts from higher density undiluted contrast in the right atrium.[45] For assessment of CIED-associated thrombus, either a prospective or a retrospective protocol may be used. Similarly, a triphasic contrast bolus technique may be used with a 50:50 contrast mix for second phase to optimize right heart chamber

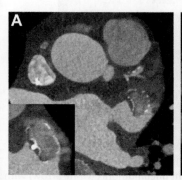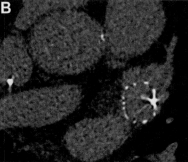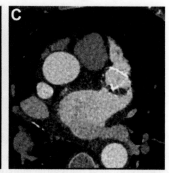

Fig. 21. Postcontrast arterial (*A*) and delayed (*B*) oblique reformatted CT images in an 88-year-old man with a tilted Watchman device resulting in a peridevice leak. (*C*) Similar findings on postcontrast delayed CT images in a different patient, a 79-year-old man, after Watchman device implantation.

visualization. A 1-minute delayed image of the heart is required.

Relevant anatomy and reporting: CIEDs can have varying numbers and types of leads. Pacemakers can have single leads (terminating in the right atrial appendage or right ventricle), dual-chamber leads (terminating in the right atrial appendage and right ventricular apex), or biventricular leads (terminating in the right atrial appendage, right ventricular apex, and left ventricular wall epicardial vein via the coronary sinus). Implantable cardioverter-defibrillators (ICDs) can be placed in isolation or combined with pacemakers (cardiac resynchronization therapy). ICD leads seem thicker than pacemaker leads when visualized on tomogram images. When evaluating for lead perforation, the distal point of each lead should be identified on axial imaging, after which multiplanar reformatted images should be used to determine if the lead tip extends beyond the epicardial fat of the relevant cardiac chamber, indicating a lead perforation (**Fig. 22**). Perforation is most likely to occur at the right ventricular apex

than the septal wall as the apex is thinner. Supportive additional findings may include the presence of hemopericardium, hemomediastinum, hemothorax, and/or pneumothorax (**Fig. 23**).

Thrombi may form anywhere along a CIED lead and may be visualized as a hypoattenuating filling defect that persists on delayed imaging (**Fig. 24**). Close inspection of the pulmonary arteries is needed to assess for pulmonary embolism.

Myocardial Tissue Evaluation

Background: Cardiac imaging can help identify causes of cardiac arrhythmias. It is particularly useful for ventricular arrhythmias to determine if the precipitant of the arrhythmia is a reversible cause, such as myocarditis, or an irreversible cause, such as infarction-related myocardial fibrosis. Determining the cause of the arrhythmia may influence decisions regarding ICD placement and assist in locating the source of arrhythmia for interventions such as ablation. Cardiac magnetic

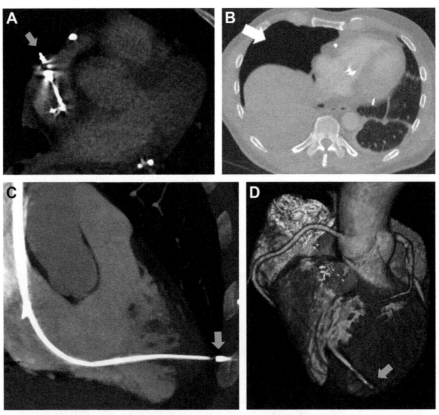

Fig. 22. Top row showing CT images of a 75-year-old man who developed chest pain after pacemaker insertion. (*A*) perforation of right atrial appendage lead (*blue arrow*) and (*B*) large right pneumothorax (*white arrow*) with a collapse of the underlying lung. The bottom row shows images of a cardiac CT of a separate patient, a 55-year-old woman, with perforation of the right ventricular lead in coronal oblique reformat (*C*) and 3D volume rendered (*D*) images (*blue arrows*).

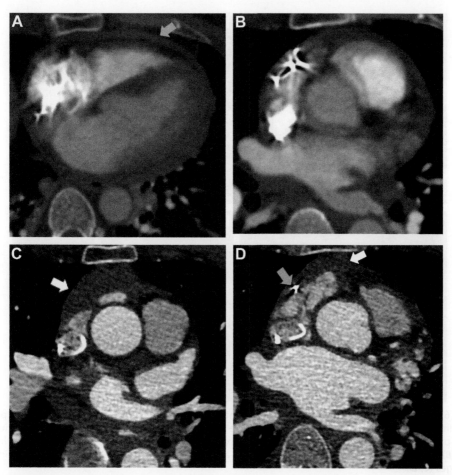

Fig. 23. A 63-year-old woman, 2 days after pacemaker insertion, presented with pleuritic chest pain. Axial CT pulmonary angiogram showing (*A*) a small hemopericardium (*green arrow*). (*B*) No obvious lead perforation or mediastinal hematoma. ECG-gated cardiac CT images (*bottom row*) of the same patient 24 hours later demonstrating (*C*) a new small mediastinal hematoma (*white arrows*) and (*D*) right atrial appendage lead perforation (*blue arrow*).

resonance (CMR) imaging is the preferred imaging modality for myocardial tissue characterization but availability can be limited depending on local resources, and some individuals may have non-CMR-compatible implants.

Role of cardiac CT for myocardial tissue evaluation: Cardiac CT has the potential to serve as an alternative to CMR for the assessment of myocardial tissue in situations where CMR is unavailable or contraindicated. Several small cohort studies have demonstrated good agreement ($\kappa = 0.89$) between these 2 modalities.[46–50]

Cardiac CT protocol for myocardial tissue characterization: For comprehensive assessment of myocardial tissue, an ECG-gated retrospective scan should be obtained, which allows accurate assessment of wall thickness at end-diastole. Larger contrast volumes (approximately 1.5 mL/ kg) are required compared with coronary CT angiography. Following arterial phase acquisition, after 8 to 10 minutes, delayed imaging of the whole heart should be obtained using ECG gating.

Relevant anatomy and reporting: Old myocardial infarction may be identified on CT imaging by the presence of thinning, fatty metaplasia (subendocardial), myocardial calcifications, and regional wall motion abnormalities.[51,52]

Enhancement on late (8–10 minutes) delayed imaging (late iodine enhancement) is suggestive of myocardial fibrosis (similar to late gadolinium enhancement on CMR). It may be characterized according to its location within the wall (eg, subendocardial, midmyocardial, or epicardial) to assist in differentiating the cause (**Fig. 25**). However, the diagnostic performance of detecting such scars relies on the reader's experience, particularly in cases with a nonischemic scar, low scar burdens, and low contrast-to-noise ratio.[53]

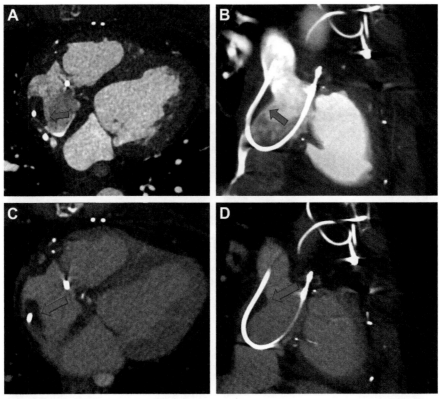

Fig. 24. A 67-year-old woman with a history of right ventricle angiosarcoma. The patient is now status postresection with implantation of a bioprosthetic tricuspid valve and PPM. There is a thrombus in the right atrium along the atrial pacemaker lead. Postcontrast cardiac CT in axial and oblique sagittal reformatted images in arterial phase (*A, B*) show a low attenuation filling defect (*blue arrows*) along the pacemaker lead, which persists on delayed images (*C, D*).

LIMITATIONS OF CARDIAC COMPUTED TOMOGRAPHY

Although cardiac CT has several strengths, there are limitations that clinicians should be familiar with.

- *Radiation exposure*: Cardiac CT exposes patients to radiation. The total amount of radiation exposure depends on the type of CT scan, body parts included, and the patient's body habitus. Nevertheless, substantial progress in CT technology, including innovations such as ECG-guided tube current modulation, prospective ECG gating, low kV techniques, and iterative reconstruction, has markedly decreased radiation exposure associated with cardiac CT scans during the preceding 2 decades.[54] By using these methodologies in conjunction, conducting cardiac CT scans on nonobese patients is feasible using doses below the submillisievert threshold. Adherence to these strategies is imperative to customize scans and curtail radiation exposure while maintaining diagnostic image quality.

- *Cost:* Cardiac CT can be expensive. The cost of a scan varies depending on the type of CT scan performed and the scanner's location.
- *Contrast reactions:* Hypersensitivity reactions to contrast are now rare, occurring in less than 1% of individuals.[55] When they occur, they are usually mild but can be severe or life threatening, requiring prompt treatment.
- *Contrast-induced acute kidney injury:* Our understanding of contrast-induced kidney injury is constantly evolving as recent evidence suggests the risk is low.[56] Nevertheless, it remains crucial to exercise specific caution when dealing with patients with compromised kidney function. In instances of severe impairment, thorough deliberation regarding the balance between potential risks and benefits holds significant importance before administering intravenous contrast. The risk of contrast-induced acute kidney injury is near 0% at eGFR (estimated glomerular filtration rate) greater than or equal to 45 mL/min/ 1.73 m^2, 0% to 2% at eGFR, 30 to 44 mL/

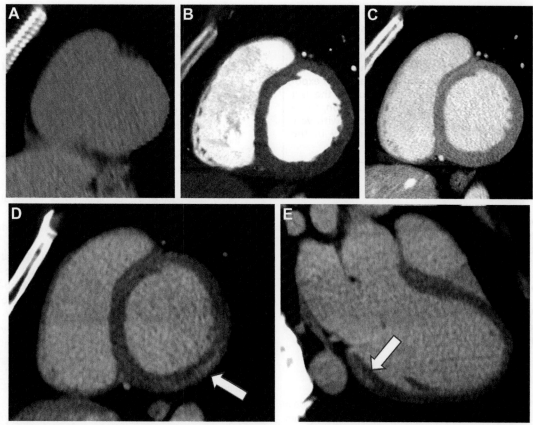

Fig. 25. Myocardial Scar on CT. ECG-gated cardiac CT of a 45-year-old man with history of ventricular tachycardia. There is no significant abnormality on short axis views of the left ventricle on noncontrast (*A*), arterial phase (*B*) and 1 minute delayed (*C*) phase. The 8-minute delayed images in short axis (*D*) and 3-chamber (*E*) views of the left ventricle demonstrate enhancement (*white arrows*) in the basal inferolateral wall likely a sequelae of prior myocarditis.

min/1.73 m^2, and 0% to 17% at less than 30 mL/min/1.73 m^2.[57]

SUMMARY

Cardiac CT is a valuable imaging technique because it provides comprehensive anatomic evaluation, which not only aids in preprocedure planning but is also helpful for postprocedure assessment of EP interventions. Despite the known risks of radiation exposure and potential costs, this noninvasive and easily accessible imaging modality will likely continue to have an exponential role in cardiac EP.

CLINICS CARE POINTS

- *Left Atrial Appendage Thrombus Evaluation*: Cardiac CT evaluates left atrial appendage

thrombi with high sensitivity and specificity (up to 98% and 100%, respectively).

- *Post-PVI Cardiac CT*: After undergoing PVI, 5% of patients may experience complications as detected by cardiac CT, with pulmonary vein stenosis being the most common (up to 4%), followed by stroke or transient ischemic attack (0.9%), and pericardial effusions with or without tamponade (0.3%).

- *Percutaneous Left Atrial Appendage Closure*: Accurate measurement of the left atrial appendage is essential for selecting the appropriate device size. A mismatch between the device and the actual measurements can result in peridevice leaks in up to 20% of the cases.

- *Complications of CIED*: About 10% of patients with CIED experience complications. Cardiac CT helps to assess for lead-associated deep vein thrombosis and lead perforation (incidences of up to 2% and 3%, respectively).

- *Limitations of Cardiac CT*: Although there are concerns about radiation exposure, advancements in CT technology, including ECG-guided modulation, prospective ECG gating, low kV techniques, and iterative reconstruction, have notably decreased radiation exposure from cardiac CT scans during the last 2 decades. When used in conjunction, these techniques can allow a cardiac CT with very low radiation exposure, potentially in the submillisievert range.

FUNDING

Dr C.P. McCarthy is supported by a grant from the National Heart, Lung, And Blood Institute of the National Institutes of Health (K23HL167659).

DISCLOSURE

Dr C.P. McCarthy has received consulting income/honorarium from Abbott Laboratories and Roche Diagnostics.

REFERENCES

1. Schnabel RB, Yin X, Gona P, et al. 50 year trends in atrial fibrillation prevalence, incidence, risk factors, and mortality in the Framingham Heart Study: a cohort study. Lancet (London, England) 2015; 386(9989):154–62.
2. Staerk L, Wang B, Preis SR, et al. Lifetime risk of atrial fibrillation according to optimal, borderline, or elevated levels of risk factors: cohort study based on longitudinal data from the Framingham Heart Study. BMJ 2018;361:k1453.
3. Scott M, Baykaner T, Bunch TJ, et al. Contemporary trends in cardiac electrophysiology procedures in the United States, and impact of a global pandemic. Heart rhythm O2 2023;4(3):193–9.
4. Heseltine TD, Murray SW, Ruzsics B, et al. Latest Advances in Cardiac CT. European cardiology 2020;15:1–7.
5. Reeves RA, Halpern EJ, Rao VM. Cardiac Imaging Trends from 2010 to 2019 in the Medicare Population. Radiology: Cardiothoracic Imaging 2021;3(5): e210156.
6. Goldfarb JW, Weber J. Trends in Cardiovascular MRI and CT in the U.S. Medicare Population from 2012 to 2017. Radiol Cardiothorac Imaging 2021; 3(1):e200112.
7. Romero J, Husain SA, Kelesidis I, et al. Detection of Left Atrial Appendage Thrombus by Cardiac Computed Tomography in Patients With Atrial Fibrillation. Circulation: Cardiovascular Imaging 2013; 6(2):185–94.
8. Echt DS, Liebson PR, Mitchell LB, et al. Mortality and Morbidity in Patients Receiving Encainide, Flecainide, or Placebo. N Engl J Med 1991;324(12): 781–8.
9. Hilberath JN, Oakes DA, Shernan SK, et al. Safety of transesophageal echocardiography. J Am Soc Echocardiogr 2010;23(11):1115–27. quiz 220-1.
10. Yu S, Zhang H, Li H. Cardiac Computed Tomography Versus Transesophageal Echocardiography for the Detection of Left Atrial Appendage Thrombus: A Systemic Review and Meta-Analysis. J Am Heart Assoc 2021;10(23):e022505.
11. Kapa S, Martinez MW, Williamson EE, et al. ECG-gated dual-source CT for detection of left atrial appendage thrombus in patients undergoing catheter ablation for atrial fibrillation. J Intervent Card Electrophysiol 2010;29(2):75–81.
12. Pinho J, Dhaenens L, Heckelmann J, et al. Left atrial appendage thrombus in acute stroke: diagnostic accuracy of CT angiography compared to transesophageal echocardiography. J Stroke Cerebrovasc Dis 2023;32(2):106936.
13. Patel A, Au E, Donegan K, et al. Multidetector row computed tomography for identification of left atrial appendage filling defects in patients undergoing pulmonary vein isolation for treatment of atrial fibrillation: comparison with transesophageal echocardiography. Heart Rhythm 2008;5(2):253–60.
14. Odutayo A, Wong CX, Hsiao AJ, et al. Atrial fibrillation and risks of cardiovascular disease, renal disease, and death: systematic review and meta-analysis. BMJ 2016;354:i4482.
15. Haïssaguerre M, Jaïs P, Shah DC, et al. Spontaneous initiation of atrial fibrillation by ectopic beats originating in the pulmonary veins. N Engl J Med 1998;339(10):659–66.
16. Kirchhof P, Camm AJ, Goette A, et al. Early Rhythm-Control Therapy in Patients with Atrial Fibrillation. N Engl J Med 2020;383(14):1305–16.
17. Wazni OM, Marrouche NF, Martin DO, et al. Radiofrequency ablation vs antiarrhythmic drugs as first-line treatment of symptomatic atrial fibrillation: a randomized trial. JAMA 2005;293(21):2634–40.
18. Raeisi-Giglou P, Wazni OM, Saliba WI, et al. Outcomes and Management of Patients With Severe Pulmonary Vein Stenosis From Prior Atrial Fibrillation Ablation. Circulation: Arrhythmia and Electrophysiology 2018;11(5):e006001.
19. Han H-C, Ha FJ, Sanders P, et al. Atrioesophageal Fistula. Circulation: Arrhythmia and Electrophysiology 2017;10(11):e005579.
20. Istratoaie S, Roşu R, Cismaru G, et al. The Impact of Pulmonary Vein Anatomy on the Outcomes of Catheter Ablation for Atrial Fibrillation. Medicina (Kaunas, Lithuania) 2019;55(11).
21. Lickfett L, Dickfeld T, Kato R, et al. Changes of pulmonary vein orifice size and location throughout the

cardiac cycle: dynamic analysis using magnetic resonance cine imaging. J Cardiovasc Electrophysiol 2005;16(6):582–8.

22. Schwartzman D, Lacomis J, Wigginton WG. Characterization of left atrium and distal pulmonary vein morphology using multidimensional computed tomography. J Am Coll Cardiol 2003;41(8):1349–57.

23. Kato R, Lickfett L, Meininger G, et al. Pulmonary vein anatomy in patients undergoing catheter ablation of atrial fibrillation: lessons learned by use of magnetic resonance imaging. Circulation 2003;107(15): 2004–10.

24. Scharf C, Sneider M, Case I, et al. Anatomy of the pulmonary veins in patients with atrial fibrillation and effects of segmental ostial ablation analyzed by computed tomography. J Cardiovasc Electrophysiol 2003;14(2):150–5.

25. Marom EM, Herndon JE, Kim YH, et al. Variations in pulmonary venous drainage to the left atrium: implications for radiofrequency ablation. Radiology 2004; 230(3):824–9.

26. Lacomis JM, Wigginton W, Fuhrman C, et al. Multi–Detector Row CT of the Left Atrium and Pulmonary Veins before Radio-frequency Catheter Ablation for Atrial Fibrillation. Radiographics 2003;23(suppl_1): S35–48.

27. Saremi F, Channual S, Abolhoda A, et al. MDCT of the S-shaped sinoatrial node artery. AJR American journal of roentgenology 2008;190(6):1569–75.

28. Benali K, Khairy P, Hammache N, et al. Procedure-Related Complications of Catheter Ablation for Atrial Fibrillation. J Am Coll Cardiol 2023;81(21):2089–99.

29. Pürerfellner H, Martinek M. Pulmonary vein stenosis following catheter ablation of atrial fibrillation. Curr Opin Cardiol 2005;20(6):484–90.

30. Pappone C, Oral H, Santinelli V, et al. Atrio-esophageal fistula as a complication of percutaneous transcatheter ablation of atrial fibrillation. Circulation 2004;109(22):2724–6.

31. Ravenel JG, McAdams HP. Pulmonary venous infarction after radiofrequency ablation for atrial fibrillation. AJR American journal of roentgenology 2002;178(3):664–6.

32. Qureshi AM, Prieto LR, Latson LA, et al. Transcatheter Angioplasty for Acquired Pulmonary Vein Stenosis After Radiofrequency Ablation. Circulation 2003; 108(11):1336–42.

33. Al-Saady NM, Obel OA, Camm AJ. Left atrial appendage: structure, function, and role in thromboembolism. Heart (British Cardiac Society) 1999;82(5): 547–54.

34. Osmancik P, Herman D, Neuzil P, et al. 4-Year Outcomes After Left Atrial Appendage Closure Versus Nonwarfarin Oral Anticoagulation for Atrial Fibrillation. J Am Coll Cardiol 2022;79(1):1–14.

35. Reddy VY, Sievert H, Halperin J, et al. Percutaneous Left Atrial Appendage Closure vs Warfarin for Atrial Fibrillation: A Randomized Clinical Trial. JAMA 2014;312(19):1988–98.

36. January CT, Wann LS, Calkins H, et al. 2019 AHA/ACC/HRS Focused Update of the 2014 AHA/ACC/HRS Guideline for the Management of Patients With Atrial Fibrillation: A Report of the American College of Cardiology/American Heart Association Task Force on Clinical Practice Guidelines and the Heart Rhythm Society in Collaboration With the Society of Thoracic Surgeons. Circulation 2019;140(2):e125–51.

37. Rajiah P, Alkhouli M, Thaden J, et al. Pre- and Postprocedural CT of Transcatheter Left Atrial Appendage Closure Devices. Radiographics 2021; 41(3):680–98.

38. Lupercio F, Carlos Ruiz J, Briceno DF, et al. Left atrial appendage morphology assessment for risk stratification of embolic stroke in patients with atrial fibrillation: A meta-analysis. Heart Rhythm 2016;13(7): 1402–9.

39. Ahmed A, Bawa D, Ukwu H, et al. PO-03-192 Intradevice leaks on post left atrial appendage occluder follow up tomographic imaging–true leak or mere incomplete endothelialization. Heart Rhythm 2023; 20(5):S394.

40. Wang YAN, Di Biase L, Horton RP, et al. Left Atrial Appendage Studied by Computed Tomography to Help Planning for Appendage Closure Device Placement. J Cardiovasc Electrophysiol 2010;21(9):973–82.

41. Lindner S, Behnes M, Wenke A, et al. Assessment of peri-device leaks after interventional left atrial appendage closure using standardized imaging by cardiac computed tomography angiography. Int J Cardiovasc Imag 2019;35(4):725–31.

42. Alkhouli M, Sievert H, Rihal CS. Device Embolization in Structural Heart Interventions: Incidence, Outcomes, and Retrieval Techniques. JACC Cardiovasc Interv 2019;12(2):113–26.

43. Kirkfeldt RE, Johansen JB, Nohr EA, et al. Complications after cardiac implantable electronic device implantations: an analysis of a complete, nationwide cohort in Denmark. Eur Heart J 2014;35(18):1186–94.

44. Kalinin R, Suchkov I, Mzhavanadze N, et al. Assessment of Coagulation Parameters as Potential Markers for Venous Thromboembolism in Patients With Cardiac Implantable Electronic Devices. Eur J Vasc Endovasc Surg 2019;58(6):e820–1.

45. Rajiah PS, Reddy P, Baliyan V, et al. Utility of CT and MRI in Tricuspid Valve Interventions. Radiographics 2023;43(7):e220153.

46. Mahnken AH, Koos R, Katoh M, et al. Assessment of myocardial viability in reperfused acute myocardial infarction using 16-slice computed tomography in comparison to magnetic resonance imaging. J Am Coll Cardiol 2005;45(12):2042–7.

47. le Polain de Waroux JB, Pouleur AC, Goffinet C, et al. Combined coronary and late-enhanced multidetector-computed tomography for delineation of the

etiology of left ventricular dysfunction: comparison with coronary angiography and contrast-enhanced cardiac magnetic resonance imaging. Eur Heart J 2008;29(20):2544–51.

48. Langer C, Lutz M, Eden M, et al. Hypertrophic cardiomyopathy in cardiac CT: a validation study on the detection of intramyocardial fibrosis in consecutive patients. Int J Cardiovasc Imag 2014;30(3): 659–67.

49. Aikawa T, Oyama-Manabe N, Naya M, et al. Delayed contrast-enhanced computed tomography in patients with known or suspected cardiac sarcoidosis: A feasibility study. Eur Radiol 2017;27(10):4054–63.

50. Esposito A, Palmisano A, Antunes S, et al. Cardiac CT With Delayed Enhancement in the Characterization of Ventricular Tachycardia Structural Substrate: Relationship Between CT-Segmented Scar and Electro-Anatomic Mapping. JACC Cardiovascular imaging 2016;9(7):822–32.

51. Winer-Muram HT, Tann M, Aisen AM, et al. Computed tomography demonstration of lipomatous metaplasia of the left ventricle following myocardial infarction. J Comput Assist Tomogr 2004;28(4):455–8.

52. Ichikawa Y, Kitagawa K, Chino S, et al. Adipose tissue detected by multislice computed tomography in patients after myocardial infarction. JACC Cardiovascular imaging 2009;2(5):548–55.

53. Palmisano A, Vignale D, Benedetti G, et al. Late iodine enhancement cardiac computed tomography for detection of myocardial scars: impact of experience in the clinical practice. La Radiologia medica 2020;125(2):128–36.

54. Hedgire SS, Baliyan V, Ghoshhajra BB, et al. Recent advances in cardiac computed tomography dose reduction strategies: a review of scientific evidence and technical developments. J Med Imag 2017; 4(3):031211.

55. Cha MJ, Kang DY, Lee W, et al. Hypersensitivity Reactions to Iodinated Contrast Media: A Multicenter Study of 196 081 Patients. Radiology 2019;293(1): 117–24.

56. McDonald RJ, McDonald JS, Bida JP, et al. Intravenous contrast material-induced nephropathy: causal or coincident phenomenon? Radiology 2013;267(1): 106–18.

57. Davenport MS, Perazella MA, Yee J, et al. Use of Intravenous Iodinated Contrast Media in Patients With Kidney Disease: Consensus Statements from the American College of Radiology and the National Kidney Foundation. Kidney medicine 2020;2(1): 85–93.

Computed Tomography Angiography for Aortic Diseases

Ishan Garg, MD[a], Jakub M. Siembida, MD[b], Sandeep Hedgire, MD[c], Sarv Priya, MD[d], Prashant Nagpal, MD[b],*

KEYWORDS

- Aorta • Aortic diseases • Acute aortic syndrome • Aortic dissection • Traumatic aortic injury
- Aneurysm • Computed tomography angiography (CTA)

KEY POINTS

- The prevalence of aortic diseases is increasing, and early detection is the key for timely management.
- Imaging plays a crucial role in identifying and planning aortic diseases.
- CT angiography is the test of choice in the majority of the patients, both for emergent and non-emergent aortic diseases due to very high accuracy and universal availability.
- Appropriate use of electrocardiogram-gating for suspected aortic root or ascending aortic diseases and standardized CTA protocols and aortic measurement methodology are cornerstone for high diagnostic accuracy for CT.
- Knowledge of imaging patterns of aortic diseases and post-treatment complications are important for Radiologists to recognize.

INTRODUCTION

Echocardiography, computed tomography angiography (CTA), and magnetic resonance angiography (MRA) stand as cornerstone imaging techniques for the diagnosis and therapeutic management of aortic pathologies.[1–3] Among these modalities, CTA has emerged as a first-line imaging modality owing to its excellent anatomic detail, widespread availability, established imaging protocols, evidence-proven indications, and rapid acquisition time.[1,4] The prevalence of aortic disease is on rise. The prevalence of aortic aneurysm has increased from 3.5 to 7.6 per 100,000 persons between 2002 and 2014.[5] The true prevalence of acute aortic syndrome (AAS) is difficult to estimate due to death before reaching hospital and differing autopsy rates across the world. While the overall incidence of AAS may be stable, the incidence of conditions that are now better understood and had higher chances of reaching the hospital like acute penetrating aortic ulcer (PAU) has increased from 0.6 to 2.6 per 100 000 person-years.[6]

Imaging is critical for the diagnosis as well as clinical classification, identification of complications, risk-stratification, prognostication, and treatment-planning for patients. The purpose of this article is to review the role of CTA in the management of various aortic pathologies, including acute aortic syndrome (AAS), aortic dissection, intramural hematoma (IMH), penetrating aortic ulcer (PAU), traumatic aortic injury (TAI), and aortic aneurysm.

Funding: This research received no external funding.
[a] Department of Internal Medicine, University of New Mexico Health Sciences Center, Albuquerque, NM, USA; [b] Department of Radiology, University of Wisconsin-Madison, Madison, WI, USA; [c] Division of Cardiovascular Imaging, Department of Radiology, Massachusetts General Hospital, Boston, MA, USA; [d] Department of Radiology, University of Iowa Carver College of Medicine, Iowa City, IA, USA
* Corresponding author. Cardiovascular and Thoracic Radiology, University of Wisconsin School of Medicine and Public Health, Madison, WI.
E-mail addresses: pnagpal@wisc.edu; drprashantnagpal@gmail.com

Radiol Clin N Am 62 (2024) 509–525
https://doi.org/10.1016/j.rcl.2024.01.001
0033-8389/24/© 2024 Elsevier Inc. All rights reserved.

AORTA: NORMAL ANATOMY AND VARIANTS

The aorta is the largest artery in the body, extending from the aortic valve annulus to the pelvis (fourth lumbar vertebra, L4), where it splits into the right and left common iliac arteries (**Fig. 1**). Morphologically aorta can be subdivided into the following segments.[2]

- Aortic root: From the aortic valve annulus to the sinotubular junction. The sinuses of Valsalva are part of the aortic root.[7]
- Ascending aorta: Extending upward from the sinotubular junction, then to the right before curving posteriorly into the aortic arch at the origin of the brachiocephalic trunk.
- Aortic arch: Extends from the origin of the brachiocephalic trunk to the ligamentum arteriosum. Since ligamentum arteriosum is not apparent on imaging in majority of patients, the origin of the left subclavian artery is frequently considered as the imaging landmark for aortic arch. The main branches of the aortic arch include the brachiocephalic trunk (which divides into the right common carotid and right subclavian artery), left common carotid, and left subclavian artery. Normal variants include the common origin of brachiocephalic trunk and left common carotid arteries (seen in around 25% of people) and left vertebral artery arising directly from the aortic arch (seen in 6% of people).[8] Other normal variants include ductus diverticulum, a remnant of ductus arteriosus which can be seen as a

focal bulge along the inner aspect of the isthmus. Awareness of this entity is important as it can be misinterpreted for a traumatic aortic pseudoaneurysm, dissection, or incomplete rupture. On imaging, the ductus diverticulum often presents with smooth margins with obtuse angles related to the adjacent aorta. In comparison, aortic pseudoaneurysm tends to have irregular margins with acute angles to the adjacent aorta.[9]

- Descending thoracic aorta extends from ligamentum arteriosum to the hiatus of the diaphragm, beyond which it continues as the abdominal aorta.
- The abdominal aorta is a retroperitoneal segment extending from the hiatus of the diaphragm to the pelvis (approximately at the level of L4), where it divides into the right and left common iliac arteries. The abdominal aorta is divided into suprarenal and infrarenal segments.

Computed Tomography Angiography of the Aorta

Echocardiography, CTA, and magnetic resonance angiography (MRA) are cornerstone imaging techniques for the diagnosis and therapeutic management of aortic pathologies.[10–12] Excellent anatomic detail, widespread availability, established imaging protocols, evidence-proven indications, familiarity among ordering providers and radiologists, and rapid acquisition time has

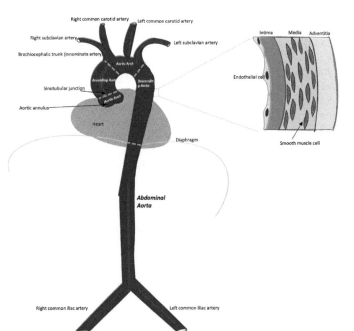

Fig. 1. Illustration showing normal aortic anatomy with wall histology (in the insert).

made computed tomography (CT) angiography (CTA) obtained using multi-detector computed tomography(MDCT) scanner, the first-line imaging modality for evaluation of acute aortic pathology with nearly 100% sensitivity and specificity.[13] Furthermore, the standardized imaging protocols for cross-sectional imaging (both CTA and magnetic resonance [MR] angiography) substantially reduce inter-operator variability, making them optimal tools for longitudinal surveillance and comparative post-treatment evaluations. The major limitations of CT include potential side effects related to exposure to a modest amount of ionizing radiation and contrast agent used in CTA.[14,15]

Imaging Protocol

A proper imaging protocol is critical for obtaining the highest quality CTA images. The CTA methodology encompasses a rapid, high-resolution volumetric isotropic CT data acquisition, including capturing pre-contrast (if needed), post-contrast (arterial, delayed phases)- based CT data; and subsequent postprocessing into 2-dimensional (2D), 3D, or 4D visual representations.[16] This sophisticated approach yields CTA images of exceptional spatial resolution appropriate for the evaluation of both the vascular anatomy and solid organs.[17]

The pre-requisite for aortic CTA examinations includes the integration of cardiac or electrocardiogram (ECG)-gating for thoracic aorta, especially for the aortic root and ascending aortic evaluation. This integration significantly mitigates motion-induced artifacts, predominantly those caused by cardiac activity, found in as much as 92% of non-gated scans.[2,16] This facilitates the examination of a near-motionless aortic root, enhancing both the diagnostic accuracy and reproducibility of aortic size measurements.

ECG-gating can be implemented in 2 ways: prospective gating, which involves a reduced radiation dose, and retrospective gating, which is associated with a higher radiation dose.[18,19] In retrospective gating, the CT images are throughout the entirety of the cardiac cycle, post which the most optimal phase is selected for reconstruction. Conversely, prospective gating captures CT scans during a predefined phase of the cardiac cycle, ensuring superior diagnostic accuracy by evaluating relatively motionless aortic root. With the advances in the CT technology, especially with dual-source CT scanners, motionless images of the aorta can also be obtained by high-pitch imaging which allows super-fast imaging practically freezing the motion even without ECG-gating.[20] The CTA imaging

protocol used at the authors' institution is summarized in **Table 1**.

Multi-detector Computed Tomography Scanner Configuration

Majority of the aortic imaging now is performed on CT scanners with detector arrays of 64 or more. Such configurations facilitate the acquisition of slices with submillimeter thickness (<1 mm), short gantry rotation durations, translating into superior temporal resolution, and rapid data collection that can cover the entire aorta in under 3 seconds. These scanners usually offer a spatial resolution ranging between 0.25 and 0.47 mm.[4,7,16] Furthermore, in urgent clinical scenarios, this expedited capture is invaluable, producing high-resolution,

Table 1
Aortic computed tomography angiography protocol at the authors' institute

Scan Range	Chest, chest and abdomen, or chest, abdomen, and pelvis—depending on the suspected or known aortic pathology. 1. Non-contrast high-pitch (pitch factor >3, if dual-source scanners) non-ECG-gated chest (non-contrast only for acute aortic syndromes and post-operative aorta) 2. Contrast-enhanced ECG-gated chest 3. Non-gated abdomen and pelvis (if chest, abdomen, and pelvis coverage)
Contrast type	Iopamidol 370 mg/mL (Bracco Diagnostic, Princeton, NJ, USA)
Contrast dose	100 mL injected at 4 mL/s
Gating	Prospective with automatic single-phase selection based on the HR (75% for HR < 75 bpm and 40% for ≥75 bpm HR)
Reconstructions	• 3.0 mm thickness with 3.0 mm interval in axial, coronal, and sagittal planes • 1 mm thickness with 0.8 mm interval for 3D postprocessing and double-oblique measurements

Abbreviations: BPM, beats per minute; ECG, electrocardiogram.

near motion-free, non-gated images when ECG or respiratory-gated CT might introduce diagnostic delays or be inaccessible.

The standard kilovolt peak (kVp) for these scanners lies between 100 and 120 kVp. For individuals with a body mass index (BMI) below 20, a lower kVp setting can be utilized, whereas a higher kVp might be requisite for those with a BMI exceeding 30. Innovations in dual-energy CT scanners can obviate the need for ECG-gating. However, while appropriate for AAS rule out examinationss, aortic examination in specific phase of the cardiac cycle (diastole or systole) is standard of care for aortic sizing and follow-up of aneurysm. Use of dual-score scanners has nonetheless led to significantly improved image quality, decreased radiation exposure, and decreased required dosage of contrast agents.[20]

Contrast Administration for Computed Tomography Angiography

To achieve optimal aortic visualization, an opacification exceeding 250 Hounsfield units (HU)—ideally surpassing 300 HU—is advised. Typically, an iodinated contrast medium is administered at a flow rate of 3 to 6 mL/s, using a total volume between 100 and 125 mL. This is subsequently followed by a 40 mL normal saline flush at a rate of 4 mL/s.[4,7] The post-contrast image acquisition is either automated through bolus tracking software or manually set using a test bolus, which typically involves 15 to 20 mL of contrast. Given the ease of use, the automated contrast bolus tracking software is preferred over the test bolus method. In addition, it involves reduced contrast doses and an enhanced signal-to-background ratio, ensuring no inadvertent opacification of parenchymal organs from test dose contrast.

While non-contrast series is desired for imaging obtained for AAS and post-operative aorta, a single arterial phase is often sufficient for aortic sizing and pre-surgical assessment.[16] For suspected acute aortic pathologies, an initial non-contrast phase can be particularly helpful for the early identification of intramural hematomas, which might otherwise be elusive on sole arterial phase imaging. This phase also aids in the preliminary evaluation of calcifications and postoperative material, which can stimulate endoleak on arterial phase.[1,7,16] Moreover, delayed phase imaging—captured 1 to 2 minutes post-contrast injection is pivotal for assessing the delayed filling of a false lumen, assessment of solid organ parenchymal enhancement in setting of dissections, slow-progressing endoleak, endovascular stent patency, and enhanced visualization of inflammatory tissues and vasculitis.

Postprocessing Techniques for Multi-detector Computed Tomography Raw Data

Several sophisticated postprocessing tools exist for the purpose of reformatting and volume rendering the raw images acquired from MDCT. Among the commonly deployed postprocessing strategies are multiplanar reconstruction (MPR), curved planar reformats (CPR), maximum intensity projection (MIP), and volume rendering (VR).[1,7,16]

Both MPR and CPR generate 2-dimensional images derived from a 3D dataset, proving invaluable for visualizing the intricate and tortuous anatomy of the aorta. This is of particular significance for visualization, preprocedural planning, and decreasing interobserver variability in the measurement of aortic pathology, such as an aortic aneurysm.

On the other hand, VR images are created from 3D data sets by utilizing predetermined density thresholds. This is particularly useful in distinguishing between intraluminal contrast and stent materials, given that stent materials usually exhibit a higher density compared to intraluminal contrast. MIP images preferentially display only the highest density pixels from the data into a single plantar image. This allows excellent visualization of a high-density material such as contrast, calcification, endograft, and collateral circulation (in scenarios with vascular occlusion or pronounced stenosis).

AORTIC SIZING AND STANDARDIZED MEASUREMENTS

The dimensions of the aortic root and the ascending aorta are influenced by factors such as age, gender, and body surface area. The use of a single cut-off value is inadvisable. Therefore, aortic diameter is frequently normalized using various indices: the aortic size index (ASI, in cm/m2), the aortic height index (AHI, in cm/m), or the cross-sectional area-to-height ratio (in cm²/m).

Regarding aortic measurements via CT or magnetic resonance (MR) imaging, the latest guidelines (2022) from the American College of Cardiology and the American Heart Association recommend estimations of the aortic diameter must be orthogonal to its long axis.[2] Oblique angle determinations can inadvertently lead to overestimations.[2] The guidelines suggest that in aorta with normal wall, the inner-edge-to-inner-edge measurements should be measured. However, in segments showcasing wall irregularities or wall disease like atherosclerosis, vasculitis, dissection, or IMH, the outer-edge-to-outer-edge (O-O) method is preferable (Fig. 2). Conversely, for graft material assessment, the inner-edge-to-inner-edge (I-I) technique aids

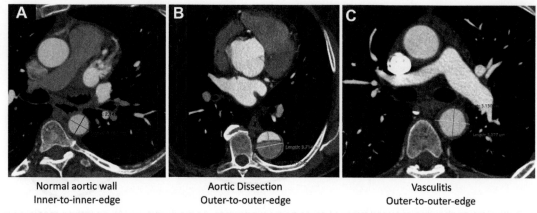

Fig. 2. Standardized methodology of measuring short-axis diameter of the aorta. In patients with normal aortic wall (A), inner-to-inner-edge measurements are recommended. While in patients with diseased aortic wall, like aortic dissection (B) or vasculitis (C), outer-to-outer-edge measurements are recommended.

in ascertaining the functional lumen and informs subsequent treatment strategies. For CT-based assessments, the Sinus of Valsalva dimensions are taken from the commissure to the opposing sinus or between sinuses, opting for the larger measurement. Both the sinus-to-sinus and inner-edge-to-inner-edge (I-I) measurements on CT & MR imaging have demonstrated considerable user confidence with minimized intra-observer and inter-observer variability.[2,4] ECG-gated triggering can help further reduce these variabilities.[4]

It is paramount to recognize that distinct imaging procedures might yield marginally different aortic dimensions. As such, maintaining the same imaging modality for successive evaluations may ensure a more consistent and reliable monitoring of aortic pathology.

COMPUTED TOMOGRAPHY IMAGING OF AORTIC DISEASES IN ADULTS
Acute Aortic Syndrome

Acute aortic syndrome (AAS) is a group of life-threatening aortic pathologies. These disorders share a defining trait, a sudden disruption in the integrity of the aortic wall. It includes conditions such as aortic dissection, intramural hematoma (IMH), penetrating aortic ulcer (PAU), traumatic aortic rupture (TAR), and ruptured aneurysm (contained or not contained).[21] The common AAS are illustrated in Fig. 3. Predominantly, the clinical manifestations of AAS include intense chest pain, often radiating to adjacent areas like the back, neck, or abdomen, coupled with signs of hemodynamic instability like shock.[21–24]

Given the urgent and potentially fatal nature of these conditions, CTA is the preferred modality for diagnosis and management, given its rapid

acquisition, excellent diagnostic accuracy, and excellent spatial-temporal resolution. For instance, according to a meta-analysis, CTA was shown to have 100% sensitivity and 98% specificity for diagnosis of traumatic aortic dissection (TAD).[25]

Aortic Dissection

Aortic dissection (AD) is the most common cause of AAS. The overall incidence of aortic dissection ranges between 0.5 and 3 cases per 100,000 person-years.[2] While it predominantly affects individuals aged 50-year-old to 70-year-old, congenital aortic diseases or connective tissue diseases might precipitate its onset earlier. Hypertension remains its primary risk factor, followed by pre-existing aortic diseases, aortic valve anomalies, familial predisposition, smoking, blunt chest trauma, and illicit drug use such as cocaine and amphetamine.[14,26,27]

It is characterized by an intimal tear, causing blood flow into the media, ultimately resulting creation of a blood-filled dissection flap. This dissection flap can expand either antegrade or retrograde along the aortic long axis. Classification of AD is based on either anatomic location (Stanford or DeBakey classification) (Fig. 4) or symptomatic duration. The more commonly used Stanford classification system divides dissections into.[2]

- Type A (more common): Involving the ascending aorta. Require urgent surgical intervention.
- Type B (less common): Not involving the ascending aorta. Managed conservatively with antihypertensive therapy or by endovascular stent repair if complicated by end-organ ischemia or persistent symptoms.[28] The endovascular stent is associated with

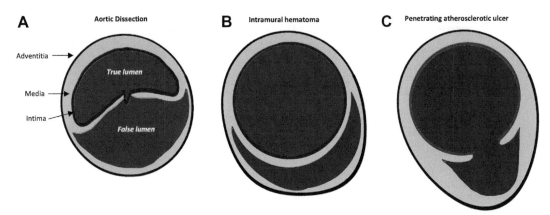

Fig. 3. Illustration showing common types of acute aortic syndromes. Aortic dissection (*A*), an intimo-medial tear leading to blood collection in aortic media, creating a clear true and false lumen. Intramural hematoma (*B*), slow leak of blood in aortic media causing aortic wall thickening, with a relatively normal-appearing aortic lumen. Penetrating atherosclerotic ulcer (*C*), intimal ulcer that allows penetration of blood into aortic media, which is typically confined to a single discrete location (vs propagation in case of aortic dissection).

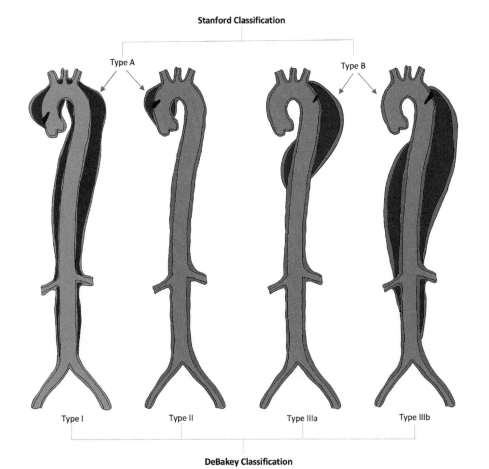

Fig. 4. Illustration showing classification of aortic dissection. The Stanford and DeBakey classification system.

reduced aorta-specific mortality but without an overall mortality benefit vis-à-vis medical management.[7]

The most common complications include.

- Aortic regurgitation (AR): Frequently concomitant with Type A AD, AR is evident in nearly half of the cases. It has multifactorial etiopathogenesis, including aortic dilatation, dissection flap extension into the Sinuses of Valsalva, and flap prolapse affecting the aortic leaflet.[29,30] Distinguishing AR and its triggers is important for apt surgical decisions and is primarily done by echocardiogram.
- Malperfusion Syndrome: Characterized by clinically manifested end-organ ischemia secondary to branch vessel obstruction. It is a poor prognostic sign associated with a 30.5% overall mortality rate, with an even worse mortality rate of 63.2% noted with mesenteric malperfusions.[2] The obstruction can be static, where the dissection flap obstructs a branch vessel, or dynamic, wherein the false lumen compresses the true lumen, compromising branch vessel perfusion.

Role of Computed Tomography Angiography in Aortic Dissection

Diagnosis and risk stratification

CTA is the most preferred imaging modality for AD, primarily due to its widespread availability in emergency departments and rapid image acquisition. CTA can help in the diagnosis of AD by identification of the dissection flap, which is a pathognomic feature of AD (**Fig. 5**). CTA can also help in differentiating the true lumen from the false lumen. Typically, the true lumen tends to be smaller, with irregular contour, contiguous with the lumen of the adjacent non-dissected aorta.[31] Conversely, the false lumen is characterized by a larger cross-sectional area on the axial image, slow blood flow (as it is not part of the aortic lumen), presence of signs like "bbeak," thrombi,and "cobwebs" (linear low-attenuation areas, representing residual dissected media fragments).[32] However, sometimes linear hypodense areas can also be seen in the true lumen from hypodense contrast coming from the hypodense false lumen along the intimal tear due to high pressure in the false lumen (**Fig. 6**). CTA affords an expansive view of the dissection, revealing its full extent, initiation tear, and surrounding mediastinal entities, vital for diagnosis and treatment planning.[33,34]

Penetrating Aortic Ulcer

An acute PAU occurs due to the ulceration of an atherosclerotic plaque deep into the arterial wall. It accounts for 2% to 7% of all AAS and affects elderly patients with severe atherosclerotic disease.[35] It is most commonly located in the descending thoracic aorta. Clinically acute PAU presents similar to aortic dissection and other AAS.[2]

Acute PAU can be associated with IMH from hemorrhage in the media and can progress to frank aortic dissection (intimomedial tear with true and false lumen), aneurysm, or rupture (penetrating through all 3 layers of the aortic wall resulting in saccular, fusiform, or pseudoaneurysm, which may ultimately rupture) based on level of penetration. Overall, rupture is uncommon.

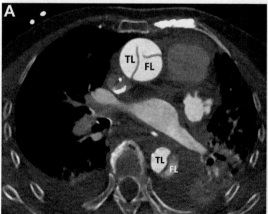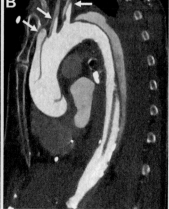

Fig. 5. Type A aortic dissection. Axial post-contrast CT image (*A*) and sagittal oblique multiplanar reformation image (*B*) showing Stanford type A aortic dissection showing dissection flap extending into the arch branches (*white arrows, B*) and the abdominal aorta. FL, false lumen; TL, true lumen.

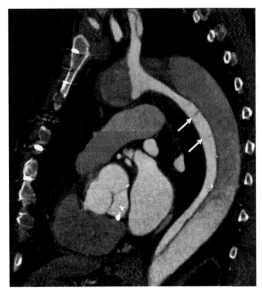

Fig. 6. Sagittal CTA image in a patient with aortic dissection showing linear low attenuation areas in the true lumen (*white arrows*). These are due to small foci of intimal tear with blood flow from false lumen to the true lumen. Note that the low attenuation of these jets match with the attenuation of the false lumen.

Role of Computed Tomography Angiography in Penetrating Aortic Ulcer

Diagnosis and risk stratification

PAUs are characterized as irregular, crater-like, contrast-enhanced-protrusion from the aortic wall[36] (**Fig. 7**). Calcified atherosclerotic plaques are frequently seen surrounding the PAUs. One of the serious associations of acute PAUs is the development of IMH, which occurs due to hemorrhage progression into the tunica media layer. CTA can identify these IMHs, offering insights into the ulcer's severity and potential complications. While PAUs share some radiological similarities with ulcerated atherosclerotic plaques, discontinuity of intimal calcification, vessel contour deformity, associated IMH, or focal peri-aortic fat stranding favor the presence of PAU. The differentiation is crucial since the treatment and prognostic implications can be significantly varied. Notably, acute PAUs exceeding 13 mm in size or with a neck diameter beyond 10 mm are at risk of aortic rupture and require immediate therapeutic intervention.[37]

Intramural Hematoma

IMH is defined by the presence of hemorrhage within the media. It can be seen in association of another aortic pathology like PAU or aneurysm, indicating extension of blood into the aortic wall or can occur in isolation as the primary AAS. IMH, when present with another aortic pathology is a marker of disease acuity. Historically, isolated IMH was believed to occur from the rupture of vasa vasorum in the aortic media. But improved imaging resolution and surgical literature has pointed to presence of small intimomedial tears that are sometimes not apparent at acute or preoperative imaging.[38] Studies have shown that an intimal microtear can be identified in 68% to 73% of patients with acute IMH.[39,40] On such patients with intimal microtear, the differentiation of IMH and AD is that AD contains 2 intimomedial tears (entry tear from the lumen into the media, and a reentry tear back into the aortic lumen) while IMH with intimomedial tear has an entry tear only.

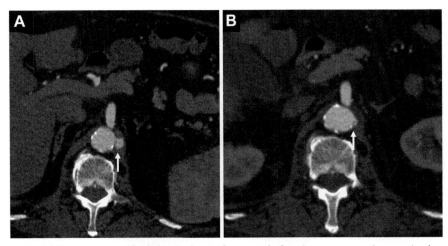

Fig. 7. Axial CTA (*A*) in a patient with abdominal pain for a week showing a penetrating aortic ulcer (*white arrow, A*) along the left lateral wall of the upper abdominal aorta. CTA obtained 5 days prior (*B*) also showing subtle intimal irregularity (*white arrow, B*) which was missed on this examination.

IMH predominantly affects the geriatric population, especially those with underlying hypertension and pronounced atherosclerotic disease.[41] The descending thoracic aorta is the most frequently involved site at 60%, with the ascending aorta and aortic arch following at 30% and 10%, respectively.[41] Intramural hematomas use the same classification system as aortic dissection. For instance, Type A IMH presents with a significant 18% rupture risk at the outset and, without surgical intervention, invariably leads to mortality.[42] In comparison, Type B IMH demonstrates a more favorable prognosis, with mortality rates standing at 4% to 6% during hospitalization and 9% at the 1-year mark, primarily managed medically.[41,43] Common complications include progression to aortic dissection, aneurysm, and rupture.

Role of Computed Tomography Angiography in Intramural Hematoma

Diagnosis and risk stratification

The hallmark of IMH on CTA is a high-attenuation crescentic or circumferential thickening of the aorta on non-contrast imaging, without a distinct dissection flap (**Fig. 8**). Therefore, the non-contrast phase of CTA is particularly invaluable in the diagnosis of IMH. Certain imaging features seen on CTA are associated with a higher risk of complications in IMH and can significantly impact treatment decisions, including focal intimal disruption (FID) (identified as contrast-filled outpouching measuring ≥3 mm, projecting from the aortic wall), increasing aortic diameter, increasing hematoma thickness, hematoma thickness of ≥10 to 13 mm (≥13 mm for Type B and ≥10 mm for Type A), and a maximum aortic diameter ranging from >45 to 50 mm (≥47–50 mm for Type B and ≥45–50 mm for Type A) are considered significant high-risk

features.[2] Intramural blood pool differs from ulcer-like projection or intimal microtear in that there is either no apparent connectivity or a very tiny link with the aortic lumen. Because there is typically a visible communication with an intercostal or bronchial artery, an intramural blood pool is more likely to form in the descending aorta and is sometimes referred to as an aortic branch artery tear or an aortic branch artery pseudoaneurysm.

Traumatic Aortic Injury

Traumatic aortic injury (TAI) is a medical emergency, with over 80% of patients dying before reaching the hospital.[44,45] TAI can be from sharp (penetrating/direct) or blunt (indirect) trauma. Penetrating aortic trauma is usually fatal. Here, we will discuss a more prevalent entity, blunt traumatic thoracic aortic injury (BTTAI).[2]

BTTAI stands as a leading cause of trauma-related mortality, surpassed only by traumatic brain injuries.[4] Of note, while traumatic injuries to the thoracic aorta are relatively common, their abdominal counterpart—Blunt Abdominal Aortic Injury—is markedly rare, representing less than 1% of blunt trauma cases.[4]

Motor vehicle accidents predominantly contribute to BTTAI, representing over 70% of the incidents. Other significant causes encompass falls from considerable heights, crush-related traumas, and pedestrian-related injuries. The pathophysiology underlying BTTAI merges various mechanisms, including rapid deceleration, the water-hammer effect leading to heightened intravascular pressure, torsional forces, and shearing forces.

Anatomically, the aortic isthmus, a transition zone between the mobile aortic arch and the more fixed descending thoracic aorta, is the most vulnerable site for BTTAI, followed by other sites

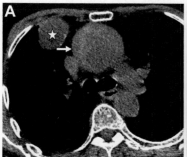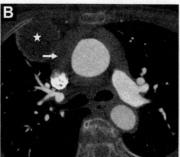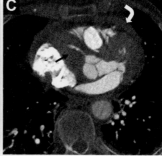

Fig. 8. Axial non-contrast CT (*A*) showing high-attenuation thickening (*white arrow, A*) of the ascending aorta in a patient with acute chest pain. Axial CTA image confirms the thickening (*white arrow, B*) and absence of a discrete true and false lumen consistent with intramural hematoma. Critical findings like extension of the intramural hematoma along the right coronary artery (*black arrow, C*) and hemopericardium (*curved block arrow, C*) are highlighted. Incidentally noted is a thymic mass (*star, A and B*) which was resected at the time of aortic surgery.

at which the aorta is relatively fixed—the aortic root, and near the diaphragmatic hiatus.[4]

Classification of Blunt Traumatic Thoracic Aortic Injury

The most widely used classification system used for grading the severity of BTTAI was developed by Azizzadeh and colleagues in 2009, and since then, it has been endorsed by the Society for Vascular Surgery clinical practice guidelines.[46,47]

- Grade 1: Intimal tear, intimal flap, or both.
- Grade 2: Intramural hematoma
- Grade 3: Aortic wall disruption with pseudo-aneurysm
- Grade 4: Aortic wall disruption with free rupture

Grade 1 and 2 BTTAIs can be managed with either a nonoperative or operative approach. In contrast, the severity of Grade 3 and 4 injuries typically necessitates prompt, definitive management using endovascular repair. The grading of BTTAI is highlighted in **Fig. 9**. Frequently, the term, "minimal aortic injury" is used for sub-centimeter intimo-medial abnormality with no external contour deformity.[4]

Role of Computed Tomography Angiography in Blunt Traumatic Thoracic Aortic Injury

Diagnosis and management

Given the universal availability and rapid acquisition, 98% sensitivity, and nearly 100% specificity for BTTAI, CTA is the preferred imaging modality for BTTAI.[48] The direct signs of BTTAI include active contrast extravasation, contained rupture (traumatic pseudoaneurysm) (**Fig. 10**), intramural thrombus, aortic dissection, and changes in aortic contour (including a sudden change in caliber known as pseudo-coarctation).[4] Minimal aortic injury frequently presents as small intimal tear and intramural hematoma. These injuries tend to resolve spontaneously in the majority of the cases (**Fig. 11**).[4] Indirect signs may include mediastinal or periaortic hematoma, retrocrural hematoma, or a small caliber of the aorta distal to the injury site. Follow-up imaging is recommended for all grades of BTTAI injury to ensure the resolution of underlying pathology or for definitive treatment planning based on the severity of the injury. Since aortic injury is typically associated with high-velocity or high-shear force injury, other traumatic injuries are also frequently present in patients with BTTAI.[4,49]

Aortic Aneurysm

An aneurysm is characterized by permanent localized dilatation of the artery, at least 50% greater than the normal luminal diameter. True aneurysms contain all 3 layers of the vessel wall. Based on morphology, the aneurysm can be fusiform (diffuse circumferential weakening of the aortic wall) and saccular aneurysms (weakening of the partial segment of the circumferential aortic wall). The incidence of thoracic aortic aneurysm (TAA) ranges from 5 to 10 per 100,000 person-years.[50] The principal site of TAA is the aortic root or the ascending aorta (60%), followed by the descending aorta (30%) and the aortic arch (10%). The incidence of abdominal aortic aneurysm (AAA) ranges from 1.3% to 8.9% in men and 1% to 2.2% in women.[51]

The onset and progression of aortic aneurysms are often influenced by a myriad of risk factors, including hypertension, tobacco use, hypercholesterolemia, genetic disorders (Marfan syndrome, Ehlers–Danlos syndrome), and trauma.[52] Aneurysms stemming from the aortic root and ascending aorta are frequently linked to genetic disorders, with fibrillin-1 deficiency being paramount and commonly correlating with the bicuspid aortic valve. In comparison, AAA often emerges as a manifestation of atherosclerosis, distinguished by cystic medial degeneration of the aortic wall.[2]

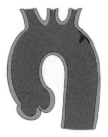 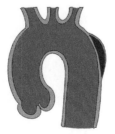 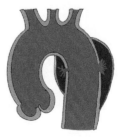 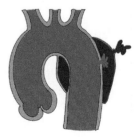

Grade 1	Grade 2	Grade 3	Grade 4
Intimal tear	Intramural hematoma	Aortic pseudoaneurysm	Free rupture

Fig. 9. Illustration highlighting blunt traumatic thoracic aortic injury (BTTAI) classification according to severity from Grade 1 to Grade 4.

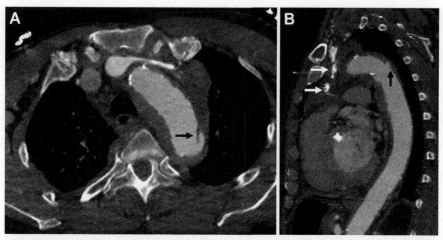

Fig. 10. Axial (*A*) and sagittal (*B*) CT angiography images in a patient with high-speed motor vehicle collision showing aortic intimal tear (*black arrows, A, B*) leading to contained rupture and periaortic hemorrhage. Also note high density contrast in the anterior mediastinum (*white arrow, B*) from left brachiocephalic vein rupture.

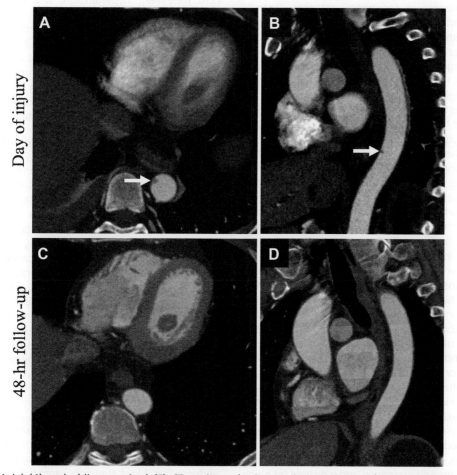

Fig. 11. Axial (*A*) and oblique sagittal (*B*) CT angiography images in a patient with motor vehicle collision showing sub-centimeter intimal irregularity (*white arrow, A, B*) along the distal descending thoracic aorta without any external contour deformity consistent with minimal aorta injury. CTA images (*C, D*) obtained after 48 h showing complete resolution of the minimal aortic injury.

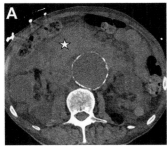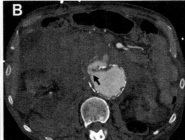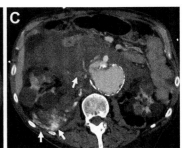

Fig. 12. Non-contrast (*A*), arterial phase (*B*), and delayed phase (*C*) CT angiography images showing hyperdense retroperitoneal hematoma (*star, A*) with disrupted intimal calcification (*black arrow, B*) and pooling of extraluminal contrast in the right periaortic region and posterior to the right kidney (*white arrows, C*) consistent with actively bleeding ruptured aortic aneurysm.

Role of Computed Tomography Angiography in Aortic Aneurysm

Screening and risk stratification

While most patients with TAA or AAA remain asymptomatic, detection often arises from incidental imaging or screening protocols. Specifically, abdominal ultrasound screening for AAA is recommended for those aged 65 to 75 years with either a history of smoking or a family history of AAA (grade 1 recommendation in men and grade 2a recommendation in women). Evidence from single and multi-center studies indicate screening benefits like notable reductions in mortality and AAA-related ruptures.[53,54] Traditionally, ultrasound-based techniques, including transthoracic echocardiography (TTE) and transesophageal echocardiography (TEE), are preferred for screening of aneurysms. However, these modalities sometimes struggle to capture all segments of the aorta in patients with large body habitus or due to normal anatomic structures obscuring the view of the aorta. In such situations, MDCT and MR imaging offer excellent alternatives for comprehensive aortic evaluation.

The most significant complications associated with aortic aneurysms include dissection and rupture. In fact, AAA rupture mortality estimates hover between 80% and 90%, underscoring the urgency of timely intervention.[55] Aortic diameter is an important prognostic indicator of aortic rupture or dissection. Typical CTA findings of AAA rupture include retroperitoneal hemorrhage, disrupted intimal calcium, frank aortic wall discontinuity, extravasated IV contrast, crescent-sign (high attenuation crescent-shaped abnormality associated with aneurysm mural thrombus/aortic wall) (**Fig. 12**), and drape sign (posterior aortic wall lacking a sharp margin and a distinct fat plane with the adjacent vertebral bodies).[56,57] While an aortic diameter of 5.5 cm often prompts elective aneurysm repair, a diverse range of factors must

be incorporated into the risk stratification process. This includes patient-specific factors like gender (women may have higher rupture risk at smaller diameter compared with men) and increasing the aortic diameter (>3 mm/year), aneurysm growth (>10 mm/year), hypertension, and inherited or family history of the aortic disease.[2,7,58] CTA can be used for serial evaluation of aortic diameter, morphology, and the aorta's branch involvement. If aortic sizing is required in a patient with contraindication to iodinated contrast, non-contrast CT or MRA should be considered.[3,59] In the authors' program, MRA is the preferred modality for patients with contraindication to iodinated contrast.

Treatment planning and post-procedure surveillance

CTA can provide important information on the landing zone (proximal and distal), characteristics of the aneurysm sac (tortuosity and angulation), the relationship of the aneurysm sac with surrounding structures (eg, compression), assessment of potential vascular access site (patency and lumen size). Such data streamline the decision-making process regarding intervention techniques (open surgical vs endovascular approach), vascular access points, and stent specifications (material, lumen, and length). As discussed later in this review, the post-endovascular aneurysm repair (EVAR) complication rate is rather high, ranging between 16% and 30%, necessitating lifelong imaging-based surveillance.

Aortitis

Infectious aortitis (mycotic aneurysm)

Infectious aortitis is an uncommon condition, typically caused by septic emboli associated with endocarditis. Most common causative organisms include bacterial causes with fungal causes may be seen in immunocompromised patients. Such infections can lead to an saccular aneurysm

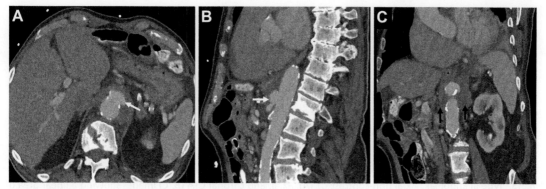

Fig. 13. Axial postcontrast CT axial (*A*), sagittal (*B*), and coronal (*C*) images in a patient with fever and abdominal pain showing a saccular "mushroom-shaped" outpouching (*white arrows–A, B*) with periaortic inflammatory soft-tissue (*black arrow, C*).

resembling a mushroom, hence its particular designation[60],[2] (**Fig. 13**). Like any other aortic aneurysms, CTA can help assess the aneurysm extent and complications including hemorrhage.

Inflammatory Aortitis

It is characterized by accumulation of inflammatory tissues in the tunica adventitia. Thoracic aortitis common causes include Takayasu arteritis and giant cell arteritis.[61] In comparison, abdominal aortitis most common cause is immunoglobulin G4–related diseases.[61] Cross-sectional imaging (CT or MR imaging) can show circumferential thickening of the vascular wall that frequently tends to involve aortic arch or arch vessels. On CT imaging, delayed images (typically obtained at 60 second) are useful to visualize enhancement of the wall thickening (**Fig. 14**). [^{18}F]Fluorodeoxyglucose (^{18}F-FDG) -PET is being increasingly used in patients with inflammatory vasculitis as active disease is associated with an increase metabolic activity.[62],[63] ^{18}F-FDG PET is excellent for follow-up of patients as metabolic activity tends to be a better marker of disease activity, rather than anatomic wall thickening in patients with aortitis.[64]

Post-procedure Monitoring

Aortic aneurysms and acute aortic syndromes are often treated by open surgery or endovascular stent graft repairs. The selected approach often depends on the location of the disease, patient's hemodynamic state, and local expertise. For instance, Type A dissections often require emergent surgical interventions.[65] During endovascular procedures such as endovascular aneurysm repair (EVAR), TEE or intravascular ultrasounds are preferred, given their real-time imaging capabilities, which are indispensable for differentiating

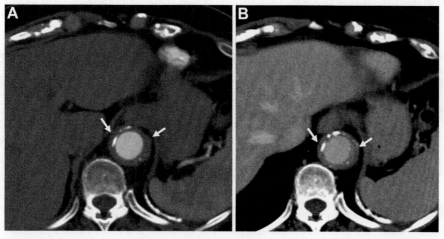

Fig. 14. Axial arterial (*A*) and delayed (*B*) phase CT angiography image in a 68-year-old patient with presumed Giant cell arteritis showing enhancing circumferential thickening of the descending thoracic aorta (*white arrows*).

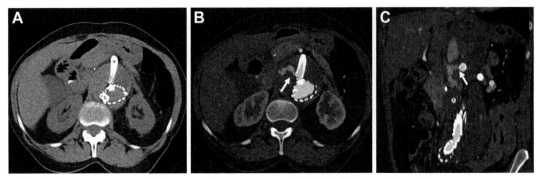

Fig. 15. Type III Endoleak. Axial non-contrast CT (*A*), axial, and coronal CTA (*B, C*) images showing a linear area of contrast enhancement along the right lateral aspect of superior mesenteric artery fenestration (*white arrow, B, C*).

lumens, selecting aorta segments devoid of protruding plaques, monitoring guide wire progress, and ensuring optimal stent graft placement.[37]

The complication rate post-EVAR is quite high, ranging from 16% to 30%, including endoleak (**Fig. 15**), stent migration, stent-graft fracture or collapse, infection (**Fig. 16**), and aneurysmal dilation of other aortic segments.[66] Endoleak is the most common complication post-EVAR, occurring in 15% to 30% of the patients within the first 30 postoperative days. Endoleak is defined as persistent blood flow outside the graft but within the aneurysm sac with contrast opacification change in degree and shape between arterial and delayed phases.[67] If untreated, this can result in continued aneurysm growth and potential rupture. Endoleak are classified into 5 types based on the origin of the blood flow to the excluded aneurysm sac.[68]

Due to the high potential for complications, especially endoleak, patients who have undergone EVAR require lifelong monitoring. This allows early identification of treatment of complications and monitoring of residual disease process. Typically, the aorta is reassessed at intervals of 1, 3, 6, and 12 months post-intervention, followed by annual surveillance check-ups.[1] Prognostic signs signifying unfavorable outcomes encompass elevated false luminal pressures, enduring patent false lumens, and augmented aortic diameter. For instance, a post-acute-phase aortic diameter surpassing 45 mm with a patent false lumen, a descending thoracic aortic diameter beyond 55 mm, or an annual growth exceeding 5 mm signifies a heightened aortic rupture risk, necessitating re-intervention.[14]

CTA is often the preferred modality for post-EVAR surveillance. It is important to remember that postoperative materials and old-calcified thrombus in the excluded portion of the aneurysm sac can often mimic an endoleak on the arterial phase. This underlines the importance of obtaining non-contrast and delayed phase imaging to help differentiate calcifications from contrast leaks. Furthermore, delayed phase imaging can aid in identifying slow-flow endoleaks, which might not be immediately obvious in the standard arterial phase. Some recent studies have shown the superiority of 4D flow-map MRA in detecting endoleaks

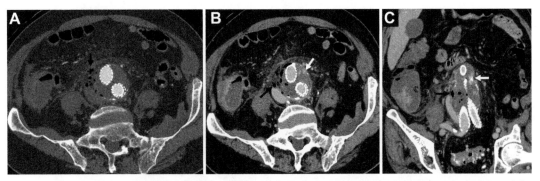

Fig. 16. Axial CTA image (*A*), axial and coronal delayed CT (*B, C*) images in a patient with sepsis showing air locules within the excluded aortic aneurysm sac and peri-aortic retroperitoneum (*black arrows–A–C*) with multiple foci of delayed contrast enhancement in the excluded aneurysm sac (*white arrows–B, C*) consistent with infected aortic graft.

when compared to traditional CTA. One of the distinct advantages of 4D flow MR imaging over CTA is its ability to differentiate between the subtypes of type II endoleaks (type IIa and IIb) based on flow patterns observed in the aortic side branches.[12,37,69] However, CTA remains the standard imaging of choice for most imaging programs given availability and need for advanced expertise for 4D Flow MRA. For most part at the authors' sites, 4D Flow MRA is used as a problem-solving tool if the precise and detailed information may help clinicians plan interventions more accurately. It is also worth noting that while TEE and intravascular ultrasound are excellent tools for surveillance of post-EVAR surveillance, however, their efficacy can be limited when visualizing through certain stent graft materials like polytetrafluoroethylene and Gore-Tex, making it challenging to detect complications like endoleaks.[1]

SUMMARY

CTA has an integral role in aortic imaging, offering a rapid, high-resolution assessment of various pathologies. Its versatility, from diagnosis to treatment planning and surveillance, is evident in conditions like acute aortic syndrome, dissection, and aneurysm, among others. With further advancements, including ECG-gated sequences, dual-energy CT, and various postprocessing techniques, CTA has become the reference standard in the management of aortic pathologies by providing excellent diagnostic accuracy while reducing the dose of radiation and contrast media.

ACKNOWLEDGMENTS

None.

DISCLOSURE

The other authors declare no conflict of interest related to this work.

REFERENCES

1. Goldstein SA, Evangelista A, Abbara S, et al. Multimodality imaging of diseases of the thoracic aorta in adults: from the American Society of Echocardiography and the European Association of Cardiovascular Imaging: endorsed by the Society of Cardiovascular Computed Tomography and Society for Cardiovascular Magnetic Resonance. J Am Soc Echocardiogr 2015;28(2):119–82.
2. Members WC, Isselbacher EM, Preventza O, et al. 2022 ACC/AHA Guideline for the diagnosis and management of aortic disease: a report of the American heart association/american college of cardiology joint committee on clinical practice guidelines. J Am Coll Cardiol 2022;80(24):e223–393.
3. Nagpal P, Grist TM. MR angiography: contrast-enhanced acquisition techniques. Magn Reson Imag Clin N Am 2023;31(3):493–501. https://doi.org/10.1016/j.mric.2023.04.007.
4. Nagpal P, Mullan BF, Sen I, et al. Advances in imaging and management trends of traumatic aortic injuries. CVIR (Cardiovasc Interventional Radiol) 2017;40:643–54.
5. McClure RS, Brogly SB, Lajkosz K, et al. Epidemiology and management of thoracic aortic dissections and thoracic aortic aneurysms in Ontario, Canada: A population-based study. J Thorac Cardiovasc Surg 2018;155(6):2254–64. https://doi.org/10.1016/j.jtcvs.2017.11.105.
6. DeMartino RR, Sen I, Huang Y, et al. Population-based assessment of the incidence of aortic dissection, intramural hematoma, and penetrating ulcer, and its associated mortality from 1995 to 2015. Circ Cardiovasc Qual Outcomes 2018;11(8):e004689. https://doi.org/10.1161/CIRCOUTCOMES.118.004689.
7. Nagpal P, Khandelwal A, Saboo SS, et al. Modern imaging techniques: applications in the management of acute aortic pathologies. Postgrad Med 2015;91(1078):449–62.
8. Berko NS, Jain VR, Godelman A, et al. Variants and anomalies of thoracic vasculature on computed tomographic angiography in adults. J Comput Assist Tomogr 2009;33(4):523–8.
9. Ann JH, Kim EY, Jeong YM, et al. Morphologic evaluation of ductus diverticulum using multi-detector computed tomography: comparison with traumatic pseudoaneurysm of the aortic isthmus. Iran J Radiol 2016;13(4).
10. Lu T-LC, Huber CH, Rizzo E, et al. Ascending aorta measurements as assessed by ECG-gated multidetector computed tomography: a pilot study to establish normative values for transcatheter therapies. Eur Radiol 2009;19:664–9.
11. Davenport MS, Perazella MA, Yee J, et al. Use of intravenous iodinated contrast media in patients with kidney disease: consensus statements from the American College of Radiology and the National Kidney Foundation. Radiology 2020;294(3):660–8.
12. Garg I, Grist TM, Nagpal P. MR angiography for aortic diseases. Magn Reson Imag Clin N Am 2023;31(3):373–94. https://doi.org/10.1016/j.mric.2023.05.002.
13. Saadi EK. Multidetector computed tomography scanning is still the gold standard for diagnosis of acute aortic syndromes. Interact Cardiovasc Thorac Surg 2010;11(3):359.
14. Erbel R, Aboyans V, Boileau C, et al. 2014 ESC guidelines on the diagnosis and treatment of aortic diseases. Kardiol Pol 2014;72(12):1169–252.

15. Roos JE, Willmann JrK, Weishaupt D, et al. Thoracic aorta: motion artifact reduction with retrospective and prospective electrocardiography-assisted multi–detector row CT. Radiology 2002;222(1):271–7.

16. Fleischmann D, Chin AS, Molvin L, et al. Computed tomography angiography: a review and technical update. Radiol Clin 2016;54(1):1–12.

17. Vernhet H, Serfaty JM, Serhal M, et al. Abdominal CT angiography before surgery as a predictor of post-operative death in acute aortic dissection. Am J Roentgenol 2004;182(4):875–9.

18. Konen E, Goitein O, Feinberg MS, et al. The role of ECG-gated MDCT in the evaluation of aortic and mitral mechanical valves: initial experience. Am J Roentgenol 2008;191(1):26–31.

19. Wu W, Budovec J, Foley WD. Prospective and retro-spective ECG gating for thoracic CT angiography: a comparative study. Am J Roentgenol 2009;193(4):955–63.

20. Nagpal P, Agrawal MD, Saboo SS, et al. Imaging of the aortic root on high-pitch non-gated and ECG-gated CT: awareness is the key. Insights Imaging 2020;11(1):51. https://doi.org/10.1186/s13244-020-00855-w.

21. Vilacosta I, San Román JA. Acute aortic syndrome. BMJ Publishing Group Ltd and British Cardiovascu-lar Society; 2001. p. 365–8.

22. Moore AG, Eagle KA, Bruckman D, et al. Choice of computed tomography, transesophageal echocardi-ography, magnetic resonance imaging, and aortog-raphy in acute aortic dissection: International Registry of Acute Aortic Dissection (IRAD). Am J Cardiol 2002;89(10):1235–8.

23. Chen C-W, Tseng Y-H, Lin C-C, et al. Aortic dissec-tion assessment by 4D phase-contrast MRI with he-modynamic parameters: The impact of stent type. Quant Imag Med Surg 2021;11(2):490.

24. Ramanath VS, Oh JK, Sundt TM III, et al. Acute aortic syndromes and thoracic aortic aneurysm. Elsevier; 2009. p. 465–81.

25. Shiga T, Wajima Zi, Apfel CC, et al. Diagnostic accu-racy of transesophageal echocardiography, helical computed tomography, and magnetic resonance imaging for suspected thoracic aortic dissection: systematic review and meta-analysis. Arch Intern Med 2006;166(13):1350–6.

26. Meszaros I, Morocz J, Szlavi J, et al. Epidemiology and clinicopathology of aortic dissection. Chest 2000;117(5):1271–8.

27. Clouse WD, Hallett JW, Schaff HV, et al. Acute aortic dissection: population-based incidence compared with degenerative aortic aneurysm rupture. Elsevier; 2004. p. 176–80.

28. Nienaber CA, Eagle KA. Aortic dissection: new fron-tiers in diagnosis and management: Part I: from eti-ology to diagnostic strategies. Circulation 2003;108(5):628–35.

29. Movsowitz HD, Levine RA, Hilgenberg AD, et al. Transesophageal echocardiographic description of the mechanisms of aortic regurgitation in acute type A aortic dissection: implications for aortic valve repair. J Am Coll Cardiol 2000;36(3):884–90.

30. La Canna G, Maisano F, De Michele L, et al. Deter-minants of the degree of functional aortic regurgita-tion in patients with anatomically normal aortic valve and ascending thoracic aorta aneurysm. Transoeso-phageal Doppler echocardiography study. Heart 2009;95(2):130–6.

31. LePage MA, Quint LE, Sonnad SS, et al. Aortic dissection: CT features that distinguish true lumen from false lumen. Am J Roentgenol 2001;177(1):207–11.

32. Williams DM, Joshi A, Dake MD, et al. Aortic cob-webs: an anatomic marker identifying the false lumen in aortic dissection–imaging and pathologic correlation. Radiology 1994;190(1):167–74.

33. Weiss G, Wolner I, Folkmann S, et al. The location of the primary entry tear in acute type B aortic dissec-tion affects early outcome. Eur J Cardio Thorac Surg 2012;42(3):571–6.

34. Erbel R, Alfonso F, Boileau C, et al. Diagnosis and management of aortic dissection: task force on aortic dissection, European society of cardiology. Eur Heart J 2001;22(18):1642–81.

35. Eggebrecht H, Plicht B, Kahlert P, et al. Intramural hematoma and penetrating ulcers: indications to en-dovascular treatment. Eur J Vasc Endovasc Surg 2009;38(6):659–65.

36. Kpodonu J, Ramaiah VG, Diethrich EB. Intravas-cular ultrasound imaging as applied to the aorta: a new tool for the cardiovascular surgeon. Ann Thorac Surg 2008;86(4):1391–8.

37. Rocchi G, Lofiego C, Biagini E, et al. Transesopha-geal echocardiography–guided algorithm for stent-graft implantation in aortic dissection. J Vasc Surg 2004;40(5):880–5.

38. Gutschow SE, Walker CM, Martinez-Jimenez S, et al. Emerging Concepts in Intramural Hematoma Imag-ing. Radiographics 2016;36(3):660–74. https://doi.org/10.1148/rg.2016150094.

39. Park KH, Lim C, Choi JH, et al. Prevalence of aortic intimal defect in surgically treated acute type A intra-mural hematoma. Ann Thorac Surg 2008;86(5):1494–500. https://doi.org/10.1016/j.athoracsur.2008.06.061.

40. Kitai T, Kaji S, Yamamuro A, et al. Detection of intimal defect by 64-row multidetector computed tomogra-phy in patients with acute aortic intramural hematoma. Circulation 2011;124(11 Suppl):S174–8. https://doi.org/10.1161/CIRCULATIONAHA.111.037416.

41. Harris KM, Braverman AC, Eagle KA, et al. Acute aortic intramural hematoma: an analysis from the International Registry of Acute Aortic Dissection. Cir-culation 2012;126(11_suppl_1):S91–6.

42. Chou AS, Ziganshin BA, Charilaou P, et al. Long-term behavior of aortic intramural hematomas and penetrating ulcers. J Thorac Cardiovasc Surg 2016;151(2):361–73. e1.

43. Tolenaar JL, Harris KM, Upchurch GR Jr, et al. The differences and similarities between intramural hematoma of the descending aorta and acute type B dissection. J Vasc Surg 2013;58(6):1498–504.

44. Fox N, Schwartz D, Salazar JH, et al. Evaluation and management of blunt traumatic aortic injury. J Trauma Nurs 2015;22(2):99–110.

45. Neschis DG, Scalea TM, Flinn WR, et al. Blunt aortic injury. N Engl J Med 2008;359(16):1708–16.

46. Azizzadeh A, Keyhani K, Miller CC III, et al. Blunt traumatic aortic injury: initial experience with endovascular repair. J Vasc Surg 2009;49(6):1403–8.

47. Lee WA, Matsumura JS, Mitchell RS, et al. Endovascular repair of traumatic thoracic aortic injury: clinical practice guidelines of the Society for Vascular Surgery. J Vasc Surg 2011;53(1):187–92.

48. Steenburg SD, Ravenel JG, Ikonomidis JS, et al. Acute traumatic aortic injury: imaging evaluation and management. Radiology 2008;248(3):748–62.

49. Nagpal P, Saboo SS, Khandelwal A, et al. Traumatic right atrial pseudoaneurysm. Cardiovasc Diagn Ther 2015;5(2):141–4. https://doi.org/10.3978/j.issn.2223-3652.2015.01.04.

50. Sampson UK, Norman PE, Fowkes FGR, et al. Global and regional burden of aortic dissection and aneurysms: mortality trends in 21 world regions, 1990 to 2010. Global Heart 2014;9(1):171–80.e10.

51. Mathur A, Mohan V, Ameta D, et al. Aortic aneurysm. Journal of Translational Internal Medicine 2016;4(1):35–41.

52. Singh K, Bønaa K, Jacobsen B, et al. Prevalence of and risk factors for abdominal aortic aneurysms in a population-based study: The Tromsø Study. Am J Epidemiol 2001;154(3):236–44.

53. Thompson SG, Ashton HA, Gao L, et al. Final follow-up of the Multicentre Aneurysm Screening Study (MASS) randomized trial of abdominal aortic aneurysm screening. Br J Surg 2012;99(12):1649–56. https://doi.org/10.1002/bjs.8897.

54. Mansoor SM, Rabben T, Hisdal J, et al. Eleven-year outcomes of a screening project for abdominal aortic aneurysm (AAA) in 65-year-old men. Vasc Health Risk Manag 2023;19:459–67. https://doi.org/10.2147/VHRM.S412954.

55. Hoornweg L, Storm-Versloot M, Ubbink D, et al. Meta analysis on mortality of ruptured abdominal aortic aneurysms. Eur J Vasc Endovasc Surg 2008;35(5):558–70.

56. Halliday KE, Al-Kutoubi A. Draped aorta: CT sign of contained leak of aortic aneurysms. Radiology 1996;199(1):41–3.

57. Arita T, Matsunaga N, Takano K, et al. Abdominal aortic aneurysm: rupture associated with the high-attenuating crescent sign. Radiology 1997;204(3):765–8.

58. Forbes TL, Lawlor DK, DeRose G, et al. Gender differences in relative dilatation of abdominal aortic aneurysms. Ann Vasc Surg 2006;20(5):564–8.

59. Kuo AH, Nagpal P, Ghoshhajra BB, et al. Vascular magnetic resonance angiography techniques. Cardiovasc Diagn Ther 2019;9(Suppl 1):S28–36. https://doi.org/10.21037/cdt.2019.06.07.

60. Sakalihasan N, Michel J-B, Katsargyris A, et al. Abdominal aortic aneurysms. Nat Rev Dis Prim 2018;4(1):34.

61. Svensson LG, Arafat A, Roselli EE, et al. Inflammatory disease of the aorta: patterns and classification of giant cell aortitis, Takayasu arteritis, and nonsyndromic aortitis. J Thorac Cardiovasc Surg 2015;149(2):S170–5.

62. Blockmans D, Stroobants S, Maes A, et al. Positron emission tomography in giant cell arteritis and polymyalgia rheumatica: evidence for inflammation of the aortic arch. Am J Med 2000;108(3):246–9.

63. Lariviere D, Benali K, Coustet B, et al. Positron emission tomography and computed tomography angiography for the diagnosis of giant cell arteritis: a real-life prospective study. Medicine 2016;95(30).

64. Veeranna V, Fisher A, Nagpal P, et al. Utility of multimodality imaging in diagnosis and follow-up of aortitis. J Nucl Cardiol 2016;23(3):590–5. https://doi.org/10.1007/s12350-015-0219-z.

65. Zindovic I, Sjögren J, Bjursten H, et al. Impact of hemodynamic instability and organ malperfusion in elderly surgical patients treated for acute type A aortic dissection. J Card Surg 2015;30(11):822–9.

66. d'Audiffret A, Desgranges P, Kobeiter DH, et al. Follow-up evaluation of endoluminally treated abdominal aortic aneurysms with duplex ultrasonography: validation with computed tomography. J Vasc Surg 2001;33(1):42–50.

67. Rand T, Uberoi R, Cil B, et al. Quality improvement guidelines for imaging detection and treatment of endoleaks following endovascular aneurysm repair (EVAR). CVIR (Cardiovasc Interventional Radiol) 2013;36:35–45.

68. Bryce Y, Rogoff P, Romanelli D, et al. Endovascular repair of abdominal aortic aneurysms: vascular anatomy, device selection, procedure, and procedure-specific complications. Radiographics 2015;35(2):593–615.

69. Koschyk DH, Nienaber CA, Knap M, et al. How to guide stent-graft implantation in type B aortic dissection? Comparison of angiography, transesophageal echocardiography, and intravascular ultrasound. Circulation 2005;112(9_supplement):I260–4.

Computed Tomography Angiography After Transcatheter and Surgical Aortic Interventions

Ayaz Aghayev, MD*, Sumit Gupta, MD, PhD, Michael Steigner, MD

KEYWORDS

• Computed tomography angiography • Surgical aortic open repair • Endovascular aortic repair

KEY POINTS

- Computed tomography angiography (CTA) plays a crucial role in assessing and monitoring the status of the postsurgical or endovascular repaired aorta.
- To ensure a comprehensive imaging assessment of the postprocedural aorta, it is essential for the diagnostic radiologist to possess a solid understanding of prevalent surgical, endovascular, and hybrid repair techniques, along with their anticipated postprocedural manifestations.
- The postprocedural aorta is susceptible to many potential complications, the detection of which relies on imaging. The nature of these complications varies according to the specific procedure undertaken.

INTRODUCTION

Presently, a diverse array of techniques are employed for aortic repair, encompassing classical surgical approaches and endovascular procedures for thoracic/abdominal aortic repair (thoracic endovascular aortic repair/endovascular aortic repair [TEVAR/EVAR]), as well as hybrid methodologies that combine elements of both. As an integral component of routine follow-up care, patients who have undergone any of these procedures necessitate assessment through computed tomography angiography (CTA) to preemptively address potential short-term and long-term complications.

Irrespective of whether the patient underwent surgical, endovascular, or hybrid aortic repair, the complexity inherent in these procedures can render their cases challenging. Therefore, it becomes imperative for the radiologist to possess a comprehensive understanding of the techniques employed and the subsequent postprocedural manifestations. This familiarity empowers them to identify any unforeseen findings or complications that might arise.

In this review article, we will cover the technical aspects of CTA acquisition, the prevalent surgical and EVAR techniques, the expected postprocedural findings, and finally, the potential complications that may manifest after the procedures.

COMPUTED TOMOGRAPHY ANGIOGRAPHY ACQUISITION

CTA is the foremost utilized imaging modality for monitoring postprocedural aortic conditions, irrespective of the procedural nature. Establishing departmental protocols becomes imperative to ensure uniformity in patient assessment, thereby facilitating the prompt identification of potential complications. Numerous parameters are amenable to standardization, with a subset of these parameters elucidated in **Table 1** for reference. The

Department of Radiology, Cardiovascular Imaging Program, Brigham and Women's Hospital, Harvard Medical School, Boston, MA 02115, USA
* Corresponding author.
E-mail address: aaghayev@bwh.harvard.edu

Radiol Clin N Am 62 (2024) 527–542
https://doi.org/10.1016/j.rcl.2024.02.002

Table 1
Multidetector computed tomographic angiography

Type of Scan	Non-gated CTA	ECG-Gated CTA
Slice thickness	Thinnest available, ideally 0.5–0.625	
Tube potential (kV)	100–120	
Collimation	64 × 0.625	
Pitch	0.8–1	
Rotation time (s)	Minimum	
Field of view (mm)	210–260	
Matrix	512 × 512	
Nonionic iodinated contrast material (mL)	120 (plus saline chaser)	
Multiphase injection protocol	Yes	
Injection rate (mL/s)	4–6 (18–20 G preferably in right arm)	
Region of interest	Chest/Chest and abdomen: Proximal descending thoracic aorta (bolus triggering) Abdomen: Distal descending thoracic aorta/proximal abdominal aorta (bolus triggering)	
Length of the scan	Thoracoabdominal aorta: Lung apices to the groin Thoracic aorta: Lung apices to upper abdomen Abdominal aorta: Lung bases to the groin	

objectives of creating a protocol are achieving adequate and homogeneous blood pool enhancement, minimizing aortic motion, administering the least amount of radiation (while maintaining diagnostic image quality), and injecting a standard amount of intravenous contrast material.

The core CTA protocol demonstrates variations influenced by institutional preferences, but it typically consists of 3 phases for patients undergoing open surgical graft repairs: (1) precontrast phase, (2) arterial phase, and (3) delayed phase. The precontrast phase is significant in evaluating hyperdense surgical materials that can resemble pseudoaneurysms or leaks. For individuals who have undergone aortic aneurysm repair with stent grafts, the delayed phase is added to evaluate the presence of endoleaks.

PROCEDURES OF THE AORTIC ROOT, ASCENDING AORTA, AND AORTIC ARCH

Aortic root and ascending aortic repairs commonly require an open surgical approach. However, when dealing with the aortic arch or proximal descending aorta, the repair becomes more complex, often necessitating a hybrid approach combining open and endovascular procedures. Moreover, a concept of zonal anatomy has emerged, classifying the aorta into 11 distinct zones. Notably, the aortic root and ascending aorta are designated as Zone 0. Moving on, Zone 1 encompasses the origin of the left common

carotid artery, while Zone 2 covers the origin of the left subclavian artery. Extending the delineation, Zone 3 spans from the distal aspect of the left subclavian artery through the initial 2 cm of the descending aorta, with Zone 4 continuing distally. Further comprehensive insight regarding zonal anatomy can be accessed through the recent guidelines published by the Society of Vascular Surgery.[1]

Table 2 serves as a comprehensive resource detailing various open surgical techniques that encompass the aortic root, ascending aorta, and aortic arch, including hybrid approaches.

In brief, for the ascending aorta, classification can be divided into *valve-sparing techniques*, which include

1. *Supracoronary graft repair*: This approach involves replacing the ascending aorta with a graft.
2. *Yacoub technique*: Although an older method, it can still be encountered. It entails creating larger/bulbous neo-sinuses of Valsalva and reimplanting coronary arteries.[2]
3. *David I and Demers-Miller (Stanford modification) techniques*: These techniques bear similarities. In David I, a single total graft is used with coronary artery reimplantation. In the Demers-Miller technique, 2 grafts are utilized—a tubular one for the ascending segment and a slightly larger one for the sinuses of Valsalva.[3]

Table 2
Open surgical techniques

Aortic Root/Ascending Aorta		Aortic Arch and Distal Repair
Valve-sparing technique	*Valve-repair technique*	
1. Supracoronary graft repair	1. Wheat procedure	1. Hemiarch repair
2. Yacoub technique	2. Bentall procedure	2. "Island Patch" technique
3. David I and Demers Miller technique	3. Modified Bentall procedure	3. Debranching technique
	4. Cabrol technique	4. Four-branched aortic graft technique
	5. Ross procedure	5. Chimney/Snorkel technique
		6. Elephant trunk technique

Procedures that incorporate *valve repair alongside ascending aortic repair* include

1. *Wheat procedure*: This combines valve replacement with a supracoronary graft while preserving the sinuses of Valsalva.[4]
2. *Bentall procedure*: A comprehensive replacement of the aortic valve, root, and ascending aorta is performed, coupled with coronary reimplantation. In this technique, coronary reimplantation takes the form of end-to-end anastomosis.[5] When the graft comprises both a valvular prosthesis and an ascending aortic graft, it is termed a *composite graft.*
3. *Modified Bentall procedure*: The entire technique is similar to the "Bentall procedure"; however, the coronary arteries are attached using a Carrel patch to prevent kinking, resulting in a trumpet-like appearance of the coronary ostia, referred to as the *coronary button.*[6]
4. *Cabrol technique*: This technique is employed when the proximal coronary arteries or aorta are unsuitable for direct anastomosis due to atherosclerosis or damage from dissection.[7] A conduit (graft or transposed vessel) from the graft is anastomosed at a relatively distal aspect of the coronary arteries. Typically, the conduit is anastomosed at the anterior aspect of the aorta with a retroaortic course, extending toward the left coronary artery.
5. *Ross procedure*: An infrequent technique employed in younger patients involves utilizing the native pulmonary valve and pulmonary artery as a homograft for the aorta.[8]

Procedures involving the *aortic arch and distally* (beyond zone 1) include

1. *Hemiarch repair*: In selected cases, the graft placed into Zone 0 can be extended to the lesser curvature of the aortic arch, which is known as the hemiarch technique.[9]

2. *"Island Patch" technique*: This technique encompasses extracting aortic branch vessels and a section of nearby native aortic tissue as a single unit, followed by their reattachment to an elliptical aperture within a surgically implanted open graft.
3. *Debranching technique*: In the debranching technique, the arch vessels are isolated and linked to tubular grafts of matching size.[10] Subsequently, these grafts are connected to either the graft on the ascending aorta or the native aorta. Three distinct debranching techniques are available. *Type I*—In this approach, the endovascular graft is positioned to land in Zone 0, spanning across the aortic arch. Debranched arch vessels are connected to the native aorta within Zone 0, utilizing a single tubular graft. Importantly, this technique eliminates the need for cardiopulmonary bypass. *Type II*—In this approach, debranched arch vessels are affixed to a repaired open graft within Zone 0, using a single tubular graft. The endovascular graft is positioned to land in Zone 0. *Type III*—In this variation, debranched arch vessels are connected to an open graft using a single tubular graft. Unlike Type II, the open graft may encompass Zones 1, 2, and 3 (the "elephant trunk" procedure). The endovascular graft resides within the open graft.
4. *Four-branched aortic graft technique*: In this technique, a prefabricated graft is utilized that has a separate origin/graft for each arch vessel, and the fourth branch at the level of the ascending aorta is used for cardiopulmonary bypass.[11]
5. *Chimney or Snorkel technique*: Within this approach, the stent grafts stemming from the arch vessel elongate toward the aortic arch. As the aortic stent graft is deployed along the aortic arch, these extensions align in a parallel fashion.[12]

6. *Elephant trunk technique*: This 2 stage open repair technique is employed for extensive thoracic aortic repairs.[13] In the initial Stage I, the procedure includes the open repair of the ascending aorta and aortic arch using an elephant trunk graft. Typically, during this initial stage, the graft extends to the unrepaired descending aorta, which remains suspended within the lumen. Traditionally, in the subsequent Stage II, the patient undergoes another open repair targeting the remaining aortic portion. Nevertheless, a recent development involves the option of endovascular repair for the remaining aortic segments, which can be carried out either during the initial stage or as a standalone procedure.

Expected Postsurgical Imaging Findings

Distinguishing synthetic polyester (such as Dacron) surgical grafts from the native aortic wall can be challenging in postcontrast images. However, their hyperattenuating density compared to the native aorta on noncontrast computed tomographic (CT) images makes differentiation more feasible (**Fig. 1**). In the inclusion technique, where the aortic wall envelops the graft, calcification of the native aortic wall may overlay the graft. Due to an escalated risk of pseudoaneurysm formation, the inclusion technique has been largely supplanted by interposition grafts.[14] Interposition grafts manifest smooth margins and a direct alignment with the native aorta, sometimes mimicking dissection flaps due to their folding nature[15] (**Fig. 2**). Moreover, since they constitute tubular structures, conventional anatomical landmarks of the aortic root, like the bulbous appearance of the sinuses of Valsalva, are absent in imaging. At anastomotic sites, reinforcement materials such as *felt rings* bolster weak points between grafts and the native aorta. Recognition of these materials in imaging aids in demarcating the extent of aortic grafts, apparent as hyperattenuating rings on both noncontrast and postcontrast CT scans (**Fig. 3**).[16] *Felt pledgets*, another reinforcement material integral to surgical procedures, predominantly serve to strengthen vascular access points within the aortic wall or other cardiac structures. Much like felt rings, these present hyperdense structures (but are noncircumferential) on CT scans, mirroring the appearance of pseudoaneurysms. Hence, comparing these findings with noncontrast images emerges as crucial for the accurate identification of these surgical components (**Fig. 4**). Similarly, *surgical sutures*, frequently used reinforcement materials, manifest as linear hyperdensities on noncontrast scans. Alternatively, automated sutures like the Cor-Knot find use in aortic root/annulus repairs, which have metallic components, making them relatively straightforward to distinguish on imaging.

In addition to the aortic graft and related materials, synthetic vascular grafts are also employed in aortic arch vessel repair. For instance, during arch repair with the stent graft, the left subclavian artery can be excluded with embolization, necessitating the use of left carotid-subclavian grafts to maintain blood flow to the left extremity. These grafts resemble aortic grafts and reinforcement materials on CTA images, albeit smaller in size. Lastly, short-side grafts often accompany cardiopulmonary bypass cannulation, attaching either to the aorta/graft or to the axillary artery. Postcontrast CT images display localized outpouching of these short-side grafts, mimicking pseudoaneurysms or aneurysms. However, the presence of

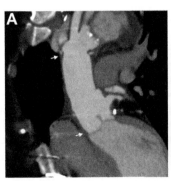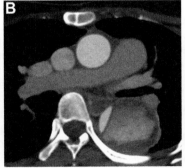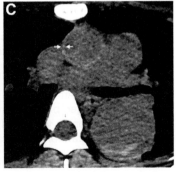

Fig. 1. A 24 year old woman with a medical history including Marfan syndrome, type A dissection, and a valve-sparing aortic root/ascending aorta repair with coronary artery reimplantation using the David I technique. An ECG-gated coronal image (*A*) from postcontrast CTA highlights the extension of the graft (*arrows*) from the valves to the arch of the aorta. Subsequently, on an axial postcontrast CTA image (*B*), the distinction between the aortic wall and the graft within the ascending aorta becomes challenging. Notably, the precontrast CTA image (*C*) reveals a hyperdense rim (*arrows*) exhibited by the graft in contrast to the native aortic wall.

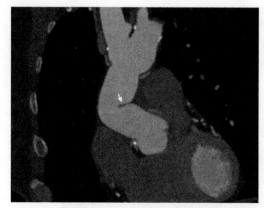

Fig. 2. A 62 year old man with an ascending aortic aneurysm underwent valve-sparing supracoronary graft repair. A coronal image from postcontrast CTA reveals a kink (*arrow*) in the graft that bears a resemblance to a dissection flap.

felt pledgets and the hyperdense rim of grafts on noncontrast images aids in distinguishing between these entities (**Fig. 5**).

Within the context of the elephant trunk technique, when solely the initial Stage I is executed, the suspended graft within the descending aorta can resemble a dissection flap. Thus, it is crucial to cross-reference with noncontrast CT scans to distinguish the distinct hyperdense border of the graft within the lumen.

Endovascular stent-graft frameworks are crafted from nitinol, imparting distinct visibility on CT scans due to their hyperattenuating struts.

Complications

Differentiating between expected postoperative imaging findings and complications becomes particularly challenging after complex surgeries.

Open Repair Complications

Hematoma and fluid collection
Following surgery, particularly in the weeks immediately following the procedure, a hematoma at the surgical site or within the pericardium, along with the presence of air or gas bubbles, is expected.[17] Over time, these accumulations of material and air

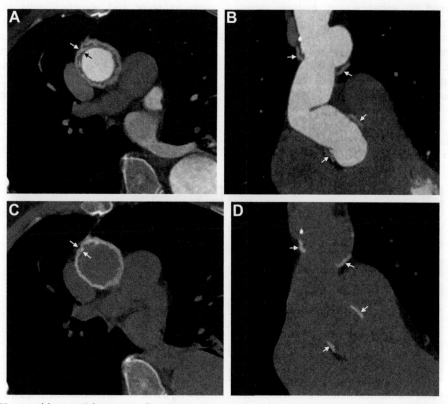

Fig. 3. A 62 year old man with an ascending aortic aneurysm, a valve-sparing supracoronary graft repair was performed. Postcontrast CTA axial and coronal images (*A, B*) reveal a circumferential hyperdensity (*arrows*) that could be misconstrued as contrast extravasation. However, the precontrast images (*C, D*) confirm the presence of the hyperdense ring (*arrows*), and any complications related to contrast extravasation/dehiscence are ruled out.

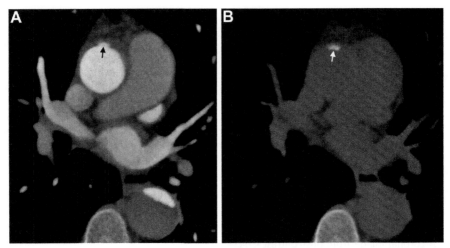

Fig. 4. A 51 year old man diagnosed with a type A dissection, a valve-sparing supracoronary graft, and hemiarch repair were performed. An axial postcontrast CTA image (*A*) displays a hyperdense structure (*arrows*) with a density similar to the contrast/iodine, creating an appearance reminiscent of a focal outpouching or pseudoaneurysm. Nonetheless, upon reviewing the axial precontrast image (*B*), the hyperdensity (*arrow*) aligns with a felt pledget positioned at the bypass cannulation site, establishing consistency in its appearance.

tend to naturally dissipate, giving way to the development of dense perigraft soft tissue thickening accompanied by enhancement. Notably, there may be a slight uptick in the collection's volume after removing surgical drains. However, developing a new collection or hematoma after the complete resolution of the initial postsurgical collection is deemed atypical and could indicate graft anastomosis failure.[18]

Infection
The appearance of new fluid accumulation or an escalation in soft tissue thickness surrounding the aortic/vascular graft can indicate an infection, particularly when correlated with clinical indicators such as fever and elevated white blood cell count.[19] In more advanced instances, air pockets within the fluid collection may become apparent due to gas-forming pathogens. Yet, distinguishing between evolving postsurgical changes and infection can be challenging on CTA scans. To delve deeper into characterization, supplementary imaging, specifically fluorodeoxyglucose positron emission tomography/computed tomography angiography (FDG-PET/CTA), can be undertaken (Fig. 6). It is important to note that the FDG-PET/

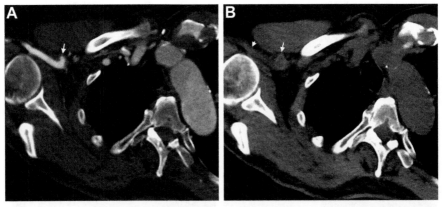

Fig. 5. A 64 year old man underwent a Wheat procedure involving aortic valve replacement and supracoronary graft repair to address a thoracic aortic aneurysm. An axial postcontrast CTA image (*A*) reveals a localized outpouching (*arrow*) in the right axillary artery. Initially suggestive of a potential pseudoaneurysm, this finding prompts caution. However, upon reviewing the pre-contrast CT image (*B*), the hyperdense border (*arrow*) around the outpouching confirms the presence of the graft from the cardiopulmonary bypass procedure rather than any alarming complications. The density can be compared to the normal axillary artery wall (*arrowhead*).

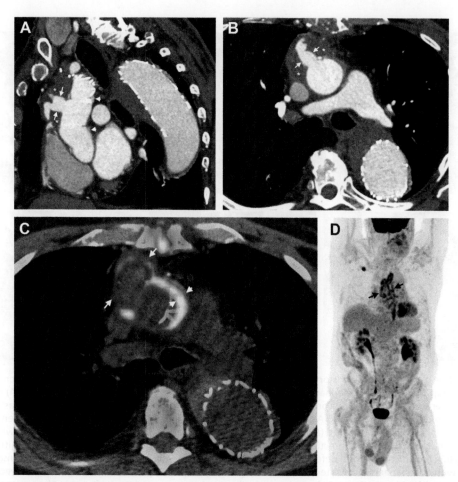

Fig. 6. A 75 year old man with a history of a remote ascending aortic aneurysm repair had type B dissection. The patient underwent a redo sternotomy, during which a type III debranching technique was employed to repair the ascending aorta, coupled with stent-graft repair for the aortic arch and descending aorta. He presented recently with recent fever, malaise, and elevated white blood cell counts. Parasagittal (*A*) and axial (*B*) postcontrast CTA images of the thoracic aorta reveal the presence of a single tubular graft (*arrows*) affixed to the ascending aortic graft (*arrowheads*). Notably, a fluid collection surrounding the debranching graft (*asterisk*) is observed in these images. Although a somewhat nonspecific finding, the clinical context suggests the possibility of an infected graft as a prominent consideration. An axial FDG-PET/CT image (*C*) depicting the graft area displays discernible FDG uptake of moderate intensity encompassing the collection (*arrows*). This uptake pattern signifies the presence of infection or an abscess. It is important to note that a moderate level of FDG uptake within the graft (*arrowheads*) aligns with expected findings on FDG-PET/CT. The maximum intensity projection image (*D*) derived from FDG-PET/CT illustrates uptake within the mediastinum surrounding the graft collection (*arrows*). This effectively eliminates alternative sources or infections as potential culprits responsible for the patient's symptoms.

CTA conducted within the initial 3 months after surgery may yield potential false-positive results.

Pseudoaneurysm

A pseudoaneurysm is a contrast-filled cavity that extends beyond the expected confines of an artery. This phenomenon arises due to a partial or complete rupture of the arterial wall while maintaining a persistent connection to the bloodstream. In this context, a pseudoaneurysm is described as an extravascular accumulation of blood or contrast material, frequently observed at locations such as the anastomosis site, cannulation site, or prosthetic valve anastomosis within the left ventricular outflow tract.[19] The precise incidence of anastomotic pseudoaneurysms remains undetermined.[20] Within aortic grafts, infection is the leading cause of pseudoaneurysm formation. Pseudoaneurysms at the anastomosis are associated with graft dehiscence. In certain cases, these 2 conditions can occur simultaneously (**Fig. 7**). As reiterated throughout the article, it is essential to establish a

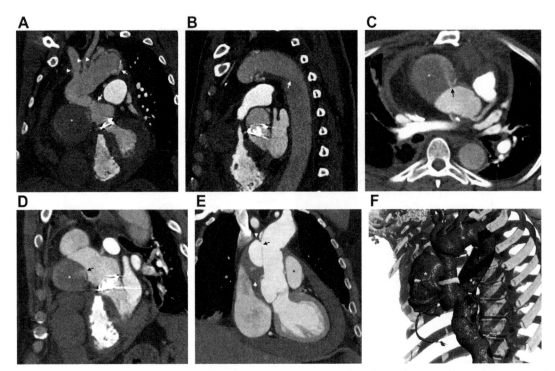

Fig. 7. A 50 year old man with a history of type A dissection underwent mechanical aortic valve replacement and open graft repair utilizing the elephant trunk technique. The postcontrast CTA parasagittal image (*A*) portrays the graft extending from the supracoronary level to the proximal descending aorta (*arrows*), with anastomosed supra-aortic branches (*arrowheads*). A large hypodense region is evident within the proximal segment of the graft (*asterisk*). A parasagittal view (*B*) through the descending aorta shows the suspended graft within the lumen, which could resemble a dissection flap. Further insights are gleaned from the axial and parasagittal views in images (*C, D*), depicting a focal defect (*arrows*) at the proximal anastomosis, which fills the hypodense region (*asterisk*) with contrast and is consistent with a pseudoaneurysm. Notably, parallel findings are observed in a 46 year old man with a history of type A dissection and valve-sparing supracoronary graft repair. The coronal view of the postcontrast CTA image (*E*) unveils a defect/graft dehiscence at the proximal anastomosis (*arrow*), accompanied by a substantial outpouching adjacent to the graft (*arrowhead*) that is consistent with a pseudoaneurysm. Remarkably, this pseudoaneurysm envelops the graft in a sizable configuration (*asterisk*). Captured in a 3D volume-rendered CTA image (*F*), the entirety of the pseudoaneurysm (*asterisk*) enveloping the graft is evident.

correlation between any hyperdensity observed in arterial phase imaging and the corresponding non-contrast images. Moreover, if accessible, including delayed images can provide valuable insights into the presence of contrast pooling.

Endovascular Repair Complications

The predominant endovascular complications include endoleak and stent migration, both of which will be thoroughly discussed in the subsequent sections.

PROCEDURES OF THE DESCENDING AORTA

The descending thoracic aorta is susceptible to a range of significant conditions, encompassing dissection, aneurysms, trauma, and aortoesophageal fistula. Some instances of descending aortic pathologies can extend from the aortic arch, a topic elaborated upon in the preceding section. This section's focus, however, is directed toward pathologies exclusively confined to the descending aorta or those extending into the abdominal aorta.

In cases of descending thoracic aortic aneurysm, as well as type B dissections involving the descending thoracic aorta, treatment options such as endovascular intervention and open graft repair are available, with a preference for the former. Nonetheless, for individuals with genetically linked thoracic aortic aneurysms and dissections, open surgical repair is generally recommended.

Endovascular repair (TEVAR) is the preferred technique in the descending thoracic aortic aneurysm.[21] The endograft must establish a secure seal at the proximal (aneurysm neck) and distal (lower end) landing zones, ensuring optimal contact with the arterial wall. Distal sealing is also crucial, with the celiac axis typically spared to avoid complications. However, in cases with sufficient collateral circulation, covering the celiac artery may be considered to gain additional seal length. Otherwise, a debranching procedure is recommended to maintain blood flow to vital organs, which may require an open approach.

Endovascular techniques for aortic dissection have the goal of sealing off the entry tear, reducing blood flow to the false lumen, and encouraging thrombosis and aortic remodeling to impede further enlargement. Notable approaches include standard TEVAR and the staged total aortic and branch vessel endovascular (STABLE) reconstruction. In the STABLE technique, a covered stent is deployed proximally to enclose the primary intimal tear, while a bare-metal stent is positioned distally to support the abdominal aortic true lumen and exert radial pressure to collapse the false lumen.[22] These endovascular methods share the common objective of sealing the intimal tear and prompting thrombosis within the false lumen, ultimately aiming to yield a more favorable outcome for patients afflicted by aortic dissection.[23]

As previously mentioned, for individuals with genetically mediated thoracic aortic aneurysms or when endovascular techniques are not an option, open repair emerges as a viable technique for addressing descending aortic pathologies. Aortic reconstruction typically entails the utilization of graft materials such as polyethylene terephthalate (PET), commonly known as Dacron, and expanded polytetrafluoroethylene (PTFE). PET, a polyester woven graft, boasts remarkable tensile strength and compliance, aiding tissue ingrowth.

Expected Postsurgical/Endovascular Findings

Expected endovascular repair findings on CTA are contingent on the underlying pathologies. For instance, in cases of aneurysms, expected imaging findings include the complete exclusion and thrombosis of the aneurysm sac. In the context of type B dissection repair, the expected imaging appearance should reflect the successful exclusion of the primary intimal tear, with no residual forward flow into it. When the left subclavian artery is embolized to establish a suitable landing zone, the vessel should demonstrate full occlusion, and any type II entry flow should be absent. It is noteworthy that the persistence of a perfused false lumen in distal aortic segments is common, and it is frequently observed that the false lumen near the distal landing zone is filled by backflow due to distal reentry tears. In imaging for open repair, reinforcement materials can be seen, especially

at the anastomosis site, as previously discussed. Additionally, to mitigate the risk of spinal cord injuries, anastomosis of the spinal artery/intercostal artery island patch is typically conducted (**Fig. 8**).

Complications

Endovascular repair complications
Endoleaks Endoleak is a frequent complication following TEVAR for thoracic aneurysms. A more comprehensive explanation of endoleak is provided in the procedures of the abdominal aorta. Notably, in thoracic cases, the major difference lies in the arteries causing the type II endoleak. Instead of lumbar or inferior mesenteric arteries, bronchial or intercostal arteries are commonly involved.

Stent migration and collapse Precise deployment is paramount to avert complications such as graft collapse and migration, often associated with the phenomenon known as "bird-beaking." The reported incidence of thoracic aortic stent-graft migration can be as high as 30%.[24] Over time, changes in neck dimension can lead to angulation or misalignment of the endograft, resulting in treatment failure due to device migration or false lumen entry flow, which increases the risk of aneurysm expansion and rupture.[23] Endograft migration is defined as a centerline length change of more than 10 mm from a fixed landmark to the proximal stent relative to the initial implantation site.[25] To effectively detect subtle stent-graft migration, it is recommended to compare the most recent study with the baseline study, especially during short-interval follow-up (**Fig. 9**). Stent-graft collapse after TEVAR can be associated with inadequate stent-graft apposition in a highly angulated aortic arch and/or excessive stent-graft oversizing.

Endograft infection/fistula formation More information concerning graft infection and its related complications, such as graft dehiscence and pseudoaneurysm, is provided in the procedures of the abdominal aorta.

Open repair complications
Much like the complications outlined for ascending aorta and arch repair above, hematomas, infections, and pseudoaneurysms are also observed in descending aortic open repair. Perianastomotic pseudoaneurysm is usually associated with graft infection, necessitating re-do surgery.

PROCEDURES OF THE ABDOMINAL AORTA

Abdominal aortic pathologies that require interventions can be categorized as aneurysms, dissection, or traumatic injuries. Most abdominal

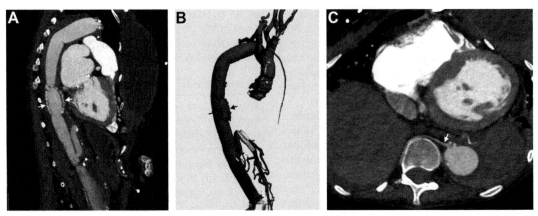

Fig. 8. A 38 year old man with Marfan syndrome and an aneurysm of the thoracoabdominal aorta underwent extensive thoracoabdominal repair with a graft with selective visceral perfusion and island patch reimplantation of T8-9 intercostal arteries. A parasagittal postcontrast CTA image (4) and a 3D volume-rendered image (B) demonstrate an island patch (white and black arrows) in the distal descending aortic graft, An axial postcontrast CTA image (C) through the level of the island patch reveals a native intercostal artery (*arrow*).

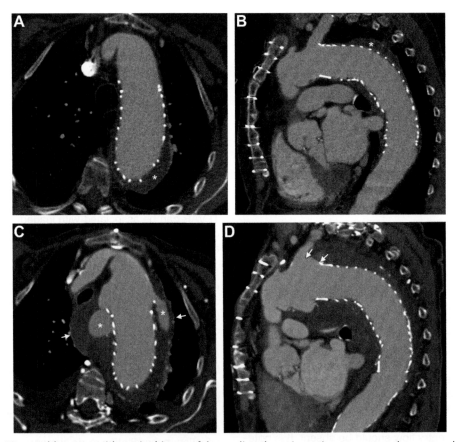

Fig. 9. A 78 year old woman with a prior history of descending thoracic aortic aneurysm underwent endovascular repair. Axial (*A*) and sagittal (*B*) postcontrast CTA images illustrate the stent graft in the descending aorta, effectively excluding the aneurysm sac (*asterisk*). However, on subsequent follow-up, an axial postcontrast CTA image (*C*) shows an expansion/aneurysm at the proximal section of the descending thoracic aorta (indicated by *arrows*), accompanied by a type I endoleak depicted by contrast leakage (*asterisk*) into the aneurysm sac. Likewise, on the follow-up sagittal postcontrast CTA image (*D*), the stent graft is observed to have migrated distally (*arrows*), differing from the depiction in the image (*B*).

aortic aneurysms (AAAs) undergo elective sur-geries when the size of the aneurysm is more than 5.5 cm or rapidly enlarges (>1 cm/y) to pre-vent fatal complications such as a rupture. For patients with an anatomy suitable for an endovas-cular approach, the recommendation is to opt for endovascular repair over open surgical repair.[26] EVAR is associated with a significant reduction in perioperative mortality compared to open AAA repair.[27] When EVAR is not an option, open surgi-cal repair can be done, which has been proven to be safe, effective in preventing aneurysm rupture, and remarkably durable.[28] Over the years, pros-thetic materials have replaced arterial homografts used in the original open repairs, but the technical approach to the operation has remained largely unchanged. Three types of grafts are available for open AAA repair: (1) polyester (eg, Dacron), (2) PTFE (eg, Gore-tex), and (3) autogenous artery or vein.

In most cases, isolated dissection in the abdom-inal aorta is managed conservatively. However, if associated complications arise, they can be treated using endovascular or open-repair ap-proaches. Similarly, for traumatic aortic injuries, the choice between endovascular and open repair depends on multiple factors, including the level of trauma/complications, availability of resources, and local expertise.

Expected Endovascular/Postsurgical Findings

Successful endovascular repair requires complete exclusion of the aneurysm from the circulatory sys-tem.[29] Expected post-EVAR CTA findings are (1) a well-positioned, patent stent graft from the infrare-nal abdominal aorta extending to the bilateral iliac arteries and excluding the aneurysm sac; (2) a completely thrombosed excluded aneurysm sac with no enhancement; (3) excluded small side-branches, including inferior mesenteric artery, lum-bar arteries, and gonadal arteries; and (4) patent renal, superior mesenteric, and celiac arteries.

Open repair procedure involves opening the AAA, removing thrombus and debris within the aorta, suturing the graft to the aorta in an end-to-end manner, and closing the graft with the aortic wall-inclusion graft repair. On immediate postsur-gical imaging, it is expected to see perigraft fluid or air. In some cases, postsurgical seroma can persist for a longer period; however, one must ensure the fluid density with no air on follow-up im-aging. Surgical materials, particularly felt rings/pledgets, are hyperintense on CTA, as discussed before; therefore, it is important to correlate with noncontrast images to differentiate from contrast leak/bleeding/pseudoaneurysm.

Complications

Endovascular repair complications
Endovascular repair complications can be catego-rized as (1) endoleak, (2) stent migration, (3) infec-tion, and (4) visceral organ ischemia.

Endoleak Endoleak is characterized by the ongoing blood flow within the excluded aneurysm sac, identifiable through contrast opacification on CTA.[30] Detecting an endoleak is crucial as it is often asymptomatic, and failure to do so can result in the progressive expansion of the aneurysm, potentially leading to rupture. The classification of endoleaks is based on the source of the leak.

A *type I endoleak* is an inadequate seal at the proximal (Ia) or distal (Ib) site.[31] This leak can either occur immediately after device placement or develop later. Timely repair of a type I endoleak is essential to prevent adverse events. On CTA im-aging, opacification of the aneurysm sac is evident during the arterial phase, and it is imperative to compare it with precontrast images to ensure that it does not overlap with calcifications (**Fig. 10**).

A *type II endoleak* occurs when there is a retro-grade flow into the sac from a patent inferior mesenteric artery, lumbar branches, or other aortic branches. Early type II endoleak is common, and the incidence gradually decreases, but some occult type II endoleaks may still emerge up to 5 years after EVAR. Spontaneous resolution of type II endoleaks is frequent, with around 60% of such endoleaks resolving within 6 months after the procedure and the rest gradually diminishing over time.[32] Interestingly, the aneurysm sac may shrink even if a type II endoleak is present. Although the significance of sac expansion with a type II endoleak is uncertain, an increase of more than 5 mm during follow-up is considered an important indicator of potential risk. Persistence of the endoleak alone does not necessarily warrant intervention. CTA images with delayed imaging are considered the gold standard for assessing type II endoleak, as it is often not visible on arterial phase images (**Fig. 11**).

A *type III endoleak* is caused by either a junctional leak or a disconnect of the endograft components (type IIIa) or holes in the endograft fabric (type IIIb). They can occur early or late after endovascular repair. Early type III endoleaks are often due to either inadequate overlap between graft compo-nents or insufficient balloon expansion at the junc-tions. Late type III endoleaks may develop months to years later, attributed to conformational changes in the aneurysm sac, endograft migration, or dila-tion of aortic and iliac attachment sites. Just like type I endoleaks, type III endoleaks necessitate

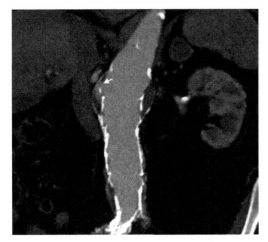

Fig. 10. A 78 year old man with abdominal and bilateral iliac aneurysm underwent stent-graft repair. In a subsequent follow-up imaging, a coronal postcontrast CTA image spanning the abdominal aorta reveals enlargement of the proximal AAA sac, accompanied by the appearance of contrast leak into the sac from the superior aspect of the graft (arrow), which is the manifestation of type I endoleak.

prompt treatment, as they can lead to rapid enlargement and rupture of the sac. A distinct mimic of type III endoleak following endovascular repair is observed with Endologix stent grafts, attributed to their unique construction, with the metallic endoskeleton within the graft cover. In some cases, a rim of contrast outside the endoskeleton can imitate a type III endoleak, but it remains well contained within the graft, a phenomenon referred to as "billowing"[33] (**Fig. 12**).

A *type IV endoleak* was described with first-generation endograft, characterized by small "blushes" in the aneurysm sac on completion of arteriography. While this issue has been typically associated with some thin polyester grafts, it is not consistently observed in all procedures, particularly with current-generation endografts.

A *type V endoleak*, also known as an endoleak of undefined origin, refers to continued aneurysm sac expansion (endotension) without a detectable leak on any imaging.

Stent migration Stent migration refers to the movement or displacement of the stent graft from its intended position within the aorta. This can happen due to various factors, such as inadequate fixation or sealing, changes in aortic anatomy, or issues related to the graft material. Stent migration can lead to complications such as endoleaks, misalignment of the graft, or reduced blood flow, necessitating further intervention to reposition or replace the stent graft. Therefore, closely monitoring for stent migration during follow-up CTA scans is essential to ensure the long-term success of the endovascular AAA repair procedure. Three-dimensional (3D) volume-rendered images of the stent graft can help cross-reference its location with respect to the vertebral bodies and identify any changes during follow-up.

Graft infection Graft infection after endovascular repair is extremely low at a rate of 0.6%.[34] Imaging features on CTA are similar to other infected endovascular grafts, including aneurysm sac wall thickening, periaortic fat stranding, periaortic lymph nodes, and air foci within the aneurysm sac (**Fig. 13**).

Visceral organ ischemia Visceral organ ischemia and infarction can occur after endovascular graft repair. Bowel ischemia may result from coverage of visceral arteries and poor collateral flow, presenting with bowel wall thickening and fat stranding in a vascular distribution, which can be easily detected in CTA studies. The incidence of bowel ischemia is 1.6% after elective repair and 15.2% after ruptured repair.[35] Similarly, infarction in solid organs such as the kidneys and spleen can be seen due to ischemia from stent coverage.

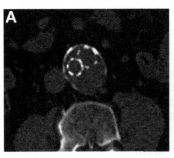
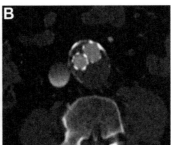
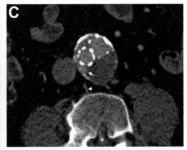

Fig. 11. A 77 year old man diagnosed with an AAA underwent stent-graft repair. While the axial noncontrast CT image (*A*) and postcontrast CTA image (*B*) exhibit no indications of endoleak or calcification within the aneurysm sac, a delayed postcontrast CTA image (*C*) demonstrates an enhancing region (*arrow*) within the excluded aneurysmal sac and the identified feeding vessel (*arrowhead*) collectively indicate a type II endoleak.

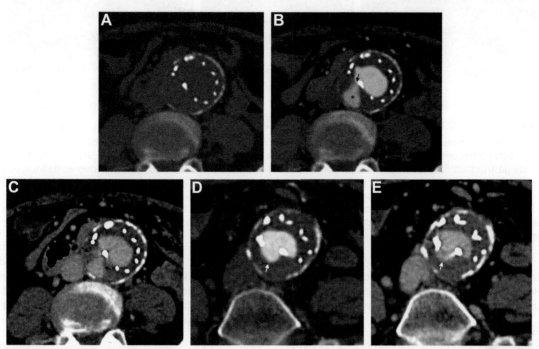

Fig. 12. A 72 year old man underwent AAA repair utilizing the Endologix stent graft. The axial noncontrast CT image (A) reveals the aneurysm sac, while the axial postcontrast arterial phase CTA image (B) illustrates contrast leakage (asterisk) originating from the defect in the fabric (arrow). This leakage enlarges (indicated by arrows) on the delayed phase CTA image (C), indicating a type III endoleak. In the same patient, a relatively lower level axial postcontrast CTA image (D) displays a focal bulging of contrast (arrow), mirrored on the axial delayed postcontrast CTA image (E). This consistency in appearance corresponds to the normal characteristics of this graft type, manifesting as a phenomenon referred to as "billowing."

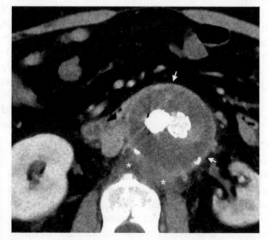

Fig. 13. A 53 year old man who underwent stent-graft repair for an AAA presented with symptoms including back pain, fever, malaise, and an elevated white blood cell count. On axial postcontrast delayed CTA image, conspicuous thickening and enhancement of the aortic sac wall (arrows) are observed, alongside evident fat stranding and edema (asterisks). In conjunction with the clinical findings, these imaging findings strongly align with the presence of an infected graft.

Open repair complications

Open repair complications can be categorized as (1) graft occlusion/thrombosis, (2) graft dehiscence, (3) pseudoaneurysm at the anastomosis, (4) graft infection, and (5) aorto-enteric fistula.

Graft occlusion/thrombosis Graft occlusion and thrombosis is an infrequent complication. Dutch Randomized Endovascular Aneurysm Repair trial reported only 3 occlusions out of 178 open repairs.[34] On imaging, particularly on CTA, it manifests as a low-density material within the graft limb and exhibits a lack of opacification on delayed imaging. Once detected, endovascular treatment options, such as employing a thrombectomy catheter, can be utilized to manage graft thrombosis effectively.

Graft dehiscence Graft dehiscence represents a rare complication of open graft repair. On CTA imaging, a significant feature to look for is contrast extravasation at the site of the anastomosis accompanied by an adjacent hematoma and pooling of contrast on delayed images. As previously mentioned, it is important to note that surgical materials, particularly felt rings/pledgets used at the

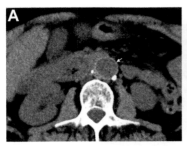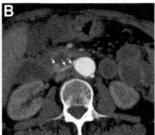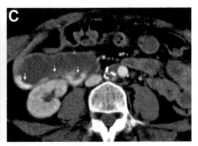

Fig. 14. A 62 year old woman exhibiting significant atherosclerotic disease throughout the abdominal aorta and lower extremities underwent aortobifemoral bypass graft utilizing a noninclusion technique. She presented with severe gastrointestinal bleeding. The axial noncontrast CT image (*A*) acquired through the abdomen delineates a hyperdense rim signifying the graft, with no native aorta enveloping it. On the axial postcontrast CTA image (*B*) captured at the same level, shows brisk contrast extravasation from the aorta to the adjacent bowel loop (*arrows*). A slightly lower-level axial postcontrast delayed CTA image (*C*) reveals a dilated duodenum containing layered contrast within its lumen (*arrows*). Collectively, these findings consistent with the diagnosis of an aortic graft-enteric fistula.

anastomosis site, appear hyperdense on CTA. Hence, a comparison with noncontrast images becomes essential for an accurate assessment.

Pseudoaneurysm at the anastomosis Pseudoaneurysm at the anastomosis is known to have some association with graft dehiscence, and in certain cases, these 2 conditions can coexist. Among the common causes of pseudoaneurysms, infection is the prevailing factor. As with dehiscence, early detection and prompt treatment are of paramount importance. On CTA imaging, the hallmark feature of a pseudoaneurysm is a new focal contrast outpouching observed at the site of the graft anastomosis.

Graft infection Graft infection is a significant complication that should be considered when a patient presents with fever, an elevated white blood cell count, and elevated inflammatory markers. On CTA, graft infection demonstrates a new fat stranding and/or hypodense collection surrounding the graft. Foci of air in the excluded perigraft space should raise concern for gas-forming organisms. Untreated infected grafts can demonstrate pseudoaneurysms or graft dehiscence, as mentioned above. As discussed in the context of thoracic grafts, it is worth noting that FDG-PET/CT can aid in distinguishing anticipated postsurgical inflammatory changes from an infected graft.

Aorto-enteric fistula Aorto-enteric fistula, or more precisely, "secondary aorto-enteric fistula," occurs after aortic graft placement, including stent grafts, noninclusion aortic graft, and inclusion-graft repairs. The exact cause of this condition remains unclear, but potential mechanisms include the pulsating motion of the graft against the bowel wall and the adhesion of an infected graft to the

bowel. The most common location reported to be in the duodenum. Clinical presentations of aorto-enteric fistula vary depending on the extent of gastrointestinal tract involvement. They may include direct fistula formation with gastrointestinal bleeding, occult fistula formation without bleeding, and indirect gastrointestinal bleeding without fistula formation. For patients suspected of having aorto-enteric fistula, concurrent CTA and endoscopy should be performed. CTA commonly reveals the presence of air within the sac or adjacent to the graft, which can indicate an aorto-enteric fistula. However, it is essential to distinguish this from infections, as the detection of adjacent bowel tethering raises concern for fistula formation. For patients experiencing active bleeding, CTA can be particularly informative, as it may demonstrate contrast extravasation to the bowel loops, with more pooling observed on delayed images (**Fig. 14**).

SUMMARY

CTA is a fundamental tool for assessing and continuously monitoring the postsurgical or endovascular repaired aortas. Achieving a comprehensive imaging evaluation of the postprocedural aorta demands that diagnostic radiologists possess a firm grasp of prevalent surgical, endovascular, and hybrid repair techniques, coupled with their expected postprocedural presentations. As the postprocedural aorta remains susceptible to a spectrum of potential complications, their early detection hinges on proficient imaging practices. The diverse nature of these complications is closely linked to the specific procedure undertaken, emphasizing the critical role of imaging in guiding clinical decision-making and patient care.

CLINICS CARE POINTS

- Recognizing expected postsurgical findings is crucial for distinguishing normal outcomes from complications, covering aspects such as graft appearance, hyperattenuating structures, and graft materials.

- Awareness of potential complications is essential. These include hematoma and fluid collection, infection, pseudoaneurysms, endoleaks, stent migration, graft infections, graft occlusion, graft dehiscence, and aortoenteric fistulas.

- Differentiating between expected postsurgical inflammatory changes and graft infections can be challenging. Imaging findings, including wall thickening, enhancement, fat stranding, and gas foci, should raise suspicion.

- Open repair procedures, including graft placement and anastomosis, require careful assessment for complications such as pseudoaneurysms, infections, graft-related issues, and imaging findings mimicking pathologies.

- Evaluation should include checking for stent migration and graft collapse, which can impact the effectiveness of the procedure.

- Always consider the clinical context when interpreting imaging findings, including patient symptoms, history, and laboratory values, to guide diagnosis and management.

REFERENCES

1. Upchurch GR Jr, Escobar GA, Azizzadeh A, et al. Society for Vascular Surgery clinical practice guidelines of thoracic endovascular aortic repair for descending thoracic aortic aneurysms. J Vasc Surg 2021;73(1S):55S–83S.
2. Yacoub MH, Gehle P, Chandrasekaran V, et al. Late results of a valve-preserving operation in patients with aneurysms of the ascending aorta and root. J Thorac Cardiovasc Surg 1998;115(5):1080–90.
3. Demers P, Miller DC. Simple modification of "T. David-V" valve-sparing aortic root replacement to create graft pseudosinuses. Ann Thorac Surg 2004;78(4):1479–81.
4. Wheat MW Jr, Wilson JR, Bartley TD. Successful Replacement of the Entire Ascending Aorta and Aortic Valve. JAMA 1964;188:717–9.
5. Bentall H, De Bono A. A technique for complete replacement of the ascending aorta. Thorax 1968;23(4):338–9.
6. Cherry C, DeBord S, Hickey C. The modified Bentall procedure for aortic root replacement. AORN J 2006;84(1):52–5, 58-70; [quiz 71-4].
7. Cabrol C, Pavie A, Gandjbakhch I, et al. Complete replacement of the ascending aorta with reimplantation of the coronary arteries: new surgical approach. J thorac Cardiovascul Surg 1981;81(2):309–15.
8. Kouchoukos NT, Masetti P, Nickerson NJ, et al. The Ross procedure: long-term clinical and echocardiographic follow-up. Ann Thorac Surg 2004;78(3):773–81 [discussion 773-81].
9. Sultan I, McGarvey J, Vallabhajosyula P, et al. Routine use of hemiarch during acute type A aortic dissection repair. Ann Cardiothorac Surg 2016;5(3):245–7.
10. Szeto WY, Bavaria JE. Hybrid repair of aortic arch aneurysms: combined open arch reconstruction and endovascular repair. Semin Thorac Cardiovasc Surg 2009;21(4):347–54.
11. Bednarkiewicz M, Khatchatourian G, Christenson JT, et al. Aortic arch replacement using a four-branched aortic arch graft. Eur J Cardio Thorac Surg 2002;21(1):89–91.
12. Kansagra K, Kang J, Taon MC, et al. Advanced endografting techniques: snorkels, chimneys, periscopes, fenestrations, and branched endografts. Cardiovascul Diag therapy 2018;8(Suppl 1):S175–83.
13. LeMaire SA, Carter SA, Coselli JS. The elephant trunk technique for staged repair of complex aneurysms of the entire thoracic aorta. Ann Thorac Surg 2006;81(5):1561–9 [discussion 1569].
14. Niederhauser U, Rudiger H, Kunzli A, et al. Surgery for acute type a aortic dissection: comparison of techniques. Eur J Cardio Thorac Surg 2000;18(3):307–12.
15. Hanneman K, Chan FP, Mitchell RS, et al. Pre- and Postoperative Imaging of the Aortic Root. Radiographics 2016;36(1):19–37.
16. Prescott-Focht JA, Martinez-Jimenez S, Hurwitz LM, et al. Ascending thoracic aorta: postoperative imaging evaluation. Radiographics 2013;33(1):73–85.
17. Green DB, Vargas D, Reece TB, et al. Mimics of Complications in the Postsurgical Aorta at CT. Radiol Cardiothorac Imaging 2019;1(4):e190080.
18. Chu LC, Johnson PT, Cameron DE, et al. MDCT evaluation of aortic root surgical complications. AJR Am J Roentgenol 2013;201(4):736–44.
19. Sundaram B, Quint LE, Patel S, et al. CT appearance of thoracic aortic graft complications. AJR Am J Roentgenol 2007;188(5):1273–7.
20. Li W, Rongthong S, Prabhakar AM, et al. Postoperative imaging of the aorta. Cardiovascular diagnosis and therapy 2018;8(Suppl 1):S45–60.
21. Makaroun MS, Dillavou ED, Kee ST, et al. Endovascular treatment of thoracic aortic aneurysms: results of the phase II multicenter trial of the GORE TAG thoracic endoprosthesis. J Vasc Surg 2005;41(1):1–9.

22. Andic M, Lescan M. Staged Hybrid Treatment with Branched Endovascular Aneurysm Repair of a Thoracoabdominal Aortic Aneurysm in the Presence of a Total Infrarenal Aortoiliac Occlusion. Vasc Specialist Int 2021;37:43.

23. Shen J, Mastrodicasa D, Al Bulushi Y, et al. Thoracic Endovascular Aortic Repair for Chronic Type B Aortic Dissection: Pre- and Postprocedural Imaging. Radiographics 2022;42(6):1638–53.

24. O'Neill S, Greenberg RK, Resch T, et al. An evaluation of centerline of flow measurement techniques to assess migration after thoracic endovascular aneurysm repair. J Vasc Surg 2006;43(6):1103–10.

25. Fillinger MF, Greenberg RK, McKinsey JF, et al, Society for Vascular Surgery Ad Hoc Committee on TRS. Reporting standards for thoracic endovascular aortic repair (TEVAR). J Vasc Surg 2010;52(4):1022–33, 1033 e15.

26. Chaikof EL, Dalman RL, Eskandari MK, et al. The Society for Vascular Surgery practice guidelines on the care of patients with an abdominal aortic aneurysm. J Vasc Surg 2018;67(1):2–77 e2.

27. Epple J, Svidlova Y, Schmitz-Rixen T, et al. Long-Term Outcome of Intact Abdominal Aortic Aneurysm After Endovascular or Open Repair. Vasc Endovascular Surg 2023. 15385744231178130.

28. Becquemin JP, Pillet JC, Lescalie F, et al. A randomized controlled trial of endovascular aneurysm repair versus open surgery for abdominal aortic aneurysms in low- to moderate-risk patients. J Vasc Surg 2011;53(5):1167–1173 e1.

29. Chaikof EL, Blankensteijn JD, Harris PL, et al. Reporting standards for endovascular aortic aneurysm repair. J Vasc Surg 2002;35(5):1048–60.

30. Cifuentes S, Mendes BC, Tabiei A, et al. Management of Endoleaks After Elective Infrarenal Aortic Endovascular Aneurysm Repair: A Review. JAMA surgery 2023. https://doi.org/10.1001/jamasurg.2023.2934.

31. Tan TW, Eslami M, Rybin D, et al. Outcomes of patients with type I endoleak at completion of endovascular abdominal aneurysm repair. J Vasc Surg 2016;63(6):1420–7.

32. Silverberg D, Baril DT, Ellozy SH, et al. An 8-year experience with type II endoleaks: natural history suggests selective intervention is a safe approach. J Vasc Surg 2006;44(3):453–9.

33. Helo N, Chang AC, Hyun C, et al. Retrospective review of billowing phenomenon-a mimic of endoleak following placement of endologix covered stent for the treatment of abdominal aortic aneurysm. Ann Vasc Surg 2017;45:239–46.

34. De Bruin JL, Baas AF, Buth J, et al. Long-term outcome of open or endovascular repair of abdominal aortic aneurysm. N Engl J Med 2010;362(20):1881–9.

35. Ultee KH, Zettervall SL, Soden PA, et al. Incidence of and risk factors for bowel ischemia after abdominal aortic aneurysm repair. J Vascul Surg 2016;64(5):1384–91.

Imaging of Visceral Vessels

Theodore T. Pierce, MD, MPH[a],*, Vinay Prabhu, MD, MS[b], Vinit Baliyan, MD[c],
Sandeep Hedgire, MD[c]

KEYWORDS

• Vasculitis • Vasculopathy • Malformations • Aneurysm • Variant • Artery • Vein • Portal

KEY POINTS

- A diverse array of inflammatory, infectious, thrombotic, neoplastic, structural, and iatrogenic diseases may affect the arterial, portal venous, and systemic venous vasculature in the abdomen and pelvis.
- Vascular abnormalities require specialized imaging protocols to optimize abnormality detection and enable conclusive characterization.
- The detection of vascular abnormalities on routine, nonvascular, imaging often requires a high index of suspicion and detailed image interrogation because characteristic findings may be less conspicuous or occult.
- Awareness and recognition of normal vascular anatomy and common variants can improve operative guidance, increase sensitivity to detect pathology, and help avoid diagnostic pitfalls.

INTRODUCTION

Although intimately involved with every organ, blood vessels are often overlooked as a cause of pathologic condition. The coexistence of systemic arteries, systemic veins, and the portal venous system in the abdomen leads to unique complexity, which requires special imaging techniques for thorough evaluation. Our goal is to understand vascular pathologic conditions, the interplay between vessels and abdominopelvic disease, and technical limitations of nondedicated imaging studies.

Imaging Technique

Abdominal vascular computed tomography (CT) and MR imaging require high spatial resolution, minimal noise, maximum contrast enhancement targeted to the vessel(s) of interest, multiphase acquisitions to characterize abnormalities, and image postprocessing (maximum intensity projection [MIP], multiplanar reformation [MPR], and curved planar reformation [CPR]) to optimize sensitivity and measurement accuracy.[1] High-resolution mitigates partial volume averaging effects to optimally assess small vessels or subtle pathology and allows generation of post hoc MPRs at the workstation. Distinct acquisitions assess arteries, portal veins (PVs), and/or systemic veins, each with different contrast timing.[2] Noncontrast and delayed phase scans troubleshoot common problems, for example, distinguishing intrinsic hyperdensity on CT or hyperintensity on MR imaging from enhancement or distinguishing contained rupture (pseudoaneurysm) from active extravasation. Other than contrast-enhanced sequences, T2-weighted, diffusion-weighted, phase contrast, and steady state free precession sequences are useful MR imaging adjuncts. Ultrasound (US) allows morphologic assessment with B-mode images and hemodynamic characterization with color and spectral Doppler. For all modalities, but particularly US and MR imaging, artifacts may lead to misdiagnosis[1,3] (Fig. 1). Routine, nonvascular, abdominal imaging may reduce conspicuity or prevent definitive characterization of vascular pathologic conditions.

[a] Department of Radiology, Harvard Medical School, Massachusetts General Hospital, White Building, Room 270, 55 Fruit Street, Boston, MA 02114, USA; [b] Department of Radiology, NYU Langone Health, 660 First Avenue, Third Floor, New York, NY 10016, USA; [c] Division of Cardiovascular Imaging, Department of Radiology, Massachusetts General Hospital-Harvard Medical School, 175 Cambridge Street, Boston, MA 02114, USA
* Corresponding author. Division of Abdominal Imaging, Department of Radiology, Massachusetts General Hospital-Harvard Medical School, 55 Fruit Street, White Building, Room 270, Boston, MA 02114.
E-mail address: ttpierce@mgh.harvard.edu

Radiol Clin N Am 62 (2024) 543–557
https://doi.org/10.1016/j.rcl.2023.12.003
0033-8389/24/© 2024 Elsevier Inc. All rights reserved.

ARTERIES

Normal Anatomy

The abdominal aorta supplies paired lumbar arteries at multiple levels posteriorly, paired renal arteries laterally, paired common iliac arteries inferiorly, and 3 visceral arteries anteriorly: the celiac artery, superior mesenteric artery (SMA), and inferior mesenteric artery (IMA; Fig. 2). In 65% to 75% of patients, the celiac artery gives rise to the left gastric artery (LGA) and then bifurcates into the common hepatic (CHA) and splenic arteries.[4] The CHA gives rise to the gastroduodenal artery (GDA) and becomes the proper hepatic artery[4]; this splits into right hepatic artery (RHA) and left hepatic artery (LHA) branches in 55% of patients.[5] Several collateral pathways interconnect the visceral arteries: pancreaticoduodenal artery (PDA) anastomosis (GDA-SMA), arc of Buhler (celiac-SMA), arc of Barkow (gastroepiploic anastomosis), marginal artery of Drummond (SMA-IMA), and arc of Riolan (SMA-IMA). Extensive collaterals connect the IMA and internal iliac arteries (IIA) via the superior and middle rectal arteries.[4]

Clinically Significant Anatomic Variants

Variant hepatic arterial anatomy (arteries from a nonstandard vessel [replaced] or supernumerary vessels supplying less than a liver lobe [accessory])[4] affects the surgical approach in liver transplantation, tumor resection, intra-arterial therapy, and other surgical situations.[5] Variants include accessory LHA (incidence 8%–13%) and replaced LHA (10%–12%) from the LGA[4] and replaced CHA

(2.5%), replaced RHA (10%–17%), or accessory RHA (6%–8%) from the SMA.[4] Combinations of these variants may be present.

The *corona mortis* is an anastomosis between external iliac or inferior epigastric vessels and the ipsilateral obturator vessel. The artero-arterial (~25% of hemipelvises) and veno-venous variants (~42%) can be injured from pelvic fractures or hip surgery resulting in life-threatening hemorrhage.[6]

A *persistent sciatic artery* (incidence 0.03%–0.06%), an embryologic remnant originating from the posterior division of the IIA, courses posterior to the ischial tuberosity and supplies the leg via the popliteal artery.[7] The artery is often dilated and tortuous from intrinsic arterial wall weakness, susceptibility to extrinsic trauma, and injury from the sacrospinal ligament and piriformis muscle during hip movement.[7] Aneurysmal dilatation (~50% of patients) leads to mural thrombus formation, distal embolization/ischemia (40% of patients with aneurysm), or occlusion (9% of patients).[7]

Genetic Syndromes

Marfan syndrome (prevalence 1:10,000–50,000) is an autosomal dominant (AD) connective tissue disease from fibrillin-1 gene mutation.[8,9] Patients are characteristically tall with long arms and digits and additional multiorgan system manifestations. Diagnostic criteria emphasize aortic root dilatation, ectopia lentis, and genetic testing.[9] Medial elastic degeneration and cystic medial necrosis most commonly lead to annuloaortic ectasia, aortic root aneurysm, and thoracic aortic dissection.[8]

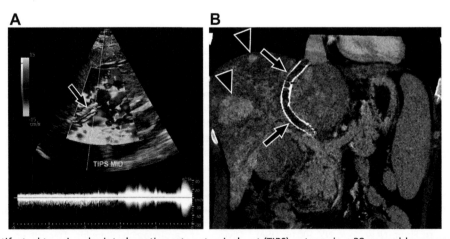

A   **B**

Fig. 1. Artifactual transjugular intrahepatic portosystemic shunt (TIPS) patency in a 28-year-old woman with BCS. (*A*) Color Doppler US image shows artifactual in-stent flow (*arrow*) due to an inappropriately elevated color gain setting, a technical pitfall for assessing vascular patency. Note the artifactual color Doppler flow in the stationary liver parenchyma and absent stent flow by spectral Doppler waveform. (*B*) Subsequently obtained contrast-enhanced CT reveals complete stent thrombosis (*arrows*). The hyperenhancing nodules (*arrowheads*) are typical of regenerative nodules in BCS.

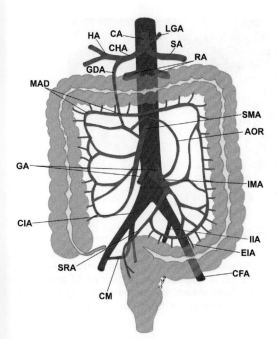

Fig. 2. Abdominal arterial anatomy. AOR, arc of Riolan; CA, celiac; CFA, common femoral; CHA, common hepatic; CIA, common iliac; CM, corona mortis; EIA, external iliac; GA, gonadal; GDA, gastroduodenal; HA, proper hepatic; IIA, internal iliac; IMA, inferior mesenteric; LGA, left gastric; MAD, marginal artery of Drummond; RA, renal; SA, splenic; SMA, superior mesenteric; SRA, superior rectal.

Patients are also at risk for abdominal aortic aneurysm (AAA), abdominal aortic dissection, and visceral artery aneurysm.[10]

Ehlers-Danlos syndrome (EDS; prevalence 1:5000–250,000[11]) is a collection of 11 distinct connective tissue diseases.[12] Vascular EDS (4% of EDS), formerly EDS type IV, is an AD defect in type III procollagen.[13,14] Vascular fragility predisposes to vascular ectasia, aneurysm, and dissection, typically multifocal, involving the aorta, head/neck, splanchnic, and iliac arteries with resulting target organ (such as renal, splenic, or brain) hemorrhage, ischemia, or infarcts[14,15] (**Fig. 3**). Aortic root involvement is uncommon.[16] Patients are at risk of uterine and intestinal rupture.[11,15] Patients often have complications as young adults, up to 80% by the age of 40 years, but are often undiagnosed at the time of their first vascular event.[15]

Loeys-Dietz syndrome (LDS; prevalence < 1:100,000) is a severe AD connective tissue disease characterized by aortic root aneurysm (98% of patients), fusiform AAA (10%), medium-sized arterial involvement (>50%), arterial tortuosity, and other multiorgan system involvement.[17,18] The leading causes of death are thoracic (67%)

and abdominal (22%) aortic dissection[17] even in nondilated aortas.[18] Aneurysms grow faster and dissection occurs at a lower threshold in LDS than Marfan syndrome.[18] Spontaneous organ rupture (spleen, bowel, and uterus) may occur.[17]

Abdominal Aorta

The abdominal aorta hosts a diverse array of inflammatory, thrombotic, degenerative, and neoplastic pathologic conditions that warrant a detailed discussion beyond the scope of this section. However, the integrated nature of the cardiovascular system necessitates brief mention of disease processes that overlap between the aorta and visceral vasculature.

Atherosclerosis, the accumulation of mural arterial plaque, is common and causes significant morbidity through visceral or lower extremity ischemia and aneurysm formation. This may affect the aorta and branch vessels. Risk factors include hypercholesterolemia, hypertension, smoking, diabetes, obesity, and diet.[19] Atherosclerosis appears as eccentric mural thickening or low attenuation filling defects and/or calcific density. Medial arterial calcification is distinct, occurring in patients with diabetes or renal dysfunction, with a predilection for branch arteries (in particular the splenic artery) and relative sparing of aorta.[20] This often appears as a "railroad track" on radiograph compared with atherosclerosis, which tends to be more spotty.

Aortic occlusion results from embolism (acute or chronic) or thrombosis (due to atherosclerosis and smoking).[21] This can be recognized by the development of extensive collaterals from the lower thoracic/upper abdominal arteries to the iliac/femoral arteries, such as the pathway of Winslow (internal mammary to inferior epigastric arteries), which supply the lower extremities in this setting[22] (**Fig. 4**). Chronic infrarenal aortic occlusion may present with characteristic symptoms, *Leriche syndrome* (buttock claudication, impotence, and/or diminished femoral pulses).[22]

Mycotic aneurysms, from infectious aortitis, are saccular or irregularly shaped outpouchings with adjacent stranding, fluid, and gas that often grow rapidly (**Fig. 5**). Distinguishing this from inflammatory aortitis can, at times, be difficult. Careful interrogation of the visceral vasculature in the setting of a suspected aortic mycotic aneurysm may identify additional sites of involvement, which can help cement the diagnosis.

Aortic Branch Vessels

SMA syndrome (Wilkie syndrome) is a controversial (prevalence 0.1%–0.3%) cause of duodenal

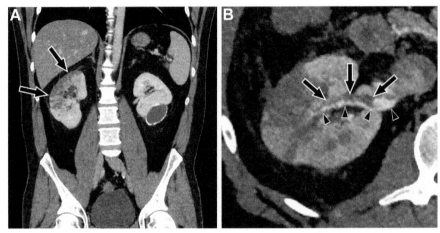

Fig. 3. Right renal artery dissection and infarct from vascular EDS in a 35-year-old man with right flank pain. (*A*) Coronal reformatted contrast-enhanced routine abdominal CT shows well-demarcated segmental right upper renal pole hypoenhancement (*arrows*) compatible with infarct. (*B*) A subsequently performed CT angiogram shows a thrombosed false lumen (*arrows*) and patent true lumen (*arrowheads*) due to segmental right renal artery dissection, which explains the renal infarct and flank pain. In a young man, these findings raise concern for underlying vasculopathy; EDS was diagnosed by genetic testing.

obstruction, typically in young women.[23] Symptoms, including abdominal pain, nausea, vomiting, and anorexia, can exacerbate weight loss and worsen the obstruction. A loss of periduodenal fat from profound rapid weight loss causes extrinsic compression of the third portion of the duodenum between the aorta and SMA. Imaging reveals duodenal obstruction, a narrow (<22°) aortomesenteric angle (AMA), and aortomesenteric distance (AMD) < 8 mm. Radiologists are cautioned to avoid overdiagnosis solely on the basis of abnormal AMA or AMD in the absence of obstruction.[23]

Median arcuate ligament (MAL) syndrome (Dunbar syndrome) consists of epigastric pain, weight loss, and celiac artery compression by the MAL.[23] Symptoms develop from chronic mesenteric ischemia, vascular steal, or celiac nerve plexus impingement.[24,25] Women (4:1) aged 30 to 50 years are most commonly affected.[24] Imaging findings, best seen on sagittal CT or MR imaging, are extrinsic narrowing of the celiac artery by the MAL, poststenotic dilatation, and up-turned or hooked distal celiac segment without significant atherosclerosis.[23] Narrowing worsens during expiration when the diaphragm rises and lifts the heart, aorta, and celiac artery cranially, pressing the celiac artery against the MAL.[24] US may show celiac stenosis and respirophasic increased celiac velocity during expiration.[23,24] The diagnosis is controversial as imaging findings exist in asymptomatic patients, the degree of narrowing and symptoms are poorly related, and surgical correction may not relieve symptoms.[23]

Fibromuscular dysplasia (FMD) is a surprisingly common (prevalence 3.34%),[26] noninflammatory and nonatherosclerotic medium-vessel arteriopathy typically involving renal (67% of patients with FMD), iliac (32%), and mesenteric arteries (22%).[27] Ninety percent of cases present in women aged 20 to 60 years.[26] Imaging findings of FMD include arterial beading, stenosis, aneurysm, dissection (including spontaneous coronary artery dissection), tortuosity, occlusion, and end organ ischemia[26,27] (**Fig. 6**). Multivessel involvement is common; however, aortic involvement is unusual.[27] Vascular findings, such as mural irregularity, may be subtle, requiring high-resolution CT angiography with MIPs, MPRs, and CPRs for detection.[27] Imaging findings of vasculitis and FMD are similar, although systemic inflammation would suggest vasculitis.[28] Multiple dissections raise the possibility of Marfan syndrome, LDS, or vascular EDS, although characteristic clinical/physical examination findings may distinguish genetic syndromes from FMD.[28]

Segmental arterial mediolysis (SAM) is a rare idiopathic noninflammatory medium vessel arteriopathy most often affecting middle-aged and elderly men.[29] SAM causes arterial dissection (71%–86%), aneurysm (43%–57%), stenosis, occlusion, spontaneous hemorrhage, and ischemia, often with multivessel involvement.[29–31] Presenting symptoms include abdominal pain (50%–74%) and hemorrhagic shock (32%) due to vessel rupture.[30,31] Visceral dissecting aneurysms, segmental mural soft tissue thickening (rind sign), and occlusion affect the renal arteries, SMA, and celiac trunk (each in half of patients) and less

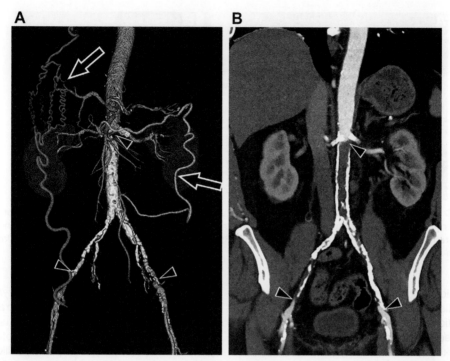

Fig. 4. Leriche syndrome in a 69-year-old man with lower extremity claudication. (*A*) Volume-rendered CT shows the extent of aortoiliac occlusion (*arrowheads*) and important arterial collateral pathways (*arrows*): in green, the abdominal portion of the pathway of Winslow (subclavian artery to internal mammary artery to superior epigastric artery to inferior epigastric artery to external iliac artery), and in yellow, the arc of Riolan (SMA to IMA). Celiac and SMA are noted in blue. (*B*) Contrast-enhanced CT angiogram CPR shows extensive atherosclerosis and occlusion of the infrarenal aorta, bilateral common iliac arteries, and bilateral external iliac arteries (*arrowheads*) with reconstitution via the inferior epigastric arteries.

frequently the hepatic, iliac, and splenic arteries.[29,30] Visceral vessel branch sites and aortic involvement are unusual. Differentiating SAM and FMD is difficult; in fact, some consider SAM an FMD-precursor,[32] an FMD-variant,[30] or the same disease as FMD.[28]

Isolated visceral arterial dissection is uncommon, occurring mostly in men.[33] Risk factors include

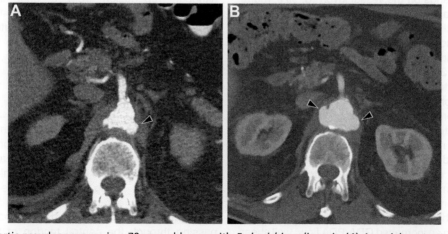

Fig. 5. Aortic pseudoaneurysm in a 79-year-old man with *Escherichia coli* sepsis. (*A*) An axial contrast-enhanced CT angiogram (CTA) image shows an aortic aneurysm with irregular contours and saccular outpouching (*arrowhead*). (*B*) A follow-up CTA shows rapid enlargement of the irregular aneurysm (*arrowheads*) compatible with an infected, or mycotic, pseudoaneurysm.

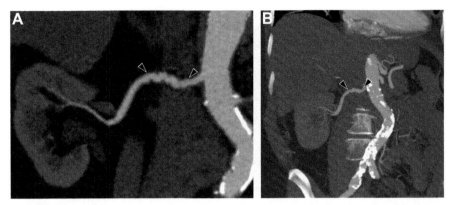

Fig. 6. FMD in a 74-year-old woman with renal artery tortuosity on chest CT. (A) Contrast-enhanced CT angiogram CPR shows right renal artery irregularity and beading (*arrowheads*), which is typical of FMD. Similar findings are demonstrated by the corresponding (B) MIP. MIPs and CPRs are useful tools to identify the subtle irregularity associated with FMD.

hypertension, trauma, secondary inflammation (ie, pancreatitis), pregnancy, vasculopathy (FMD, SAM, cystic medial necrosis, and atherosclerosis), and connective tissue disorders.[33,34] The SMA is the most likely splanchnic artery to dissect. Visceral arterial dissection, similar to that for the aorta, includes an intraluminal tissue flap (**Fig. 7**), which may be occult due to small vessel size or complete false lumen thrombosis. Other clues include aneurysmal dilation, perivascular fat stranding, and mural nonenhancing low density (the thrombosed false lumen).[34] In the setting of bowel ischemia/infarction, mesenteric dissection may require anticoagulation, endovascular treatment, or surgical intervention.[34]

Visceral artery aneurysms involve the splenic (~35%; **Fig. 8**), celiac (~30%), hepatic (13%–20%), and PDA (2%–10%) arteries.[35,36] Management depends on the vessel involved, size, mural integrity, and cause. Causes of true aneurysms include atherosclerosis, FMD, cystic medial necrosis, and portal hypertension.[35] The principal risk, aneurysm rupture, is considered low when less than 2 cm.[35] Some suggest following aneurysms up to 2.5 cm by imaging every 1 to 3 years because change in size is uncommon.[36] Patients who are pregnant or planning pregnancy undergo splenic artery aneurysm repair regardless of size due to the maternal (75%) and fetal (95%) mortality associated with rupture.[35,36] PDA and GDA aneurysms are repaired due to risk of rupture (~20%) despite small size (20% of ruptured aneurysms are <20 mm).[36,37] PDA/GDA aneurysms often occur with celiac artery narrowing or occlusion resulting in an increased GDA/PDA flow, wall shear stress, and rupture risk.[36]

Pseudoaneurysms result from inflammation (ie, pancreatitis), trauma, or infection.[35] Percutaneous biopsy may cause both pseudoaneurysm and arteriovenous fistula. Treatment is warranted at any size given the potential for rupture even when less than 1 cm.[36,37] Notably, mycotic aneurysms occur at vessel branch points, unlike aneurysms related to connective tissue disorders, SAM, or FMD.

Bowel ischemia, a serious condition with high associated mortality, may be related to arterial or venous (see later discussion) insufficiency. Chronic arterial ischemia is seen with extensive atherosclerosis. Acute arterial insufficiency can be subdivided as occlusive (ie, thrombosis, thromboembolism, or dissection) or nonocclusive (ie, hypotension). Ileus (fluid-filled dilated bowel without a transition point), although nonspecific, is the earliest sign of ischemia. In arterial insufficiency, the bowel wall is thin and hypoenhancing, although reperfusion from a prior ischemic episode may lead to bowel wall thickening and hyperenhancement.[38] Pneumatosis intestinalis and portal venous gas (PVG) are late findings (described in later discussion).

SYSTEMIC VEINS
Normal Anatomy

The inferior vena cava (IVC) drains organs below the level of diaphragm[39] (**Fig. 9**). The confluence of the right and left common iliac veins at the L5 vertebral level form the inferior IVC, which continues cranially along the right anterolateral aspect of the vertebral column, draining the lumbar, right gonadal, renal, and hepatic veins, before passing through the central tendon of the diaphragm at the T8 vertebral level. Other smaller tributaries include inferior phrenic and suprarenal veins.[39]

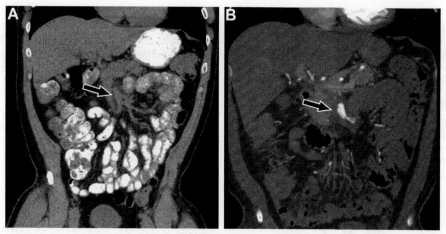

Fig. 7. SMA dissection in a 58-year-old man undergoing follow-up imaging for diverticulitis. (*A*) Noncontrast coronal CT shows subtle perivascular stranding (*arrow*) adjacent to the SMA. (*B*) Subsequently performed contrast-enhanced CT angiogram shows a dilated SMA with an intraluminal flap compatible with visceral artery dissection, which can predispose to visceral ischemia or rupture and life-threatening bleeding.

Clinically significant anatomic variants

Congenital systemic venous variants affect 4% of the population.[40] *Left IVC* (prevalence 0.2%–0.5%) describes drainage of a left-sided infrarenal segment into the left renal vein (LRV) and absence of the normal infrarenal IVC.[40] *Double IVC* (prevalence 0.2%–0.3%) is coexistence of right and left infrarenal IVC segments with drainage of the left segment via the LRV.[40] Both variants affect IVC filter placement and other surgical planning. *Absent hepatic IVC with azygos continuation* is asymptomatic but important in planning cardiopulmonary bypass and right heart catheterization.[41] Renal vein anomalies include retro-aortic (prevalence:

1.7%–3.4%) and circumaortic (prevalence: 2.4%–8.7%) variants; relevant for nephrectomy planning and potential misdiagnosis as lymphadenopathy on imaging.

Venous Thrombosis, Compression, and Occlusion

Budd-Chiari syndrome (BCS) results from partial or complete hepatic vein obstruction, most commonly from hypercoagulability and thrombosis. This leads acutely to liver congestion, hypoperfusion, and portal hypertension and subsequently to hepatocyte dysfunction, necrosis, fibrosis, and cirrhosis.[42] Hepatic vein or IVC thrombosis is a key finding.

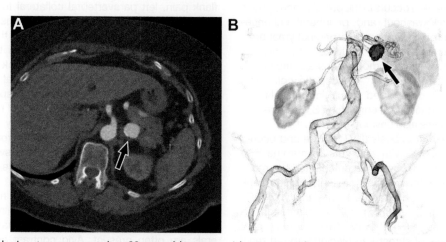

Fig. 8. Splenic artery aneurysm in a 66-year-old woman with prominent flow voids on lumbar spine MR imaging. (*A*) Axial contrast-enhanced CT image at the level of the celiac artery shows a 2.4 cm arterially enhancing lesion (*arrow*) adjacent to the pancreas. (*B*) 3D volume rendering depicts the relationship of the aneurysm (*arrow*) to splenic artery. Avoiding misdiagnosis as a pancreatic mass is critical to avoid catastrophic inadvertent aneurysm biopsy.

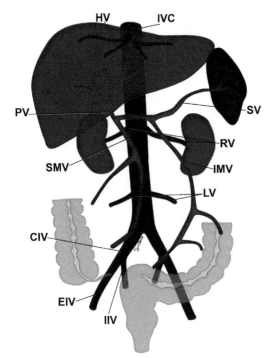

Fig. 9. Abdominal Venous Anatomy: CIV, common iliac; EIV, external iliac; HV, hepatic vein; IIV, internal iliac; IMV, inferior mesenteric vein; IVC, inferior vena cava; LV, lumbar; PV, portal; RV, renal; SMV, superior mesenteric; SV, splenic.

Acute BCS manifests as parenchymal low attenuation on CT and T1 hypointensity/T2 hyperintensity on MR imaging. The peripheral liver shows decreased arterial enhancement compared with the central parenchyma and caudate lobe.[43] A "flip-flop" pattern occurs in the portal venous phase with central washout and peripheral enhancement.[43] Chronic BCS leads to parenchymal atrophy/fibrosis sparing the caudate lobe, venous collateral formation, homogeneous enhancement, and persistent edema.[44] Intrahepatic collaterals seem as comma-shaped branching vessels and are highly suggestive of chronic BCS. Large regenerative nodules also develop (see Fig. 1).

Renal vein thrombosis (RVT) is rare and occurs mostly in adults with nephrotic syndrome and newborns with hypovolemia or inherited thrombophilia.[45] Symptoms, when present, include flank pain, hematuria, and acute kidney injury.[45] RVT, a serious complication of renal transplantation, affects less than 5% of grafts. Symptoms present within 7 days of surgery and include abrupt renal failure and swelling/tenderness of the graft. Early recognition is critical to save the graft.[46] B-mode US findings, enlarged and hypoechoic kidney in 90% of patients, are nonspecific. Color Doppler shows reduced or absent venous flow, increased arterial resistive index, and diastolic flow reversal. Computed tomography venography (CTV) and contrast-enhanced magnetic resonance venography identify intravenous thrombus but may be contraindicated due renal dysfunction.[47] Delayed renal contrast excretion may be present.

Iliocaval deep venous thrombosis (DVT), often related to extension of lower extremity clot, predisposes to pulmonary embolism and postthrombotic syndrome.[48] Risk factors include a hypercoagulability, malignancy, venous stasis, extrinsic compression, and IVC filters.[49] CTV is preferred to diagnose pelvic DVT.[49] Mixing artifact and limited systemic venous enhancement on portal venous phase CT, may mimic or obscure DVT, respectively. Iliocaval thrombosis may present with subtle perivascular inflammatory changes.

May-Thurner syndrome (iliac vein compression syndrome) is left common iliac vein compression by the right common iliac artery[50] (or left common iliac artery in the variant form) leading to left lower extremity swelling and thrombogenesis. Women (5:1) aged 10 to 40 years are mainly affected.[50] Imaging findings include left iliac vein compression ($\geq$50% narrowing), cross pelvic collaterals, left internal iliac vein flow reversal on time of flight MR imaging, and venous thrombosis.[50] Correct diagnosis is difficult without measurement of a pressure gradient because compression alone is common (25% of patients) and may resolve simply with hydration.[50]

Nutcracker anatomy is LRV compression by the SMA and aorta (anterior nutcracker) or retroaortic LRV compression by the aorta and spine (posterior nutcracker). "Nutcracker syndrome" requires symptoms such as hematuria, proteinuria, left flank pain, left paravertebral collateral formation, and left gonadal vein reflux.[23] CT findings include abrupt narrowing of the LRV between the aorta and SMA (beak sign) with dilatation of the hilar LRV. Doppler US shows an elevated peak velocity at the narrowing compared with the renal hilum; a ratio greater than 4.7 is sensitive and specific.[23] Catheter venography shows a renocaval pressure gradient greater than 3 mm Hg.[23] Many patients with positive imaging findings are asymptomatic.[23] Symptoms can coexist with SMA syndrome because the LRV and third part of duodenum are in close proximity.[23]

Superior vena cava (SVC) obstruction may present with indirect abdominal findings. Prominent azygos, hemiazygos, and abdominal wall collaterals are often present. Avid contrast enhancement of the quadrate lobe of the liver results from communication between superficial epigastric veins and left PV,[51] the cross-sectional equivalent of the nuclear medicine "*hot quadrate sign*"

(Fig. 10). The subdiaphragmatic liver may also avidly enhance due to inferior phrenic vein to hepatic subcapsular vein connections.[51]

Oncologic conditions of the systemic veins

IVC Leiomyosarcoma, although rare, is the most common primary IVC tumor affecting women (3:1) aged 40 to 60 years.[40] One-third of tumors demonstrate intraluminal growth and mimic bland thrombi, whereas the remaining grow extraluminally and must be differentiated from other retroperitoneal masses.[40] On CT, an imperceptible IVC suggests caval origin, whereas displacement of the IVC (negative embedded IVC sign) suggests extracaval origin.[52]

Tumor thrombus extending into the IVC is seen with renal cell carcinoma in 4% to 10% of tumors.[53] Imaging shows IVC luminal expansion by soft tissue, internal vascularity (parenchymal enhancement), cellularity (diffusion restriction), and metabolism (fluorodeoxyglucose uptake).[54] Typically, tumor thrombus is easily pulled from the IVC during surgery, although rarely mural invasion necessitates segmental IVC resection.[40] Supradiaphragmatic extension requires intraoperative cardiopulmonary bypass, sternotomy, and corresponds to worse outcomes. Although the PV is more typically invaded in hepatocellular carcinoma (HCC), hepatic vein invasion occurs in 4.0% to 5.9% cases.[40] Complications include BCS, distant metastasis, and worse prognosis. Adrenocortical carcinoma, although rare, is associated with IVC extension in 30% of cases, more commonly on the right and in tumors greater than 9 cm in size.[55]

Inferior vena cava filter complications

IVC filter complications include caval thrombosis (2%–30%); tilting, fragmentation, and embolization; IVC perforation (20%); and adjacent organ injury.[56] Excessive filter tilting, greater than 15°, reduces thrombus filtering ability and impairs retrieval. IVC perforation, a filter component greater than 3 mm beyond the IVC wall, may cause arterial injury, bowel perforation, or retroperitoneal hematoma. Filter migration (incidence <4.5%) is movement greater than 2 cm from initial placement site.[56] Filters may embolization to a distant site, typically the right atrium, with complications including atrial perforation, cardiac tamponade, or myocardial infarction.[57]

PORTAL VEINS
Normal Anatomy

The superior mesenteric vein (SMV) and splenic vein converge to form the PV, which divides into right and left branches to supply the liver. The SMV drains the small bowel via jejunal/ileal veins and right colon via right/middle colic veins. The inferior mesenteric vein (IMV) drains the left colon and upper rectum into the splenic vein (40%), SMV (40%), or splenoportal confluence (20%). The splenic vein drains the spleen and gastric fundus (short gastric veins). Other PV tributaries are as follows: left and right gastric veins, cystic veins, and Sappey veins.

Clinically significant variants

Congenital extrahepatic portosystemic shunt (CEPS), *Abernethy malformation*, includes 3 types:

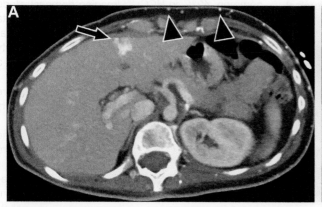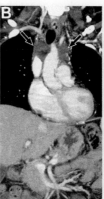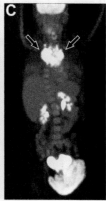

Fig. 10. Hot quadrate sign in a 30-year-old woman with Hodgkin lymphoma. (*A*) Axial contrast-enhanced CT image shows a wedge-shaped hyper-enhancement (*arrow*) in the anterior left liver lobe (the hot quadrate). This location and the presence abdominal wall collateral vessels (*arrowheads*) suggest SVC obstruction. (*B*) Coronal contrast-enhanced chest CT shows upper mediastinal lymphadenopathy (*arrows*) resulting in SVC obstruction. (*C*) Fluorodeoxyglucose-positron emission tomography MIP shows corresponding lymph node radiotracer uptake (*arrows*), consistent with the known lymphoma diagnosis.

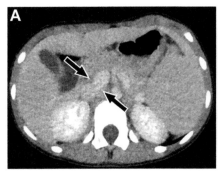
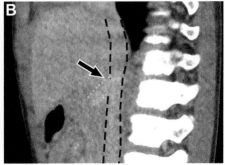

Fig. 11. Abernethy syndrome in a 6-year-old girl with liver failure. (*A*) Axial contrast-enhanced CT shows communication of the main PV with the IVC (*arrows*). The end-to-side connection, compatible with type 1 Abernethy syndrome, is shown on the sagittal (*B*) reformatted image (*arrow*). The IVC is outlined in dark blue and the main PV in light blue.

1a—Splenic vein and SMV drain to the IVC, 1b—PV drains to the IVC (**Fig. 11**), and 2—side-to-side portocaval shunt.[58] Large volume shunting leads to hepatopulmonary syndrome and hepatic encephalopathy.[58] Associated congenital anomalies, especially with type 1 CEPS, include chromosomal (eg, Down syndrome), cardiovascular, gastrointestinal, genitourinary, and skeletal defects.[58] CEPS leads to hepatic regenerative nodular hyperplasia, focal nodular hyperplasia, adenomas, and hepatoblastoma.[58] HCC may develop; however, typical imaging features (arterial hypervascularity and delayed washout) may not be seen.

Portomesenteric Venous Thrombosis and Occlusion

Portal vein thrombosis (PVT), although generally rare, affects 15% of cirrhotic patients.[59] Acute PVT presentation includes sudden onset abdominal pain, nausea, vomiting, and fever, whereas chronic PVT is asymptomatic or has signs of portal hypertension.[59] Imaging of acute PVT shows a nonenhancing intraluminal filling defect, often emanating from the main PV and extending distally (unlike tumor thrombus). Chronically, the main PV is replaced by periportal collaterals (*cavernoma/cavernous transformation*) and may not be identifiable. Sequela of portal hypertension (ascites, splenomegaly, and variceal bleeding) may be present. Periportal collaterals can compress/obstruct the biliary tree, known as portal cholangiopathy.[59] Hepatic infarction is uncommon due to dual hepatic blood supply. Chronic PVT is differentiated from CEPS by the presence of portal cavernoma, calcified thrombus, and portal hypertension.[58]

Portal vein tumor thrombus (6.5%–44% of patients with HCC[60]) affects tumor staging, prognosis, and treatment approach (ie, precluding transplant), necessitating differentiation from bland PVT (also common, 42%, in HCC).[60] Imaging demonstrates

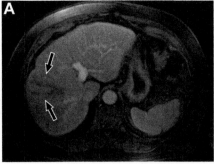
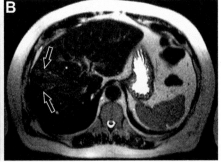

Fig. 12. PV tumor thrombus in a 74-year-old man with hemochromatosis initially suspected on chest CT. (*A*) Contrast-enhanced fat suppressed T1-weighed MR image shows branching expansile hypo-enhancing structures replacing the peripheral right PV branches (*arrows*). (*B*) Corresponding T2-weighted image shows increased signal in the expanded right PV branches. Enhancement, expansion, edema, and peripheral location favor tumor thrombus rather than bland thrombus. The infiltrating liver mass was difficult to see by MR imaging; however, biopsy confirmed a diagnosis of HCC.

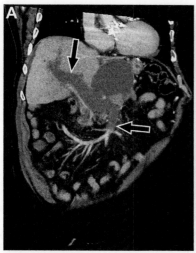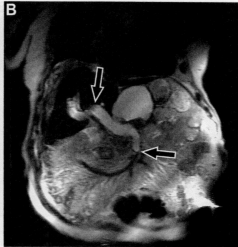

Fig. 13. PPVF in a 79-year-old man with altered mental status. (*A*) Coronal contrast-enhanced CT image shows nonenhancing fluid density material replacing the main PV and upper SMV (*arrows*). The subsequently acquired T2-weighted MR image (*B*) shows this structure has corresponding fluid signal intensity. Low density/fluid intensity in the PV reflects fistulation of a pancreatic pseudocyst into the PV. Bland thrombus is typically higher density on CT and lower signal intensity on MR imaging. Tumor thrombus would demonstrate enhancement. The biliary tree is anatomically distinct.

an expansile enhancing soft tissue-filling defect within the PV often growing centripetally from the periphery of the liver (**Fig. 12**). Arterial flow in thrombus is highly specific of PV tumor thrombus in HCC.[60] Diffusion-weighted imaging signal of bland and tumor thrombus differ,[60] although substantial overlap in apparent diffusion coefficient values exist.[61]

Pseudocyst-portal vein fistula (PPVF) is a rare complication of pancreatitis where a pancreatic pseudocyst invades the PV.[62] The major risk factor is alcohol consumption. The pathophysiology is unclear, although some postulate that pancreatic enzymes degrade the PV wall after PV thrombosis causing pseudocyst fistulation. PPVF appears as a fluid attenuating (CT) or intensity (MR imaging) nonenhancing PV[62] (**Fig. 13**). Findings of chronic PVT may be present (cavernoma, portal hypertension, and portal cholangiopathy). PPVF is easily misdiagnosed as PVT, tumor thrombus, or biliary ductal dilatation (due to fluid characteristics). In some cases, the extravascular pseudocyst may resolve, further confounding diagnosis.

Mesenteric vein thrombosis accounts for 5% to 20% of bowel ischemia, often in the setting of hypercoagulability, portal hypertension, or recent surgery. In addition to intraluminal mesenteric venous filling defect, mesenteric fat stranding and ascites are often present due to vascular congestion. Unlike arterial ischemia, the bowel wall is markedly thickened, which may be low density from edema or hyperattenuating from intramural

hemorrhage[63] (**Fig. 14**). Pneumatosis intestinalis and PVG are late findings (described in later discussion).

Aneurysm/varix

Portal venous aneurysm (prevalence 0.6–4.3:1000) is a focal saccular or fusiform dilatation significantly larger than adjacent segments or greater than 20 mm.[64] PV aneurysms most commonly affect the main PV and splenoportal confluence and are associated with cirrhosis and portal hypertension.[64] Although often asymptomatic, rupture, compression of adjacent structures, PVT, and portal hypertension can result.

Portal venous gas

PVG has a high mortality (56%–90%) due to frequent association with bowel necrosis (72%),[65] although early detection and treatment can decrease mortality.[66] Intramural bowel gas, pneumatosis intestinalis, from bowel necrosis can dissect into draining veins and lead to PVG. PVG is apparent on radiograph (branching intrahepatic lucency), US (nondependent echogenic flowing intravascular particles), and CT (intravascular gas within the mesenteric veins or PV).[65] Pneumobilia mimics PVG; however, PVG is typically peripheral while pneumobilia is central; tracing the respective structures on sequential images is helpful.[65] Notably, numerous benign causes of PVG exist.[65]

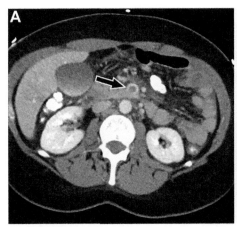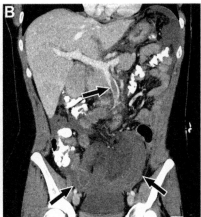

Fig. 14. SMV thrombosis and bowel ischemia in a 44-year-old woman with abdominal pain and bloody diarrhea. (*A*) Axial contrast-enhanced CT shows a partially occlusive filling defect within the SMV (*arrow*) compatible with thrombus. The extent of thrombosis is shown on (*B*) the coronal reformatted image (*top arrow*). Inferiorly, there is marked segmental small bowel wall thickening (*bottom arrows*), mural edema, and mesenteric fat stranding compatible with venous bowel ischemia.

SUMMARY

The abdominal vasculature provides unique avenues for disease spread, hosts numerous vessel-specific pathologic entities, and requires demanding technical considerations for evaluation optimization, all of which predispose to misdiagnosis and underdiagnosis. This review empowers radiologists to confidently identify vascular pathologic condition and raises awareness of uncommon but clinically important diseases of the abdominal vasculature.

CLINICS CARE POINTS

- Dedicated vascular imaging protocols require high spatial resolution, low noise, careful contrast timing, and advanced postprocessing for pathology detection and characterization. Multiphase acquisitions are frequently required.

- Arterial anatomic variants can complicate surgical planning and predispose to traumatic injury (corona mortis or persistent sciatic artery).

- Marfan syndrome, Ehlers-Danlos syndrome, and LDS are important genetic vascular diseases that predispose to aneurysm formation, dissection, and vascular rupture.

- FMD, which predisposes to dissection, is a common systemic vasculopathy with subtle features that may be overlooked.

- Visceral artery aneurysms have a low risk for rupture when less than 2 cm, except of PDA/GDA aneurysms.

- Correct diagnosis of venous compression and thrombotic syndromes require caution to avoid misdiagnosis, such as mistaking mixing artifact for thrombosis or mistaking iliac vein compression in the setting of dehydration for May-Thurner syndrome.

- Distinguishing PV thrombus from tumor thrombus is critical for the proper staging of HCC.

- PPVF is an uncommon complication of pancreatitis that can be easily mistaken for biliary ductal dilatation, PV thrombus, or PV tumor thrombus.

- PVG can herald life-threatening bowel ischemia, whereas several benign causes also exist.

ACKNOWLEDGMENTS

This review was presented as an educational exhibit at the 2019 Radiological Society of North America Conference. We thank Susanne Loomis for her contribution of several artistic renderings and Radhika Barve for her assistance with the article preparation.

DISCLOSURE

Dr T.T. Pierce discloses equity and a consultant agreement with AutonomUS Medical Technologies Inc.; ongoing research support from General Electric, United States, the US Department of Defense, United States, and the National Institutes of Health, United States; prior research support from the Society of Abdominal Radiology, United States and American Roentgen Ray Society, United States; honoraria from the Massachusetts Society of Radiologic Technologists and Zhejiang Medical Association; and royalties from Elsevier Inc. No funding was received to assist with the preparation of the article. Dr V. Prabhu, Dr V. Baliyan, and Dr S. Hedgire have nothing to disclose.

REFERENCES

1. Murphy DJ, Aghayev A, Steigner ML. Vascular CT and MRI: a practical guide to imaging protocols. Insights Imaging 2018;9(2):215–36.
2. Bae KT. Intravenous contrast medium administration and scan timing at CT: considerations and approaches. Radiology 2010;256(1):32–61.
3. Campbell SC, Cullinan JA, Rubens DJ. Slow flow or no flow? Color and power Doppler US pitfalls in the abdomen and pelvis. Radiographics 2004;24(2):497–506.
4. Walker TG. Mesenteric vasculature and collateral pathways. Semin Intervent Radiol 2009;26(3):167–74.
5. Sahani D, Mehta A, Blake M, et al. Preoperative hepatic vascular evaluation with CT and MR angiography: implications for surgery. Radiographics 2004;24(5):1367–80.
6. Noussios G, Galanis N, Chatzis I, et al. The Anatomical Characteristics of Corona Mortis: A Systematic Review of the Literature and Its Clinical Importance in Hernia Repair. J Clin Med Res 2020;12(2):108–14.
7. van Hooft IM, Zeebregts CJ, van Sterkenburg SM, et al. The persistent sciatic artery. Eur J Vasc Endovasc Surg 2009;37(5):585–91.
8. Ha HI, Seo JB, Lee SH, et al. Imaging of Marfan syndrome: multisystemic manifestations. Radiographics 2007;27(4):989–1004.
9. Loeys BL, Dietz HC, Braverman AC, et al. The revised Ghent nosology for the Marfan syndrome. J Med Genet 2010;47(7):476–85.
10. Awais M, Williams DM, Deeb GM, et al. Aneurysms of medium-sized arteries in Marfan syndrome. Ann Vasc Surg 2013;27(8):1188.e5-7.
11. Eagleton MJ. Arterial complications of vascular Ehlers-Danlos syndrome. J Vasc Surg 2016;64(6):1869–80.
12. Malfait F, Francomano C, Byers P, et al. The 2017 international classification of the Ehlers-Danlos syndromes. Am J Med Genet C Semin Med Genet 2017;175(1):8–26.
13. Beighton P, De Paepe A, Steinmann B, et al. Ehlers-Danlos syndromes: revised nosology, Villefranche, 1997. Ehlers-Danlos National Foundation (USA) and Ehlers-Danlos Support Group (UK). Am J Med Genet 1998;77(1):31–7.
14. Zilocchi M, Macedo TA, Oderich GS, et al. Vascular Ehlers-Danlos syndrome: imaging findings. AJR Am J Roentgenol 2007;189(3):712–9.
15. Chu LC, Johnson PT, Dietz HC, et al. Vascular complications of Ehlers-Danlos syndrome: CT findings. AJR Am J Roentgenol 2012;198(2):482–7.
16. Chu LC, Johnson PT, Dietz HC, et al. CT angiographic evaluation of genetic vascular disease: role in detection, staging, and management of complex vascular pathologic conditions. AJR Am J Roentgenol 2014;202(5):1120–9.
17. Johnson PT, Chen JK, Loeys BL, et al. Loeys-Dietz syndrome: MDCT angiography findings. AJR Am J Roentgenol 2007;189(1):W29–35.
18. Loughborough WW, Minhas KS, Rodrigues JCL, et al. Cardiovascular Manifestations and Complications of Loeys-Dietz Syndrome: CT and MR Imaging Findings. Radiographics 2018;38(1):275–86.
19. Rafieian-Kopaei M, Setorki M, Doudi M, et al. Atherosclerosis: process, indicators, risk factors and new hopes. Int J Prev Med 2014;5(8):927–46.
20. Hendriks EJ, Beulens JW, de Jong PA, et al. Calcification of the splenic, iliac, and breast arteries and risk of all-cause and cardiovascular mortality. Atherosclerosis 2017;259:120–7.
21. Surowiec SM, Isiklar H, Sreeram S, et al. Acute occlusion of the abdominal aorta. Am J Surg 1998;176(2):193–7.
22. Hardman RL, Lopera JE, Cardan RA, et al. Common and rare collateral pathways in aortoiliac occlusive disease: a pictorial essay. AJR Am J Roentgenol 2011;197(3):W519–24.
23. Lamba R, Tanner DT, Sekhon S, et al. Multidetector CT of vascular compression syndromes in the abdomen and pelvis. Radiographics 2014;34(1):93–115.
24. Kim EN, Lamb K, Relles D, et al. Median Arcuate Ligament Syndrome-Review of This Rare Disease. JAMA Surg 2016;151(5):471–7.
25. Weber JM, Boules M, Fong K, et al. Median Arcuate Ligament Syndrome Is Not a Vascular Disease. Ann Vasc Surg 2016;30:22–7.
26. Shivapour DM, Erwin P, Kim E. Epidemiology of fibromuscular dysplasia: A review of the literature. Vasc Med 2016;21(4):376–81.
27. Bolen MA, Brinza E, Renapurkar RD, et al. Screening CT Angiography of the Aorta, Visceral Branch Vessels, and Pelvic Arteries in Fibromuscular Dysplasia. JACC Cardiovasc Imaging 2017;10(5):554–61.
28. Varennes L, Tahon F, Kastler A, et al. Fibromuscular dysplasia: what the radiologist should know: a pictorial review. Insights Imaging 2015;6(3):295–307.
29. Alhalabi K, Menias C, Hines R, et al. Imaging and clinical findings in segmental arterial mediolysis (SAM). Abdom Radiol (NY) 2017;42(2):602–11.
30. Naidu SG, Menias CO, Oklu R, et al. Segmental Arterial Mediolysis: Abdominal Imaging of and Disease Course in 111 Patients. AJR Am J Roentgenol 2018;210(4):899–905.

31. Kalva SP, Somarouthu B, Jaff MR, et al. Segmental arterial mediolysis: clinical and imaging features at presentation and during follow-up. J Vasc Interv Radiol 2011;22(10):1380–7.

32. Baker-LePain JC, Stone DH, Mattis AN, et al. Clinical diagnosis of segmental arterial mediolysis: differentiation from vasculitis and other mimics. Arthritis Care Res 2010;62(11):1655–60.

33. Takayama T, Miyata T, Shirakawa M, et al. Isolated spontaneous dissection of the splanchnic arteries. J Vasc Surg 2008;48(2):329–33.

34. Jung SC, Lee W, Park EA, et al. Spontaneous dissection of the splanchnic arteries: CT findings, treatment, and outcome. AJR Am J Roentgenol 2013;200(1):219–25.

35. Pasha SF, Gloviczki P, Stanson AW, et al. Splanchnic artery aneurysms. Mayo Clin Proc 2007;82(4):472–9.

36. Corey MR, Ergul EA, Cambria RP, et al. The natural history of splanchnic artery aneurysms and outcomes after operative intervention. J Vasc Surg 2016;63(4):949–57.

37. Shukla AJ, Eid R, Fish L, et al. Contemporary outcomes of intact and ruptured visceral artery aneurysms. J Vasc Surg 2015;61(6):1442–7.

38. Fitzpatrick LA, Rivers-Bowerman MD, Thipphavong S, et al. Pearls, Pitfalls, and Conditions that Mimic Mesenteric Ischemia at CT. Radiographics 2020;40(2):545–61.

39. Tucker WD, Burns B. Anatomy, abdomen and pelvis, inferior vena cava. Treasure Island (FL): StatPearls; 2020.

40. Smillie RP, Shetty M, Boyer AC, et al. Imaging evaluation of the inferior vena cava. Radiographics 2015;35(2):578–92.

41. Liu Y, Guo D, Li J, et al. Radiological features of azygos and hemiazygos continuation of inferior vena cava: A case report. Medicine (Baltim) 2018; 97(17):e0546.

42. Valla DC. Hepatic vein thrombosis (Budd-Chiari syndrome). Semin Liver Dis 2002;22(1):5–14.

43. Torabi M, Hosseinzadeh K, Federle MP. CT of nonneoplastic hepatic vascular and perfusion disorders. Radiographics 2008;28(7):1967–82.

44. Cura M, Haskal Z, Lopera J. Diagnostic and interventional radiology for Budd-Chiari syndrome. Radiographics 2009;29(3):669–81.

45. Zhang LJ, Zhang Z, Li SJ, et al. Pulmonary embolism and renal vein thrombosis in patients with nephrotic syndrome: prospective evaluation of prevalence and risk factors with CT. Radiology 2014; 273(3):897–906.

46. Akbar SA, Jafri SZ, Amendola MA, et al. Complications of renal transplantation. Radiographics 2005; 25(5):1335–56.

47. Asghar M, Ahmed K, Shah SS, et al. Renal vein thrombosis. Eur J Vasc Endovasc Surg 2007;34(2): 217–23.

48. Kolbel T, Lindh M, Holst J, et al. Extensive acute deep vein thrombosis of the iliocaval segment: midterm results of thrombolysis and stent placement. J Vasc Interv Radiol 2007;18(2):243–50.

49. Sheth S, Fishman EK. Imaging of the inferior vena cava with MDCT. AJR Am J Roentgenol 2007; 189(5):1243–51.

50. Zucker EJ, Ganguli S, Ghoshhajra BB, et al. Imaging of venous compression syndromes. Cardiovasc Diagn Ther 2016;6(6):519–32.

51. Sheth S, Ebert MD, Fishman EK. Superior vena cava obstruction evaluation with MDCT. AJR Am J Roentgenol 2010;194(4):W336–46.

52. Webb EM, Wang ZJ, Westphalen AC, et al. Can CT features differentiate between inferior vena cava leiomyosarcomas and primary retroperitoneal masses? AJR Am J Roentgenol 2013;200(1):205–9.

53. Staehler G, Brkovic D. The role of radical surgery for renal cell carcinoma with extension into the vena cava. J Urol 2000;163(6):1671–5.

54. Karande GY, Hedgire SS, Sanchez Y, et al. Advanced imaging in acute and chronic deep vein thrombosis. Cardiovasc Diagn Ther 2016;6(6): 493–507.

55. Zhang L, Yang G, Shen W, et al. Spectrum of the inferior vena cava: MDCT findings. Abdom Imaging 2007;32(4):495–503.

56. Grewal S, Chamarthy MR, Kalva SP. Complications of inferior vena cava filters. Cardiovasc Diagn Ther 2016;6(6):632–41.

57. Grassi CJ, Swan TL, Cardella JF, et al. Quality improvement guidelines for percutaneous permanent inferior vena cava filter placement for the prevention of pulmonary embolism. J Vasc Interv Radiol 2003;14(9 Pt 2):S271–5.

58. Ghuman SS, Gupta S, Buxi TB, et al. The Abernethy malformation-myriad imaging manifestations of a single entity. Indian J Radiol Imaging 2016;26(3): 364–72.

59. Ponziani FR, Zocco MA, Campanale C, et al. Portal vein thrombosis: insight into physiopathology, diagnosis, and treatment. World J Gastroenterol 2010; 16(2):143–55.

60. Catalano OA, Choy G, Zhu A, et al. Differentiation of malignant thrombus from bland thrombus of the portal vein in patients with hepatocellular carcinoma: application of diffusion-weighted MR imaging. Radiology 2010;254(1):154–62.

61. Sandrasegaran K, Tahir B, Nutakki K, et al. Usefulness of conventional MRI sequences and diffusion-weighted imaging in differentiating malignant from benign portal vein thrombus in cirrhotic patients. AJR Am J Roentgenol 2013;201(6):1211–9.

62. Alessandrino F, Strickland C, Mojtahed A, et al. Clinical and cross-sectional imaging features of spontaneous pancreatic pseudocyst-portal vein fistula. Clin Imaging 2017;44:22–6.

63. Lee SS, Ha HK, Park SH, et al. Usefulness of computed tomography in differentiating transmural infarction from nontransmural ischemia of the small intestine in patients with acute mesenteric venous thrombosis. J Comput Assist Tomogr 2008;32(5): 730–7.

64. Koc Z, Oguzkurt L, Ulusan S. Portal venous system aneurysms: imaging, clinical findings, and a possible new etiologic factor. AJR Am J Roentgenol 2007;189(5):1023–30.

65. Abboud B, El Hachem J, Yazbeck T, et al. Hepatic portal venous gas: physiopathology, etiology, prognosis and treatment. World J Gastroenterol 2009; 15(29):3585–90.

66. Wiesner W, Mortele KJ, Glickman JN, et al. Pneumatosis intestinalis and portomesenteric venous gas in intestinal ischemia: correlation of CT findings with severity of ischemia and clinical outcome. AJR Am J Roentgenol 2001;177(6): 1319–23.

Moving?

Make sure your subscription moves with you!

To notify us of your new address, find your **Clinics Account Number** (located on your mailing label above your name), and contact customer service at:

Email: journalscustomerservice-usa@elsevier.com

800-654-2452 (subscribers in the U.S. & Canada)
314-447-8871 (subscribers outside of the U.S. & Canada)

Fax number: 314-447-8029

Elsevier Health Sciences Division
Subscription Customer Service
3251 Riverport Lane
Maryland Heights, MO 63043

*To ensure uninterrupted delivery of your subscription, please notify us at least 4 weeks in advance of move.

Printed and bound by CPI Group (UK) Ltd, Croydon, CR0 4YY

08/05/2025

01864747-0020